MALARIA

Volume 3

MALARIA

Volume 3
Immunology and Immunization

Edited by

Julius P. Kreier

Department of Microbiology
The Ohio State University
College of Biological Sciences
Columbus, Ohio

ACADEMIC PRESS 1980
A SUBSIDIARY OF HARCOURT BRACE JOVANOVICH, PUBLISHERS
New York   London   Toronto   Sydney   San Francisco

ACADEMIC PRESS, INC.
111 Fifth Avenue, New York, New York 10003

United Kingdom Edition published by
ACADEMIC PRESS, INC. (LONDON) LTD.
24/28 Oval Road, London NW1 7DX

Library of Congress Cataloging in Publication Data
Main entry under title:

Malaria.

Includes bibliographies and index.
CONTENTS: v. 2. Pathology, vector
studies and culture.--v. 3. Immunology, immunopathology
and immunization.
1. Malaria. I. Kreier, Julius P. [DNLM: 1.
Malaria--Congresses. WC750 R432]
QR201.M3R47   616.9'362   80-19569
ISBN 0-12-426103-5 (v. 3)

PRINTED IN THE UNITED STATES OF AMERICA

80 81 82 83   9 8 7 6 5 4 3 2 1

Contents

Appendix 5 The Agency of International Development Program for Malaria Vaccine Research and Development
Edgar A. Smith and James M. Erickson

Appendix 6 The Great Neglected Diseases of Mankind
Kenneth S. Warren

Index

List of Contributors

Numbers in parentheses indicate the pages on which the authors' contributions begin.

J. C. Armstrong (317), Department of Immunoparasitology, Naval Medical Research Institute, Bethesda, Maryland 20014

R. L. Beaudoin (317), Department of Immunoparasitology, Naval Medical Research Institute, Bethesda, Maryland 20014

Robert G. Brackett (325), Clinical Immunology, Biological Research and Development, Warner-Lambert/Parke Davis Company, Detroit, Michigan 48232

Richard Carter (263), Laboratory of Parasitic Disease, National Institutes of Health, Bethesda, Maryland 20014

A. H. Cochrane (163), Department of Microbiology, Division of Parasitology, New York University Medical Center, New York, New York 10016

Carter L. Diggs (299), Department of Immunology, Walter Reed Army Institute of Research, Washington, D.C. 20012

James M. Erickson (331), Malaria Research Office of Health, Development Support Bureau, Agency for International Development, Washington, D.C. 20523

Theodore J. Green (111), Warner-Lambert/Parke Davis Company, Detroit, Michigan 48232

Robert W. Gwadz (263), Laboratory of Parasitic Diseases, National Institutes of Health, Bethesda, Maryland 20014

Joseph Hamburger (1), Department of Protozoology, The Hebrew University, Hadassah Medical School, Jerusalem, Israel

Thomas W. Holbrook (203), Department of Laboratory Medicine, Medical University of South Carolina, Charleston, South Carolina 29403

Julius P. Kreier (1, 111), Department of Microbiology, The Ohio State University, College of Biological Sciences, Columbus, Ohio 43210

E. McConnell (317), Department of Immunoparasitology, Naval Medical Research Institute, Bethesda, Maryland 20014

J. H. E. Meuwissen (67), Department of Medical Parasitology, University of Nijmegen, Geert Grooteplein Zuid 24, Nijmegen, The Netherlands

E. H. Nardin (163), Department of Microbiology, Division of Parasitology, New York University Medical Center, New York, New York, 10016

R. S. Nussenzweig (163), Department of Microbiology, Division of Parasitology, New York University Medical Center, New York, New York 10016

Karl H. Rieckmann (321), Division of Tropical and Geographic Medicine, University of New Mexico School of Medicine, Albuquerque, New Mexico 87131

W. A. Siddiqui (231), Department of Tropical Medicine and Medical Microbiology, University of Hawaii, Honolulu, Hawaii 96816

Edgar A. Smith (331), Technical Assistance Bureau, Agency for International Development, Department of State, Washington, D.C. 20523

J. P. Verhave (67), Department of Medical Parasitology, University of Nijmegen, Geert Grooteplein Zuid 24, Nijmegen, The Netherlands

A. Voller (67), Nuffield Institute of Comparative Medicine, Zoological Society of London, Regents Park, London NW1 4RY, England

Kenneth S. Warren (335), Health Sciences, The Rockefeller Foundation, New York, New York 10036

Preface

The last major effort to review our knowledge of malaria was by Mark F. Boyd whose ''Malariology'' published by W. B. Saunders of Philadelphia in 1949 is still a valuable resource. The exquisite volume ''Malaria Parasites and other Haemosporida'' by P. C. C. Garnham published by Blackwell Scientific Publication of Oxford in 1966 is also a valuable review of malariology but in the author's words ''is about malaria parasites and not malaria.''

This three-volume treatise is appearing in a period of rising activity in malaria research. In the 1950s and 1960s and even into the 1970s funds for this research were scarce and only the hardiest of individuals remained in the field. At present malaria research is again receiving the attention it deserves. The mistaken belief common in the 1950s and 1960s that malaria would soon be eradicated by vector control and chemotherapy and that research was therefore rather pointless has been abandoned in the face of a widespread resurgence of this disease.

A variety of national and international agencies are now funding malaria research. Many individuals attracted by the possibility of funding are turning their efforts to malaria research. Biochemists, immunologists, biophysicists, and molecular biologists among others are entering the field. Many of these individuals, skilled in their specialities, know little or nothing about malaria. It is perhaps to such individuals particularly that this broad review of malariology will be of most value. Even those of us who have worked in some aspects of malaria research for some time may find the reviews of the state of the art in areas other than our own speciality of interest. Those of us actively working in a particular area may find few new facts in the reviews of the areas of our own speciality. I have, however, encouraged the authors to write critical reviews and to relate the facts reported in the literature to each other. Interpretation and speculation are discouraged by the reviewers of most scientific journals in the United States. A

Contents of Volumes 1 and 2

Contents of Babesiosis

1

The Isolation of Malaria Parasites and Their Constituents*

Joseph Hamburger and Julius P. Kreier

I. INTRODUCTION

The malaria parasite is a complex eukaryotic organism. It is described by the morphologist in terms of plasma membranes, pelicule complexes, microtubules, nuclei, ribosomes, and a multitude of other structures; the biochemist talks about proteins, lipids, and carbohydrates; the physiologist discusses enzymes, and the immunologist and serologist are concerned with antigens. They are all of course talking about the components of the same organism, only their terminology is different, reflecting their specific interests and training. Despite the differences in terminology they all require sufficient quantities of the parasite and its constituents in forms suitable for their specific purposes.

Until recently the only source of parasites was the infected host. Practically speaking this source still remains a dominant one. However, the recent development of continuous *in vitro* culture of *Plasmodium flaciparum* is important and will soon lead, no doubt, to large-scale production of the blood forms *in vitro*.

The problem of obtaining sufficient quantities of the parasite is complicated by

---

*This chapter is a revised version of a review by J. P. Kreier published in 1977 in the *Bulletin of the World Health Organization* **55**, 317–331.

its complex life cycle. The malaria parasite develops in two hosts, an invertebrate and a vertebrate. It exists in a variety of morphologically distinct forms in both hosts. In each host a variety of organ and cell systems are parasitized. Furthermore, in the vertebrate host, malaria parasites develop intracellularly, while in the invertebrate host they develop extracellularly but are nevertheless closely associated with the host's tissues. While all the stages of the parasite may share common components, each stage also has unique characteristic components. Thus, even if it were possible to overcome the problems caused by the parasite's intimate association with its host, it would still be necessary to separate parasites by stage of development before even attempting to separate the components specific to each stage. Another complication is added to the antigenic analysis of the parasites by the existence of antigenic variation.

In this chapter, which is an extension of a previous review by Kreier (1977), we will attempt to summarize the literature describing various attempts to isolate malaria parasites and their constituents, and to provide the reader with basic information on the various separatory techniques. Special emphasis will be given to the uses of isolated plasmodia and their constituents in immunological studies. There are a number of reviews and reports available which contain sections on isolation and fractionation of malaria parasites and provide information on the implications of these techniques on immunological, biochemical, and physiological studies (Agency for International Development, 1976; Brown, 1969; Fife, 1971, 1972; McGregor, 1971; Rodgers, 1969; World Health Organization, 1975; Zuckerman, 1969, 1970; Zuckerman and Ristic, 1968; Kreier, 1977).

II. ISOLATION OF PLASMODIA AND THEIR CONSTITUENTS

A. General Considerations

Asexual stages of plasmodia develop and exist intracellularly in the vertebrate host, except for merozoites which are specialized for passage from one cell to another and exist extracellularly for short periods of time. Intracellular plasmodia are found in erythrocytes or as exoerythrocytic forms in liver parenchymal cells of mammals and in cells of the lymphoid–macrophage system in avian hosts.

In order to harvest intracellular malaria parasites it is necessary to disrupt the host cell and then to achieve separation of the parasite from host cell constituents while causing minimal damage to the parasite. Keeping within these requirements presents the main technical problem in harvesting intracellular malaria parasites. The presence of nucleated cells (e.g., avian erythrocytes and leukocytes) in the starting material presents an additional problem, as the parasites adhere to the sticky DNA liberated from these cells during the process of freeing the plasmodia. It should also be borne in mind that soluble plasmodial constituents that might be located between the parasite and the host cell membrane are washed out following separation of the parasite from the host cell.

There is a very extensive literature on procedures for obtaining plasmodia from parasitized red blood cells. In some approaches the parasitized erythrocytes and the contained parasites are disrupted, and then various separation techniques are used to obtain parasite components from the mixture. Other approaches are designed to release morphologically intact parasites from the red cells and then to separate the parasites from erythrocyte debris before disruption of the parasites and fractionation of their constituents are undertaken. Practically all the procedures used for obtaining plasmodial constituents are variations of several distinct techniques; these are hypotonic lysis, lysis by freezing and thawing, lysis by subjecting the erythrocytes to shearing forces, lysis with agents such as saponin, ammonium chloride, or antiserum and complement, lysis by sudden decreases in pressure, lysis by ultrasound, and the most recent procedure, cultivation of parasitized erythrocytes to permit maturation of the parasites and their subsequent spontaneous release.

B. Isolation of Erythrocytic Parasites

1. Obtaining Infected Blood

Malaria parasites have various degrees of host specificity and pathogenicity which affect the level of parasitemia obtained in any species, probably by determining the degree and speed of the host in acquiring protective immunity. The degree of infection with a given parasite may be affected by factors such as age, sex, and genetic strain of the host (Zuckerman and Yoeli, 1954; Eling et al., 1977; Miller, 1976). Certain plasmodium–host combinations do not permit the development of parasitemia high enough for the ready harvesting of sufficient plasmodial material for study. A most common approach for increasing the degree of parasitemia in relatively nonpermissible hosts is splenectomy. The degree of infection with *P. berghei*, which preferentially develops in reticulocytes, can be increased by rendering the host polyreticulocytemic. For example, adult rats which normally develop a low and transient parasitemia will develop a fulminating parasitemia following intraperitoneal injection of phenylhydrazine (3 mg/100 g body weight) at days 5 and 3 before infection (Kreier et al., 1976). For the purpose of harvesting erythrocytic stages of malaria parasites the investigator should ideally try to obtain a host which is highly susceptible to the infection, i.e., one which will allow rapid multiplication of the parasites. Such a host should not develop the type of acquired immunity which interferes with rising parasitemia.

A most economical and convenient source of erythrocytes infected with plasmodia for laboratory study is the blood of rodents infected with one of the various rodent plasmodia. The skills and knowledge needed for isolation and fractionation of plasmodia can easily be acquired using plasmodia grown in rodents. Avian plasmodia are less suitable for the study of isolation and fractionation of plasmodia, as the presence of the erythrocyte nucleus and its contained DNA complicate separation procedures (Sherman and Hull, 1960; Sherman, 1964). Parasitized erythrocytes can also be obtained from monkeys infected with their respective malarias if desired (Coatney *et al.*, 1971). Experimental infections with human plasmodia have been reported in the chimpanzee (Bray, 1957, 1960; Rodhain and Jadin, 1964), the gibbon (Ward *et al.*, 1965; Ward and Cadigan, 1966), the owl monkey (Young *et al.*, 1966; Richards and Voller, 1969; Hickman, 1969), and a few other simian species. The use of nonhuman primates in which experimental infections with human malaria parasites may be induced has provided an important source of human plasmodia for biochemical and immunological studies. However, the rarity and cost of nonhuman primates and their poor adaptation to laboratory conditions are a serious limitation to their extensive use of malaria research.

Human plasmodia may also be collected from infected human blood. Early studies used antigens harvested from plasmodia in the peripheral blood of paretics infected with *P. vivax* (Heidelberger *et al.*, 1946). Zuckerman *et al.* (1967) described in detail a method for the collection of *P. falciparum* from the peripheral blood of West African children. An important source of *P. falciparum* constituents is the infected placenta which, unlike peripheral blood, may have a high proportion of parasitized erythrocytes containing large trophozoites or schizonts of *P. falciparum*. Plasmodial constituents from infected placentas were employed in the 1920s for precipitation tests (Taliaferro, 1930). More recently, antigens prepared from highly infected placental blood (McGregor *et al.*, 1966) were employed extensively for antigenic analysis and seroepidemiological studies of *P. falciparum*. *Plasmodium falciparum* can now be obtained by continuous culture of parasitized human erythrocytes (Trager and Jensen, 1976). Conditions for large-scale production are being investigated. The potential importance of this source of plasmodial material cannot be overemphasized.

2. Preparation of Parasitized Erythrocytes

Blood collected from infected animals or humans which is to be used for harvesting plasmodia may be subjected to certain preliminary treatments to remove unwanted blood components and to increase the proportion of parasitized erythrocytes or to select erythrocytes parasitized with given stages of the parasite. An integral part of these treatments is the removal of plasma by centrifugation and washing. The buffy coat may be removed from the packed red cell mass after centrifugation to reduce the number of platelets and leukocytes (Zuckerman *et al.*, 1967), at the risk of losing many schizont-containing cells which are of low specific gravity (Miller and Chien, 1971; McAlister and Gordon, 1976) and are located immediately underneath the buffy coat (Eaton, 1939; Brown *et al.*, 1968).

Leukocytes may be removed by suspending the washed blood cells in several volumes of dextran solution and allowing the mixture to sediment in a graduated cylinder. The leukocytes which remain in suspension are then discarded (Zuckerman *et al.*, 1967; Langer *et al.*, 1967). Final concentrations of 3.5 and 3.6% dextran of an average molecular weight of 193,000 (Langer *et al.*, 1967) or 115,000 (Zuckerman *et al.*, 1967) have been used for this purpose. Sedimentation velocity centrifugation of washed blood layered on a 10% dextran solution (MW 500,000) has also been employed (Levy and Chow, 1973). During sedimentation velocity centrifugation on a sucrose gradient of specific gravity ranging from 1.055 to 1.096 (0.25–0.7 M sucrose) the specific gravity of the leukocytes increased, and this resulted in greatly enhanced sedimentation as compared with erythrocytes (Williamson and Cover, 1966). Sucrose, however, exerts a strong osmotic pressure on the erythrocyte and may be harmful to the parasite. The osmotic effects of density gradients are least in gradients made with large molecules such as dextran. Wallach and Conley (1977) recently used a Ficoll–Hypaque solution of density 1.08 g/ml in a one-step gradient for removing leukocytes from *P. knowlesi*-infected blood. After centrifugation the white blood cells accumulated above the Ficoll–Hypaque layer, while the parasitized erythrocytes accumulated in the pellet, which was leukocyte-free. Leukocytes were also removed after releasing the parasites from parasitized erythrocytes. This was done by filtration through a Millipore filter of 5-μm pore size (Brown *et al.*, 1966).

In a comparative study on several methods for removing leukocytes it was found that the most efficient procedure was passage of the diluted blood through a column of a filter-paper powder (Homewood and Neame, 1976). This method was introduced in the mid-1950s by Fulton and Grant (1956). Later studies confirmed its effectiveness and demonstrated that passage through a filter-paper powder column did not reduce the infectivity of parasitized erythrocytes (Richards and Williams, 1973). Whatman's CF12 (Baggaley and Atkinson, 1972) or CF11 (Richards and Williams, 1973) filter-paper powder was used with good results. The powder is packed in a siliconized glass column or in a syringe. Proper packing and the use of properly premeasured amounts of powder, as well as passage of the blood through the column under properly controlled pressure, have been mentioned as important factors to be considered when using the procedure (Richards and Williams, 1973; Baggaley and Atkinson, 1972). When blood, diluted in an appropriate medium, is passed directly through the dry powder, hemolysis occurs (Richards and Williams, 1973). Hemolysis can be avoided by thoroughly wetting the column before use. The ability of the column to retain leukocytes is limited, consequently, overloading and excessive washing will result in passage of leukocytes.

While methods such as removal of the buffy coat, sedimentation in dextran, and sedimentation velocity centrifugation on a sucrose gradient remove, at best, about 75% of the leukocytes, the filter-paper column removes over 99% (Richards and Williams, 1973; Baggaley and Atkinson, 1972). The filter-paper column can be prepared over a layer of glass beads for combined removal of platelets and leukocytes (McAlister and Gordon, 1976; Scheibel and Miller, 1969a). Injection of adenosine diphosphate shortly before bleeding or its addition to the blood *in vitro* will promote clumping of the platelets and will facilitate their removal by the column (McAlister and Gordon, 1976; Scheibel and Miller, 1969a).

Before one attempts to separate the parasites from the host cells, it may be desirable to increase the proportion of parasitized erythrocytes relative to uninfected ones or to separate the parasitized erythrocytes by stage of development of the parasites. The procedures usually used to concentrate parasitized red cells are based on density differences between parasitized erythrocytes and unparasitized ones. The more parasites a red cell contains and the larger the contained parasites, the lower the density of the host cell–parasite complex. Some plasmodia cause the red cell to enlarge by inhibition of water, thereby decreasing its density, and some plasmodia preferentially infect the reticulocytes which are lighter than the normocytes. All these factors affect the density of parasitized erythrocytes (Miller and Chien, 1971). Eaton (1938) collected schizont-containing rhesus erythrocytes by allowing infected blood to settle slowly. The schizont-containing cells were present in increased concentration just under the buffy coat. More modern procedures for the separation of parasitized erythrocytes involve sedimentation or sedimentation velocity centrifugation, and equilibrium centrifugation in solutions of high density. Solutions for density centrifugation may be made from sucrose (Williamson and Cover, 1966), human albumin (Ferrebee and Geiman, 1946), bovine albumin (Rowley *et al.*, 1967; Siddiqui *et al.*, 1978a,b; Eisen, 1977), Ficoll (Lund and Powers, 1976), Ficoll–Hypaque (Wallace and Conley, 1977), Stractan II (McAlister and Gordon, 1976), Plasmagel (Pasvol *et al.*, 1978), or Physiogel (Reese *et al.*, 1978). In recent studies, Lund and Powers (1976) concentrated schizont-containing erythrocytes parasitized with *P. knowlesi* on a discontinuous Ficoll gradient. After centrifugation at 10,000 *g* for 30 minutes many schizont-containing cells were found in a layer at the interface of the 20 and 25% Ficoll bands. McAlister and Gordon (1976) separated *P. berghei*-parasitized erythrocytes by stage of development on a discontinuous gradient of Stractan II (an arabinogalactan). The infected erythrocytes were centrifuged at 50,000 *g* for 45 minutes. Schizont-containing cells had a specific gravity of less than 1.043 g/ml, those containing trophozoites and multiple ring forms had a specific gravity between 1.081 and 1.031, and uninfected cells and those containing very small rings had specific gravities greater than 1.091. Wallach and Conley (1977) obtained a preparation containing 99%

schizont-infected erythrocytes from monkey blood originally containing only 10–30% schizont-infected erythrocytes. They did it by centrifugation of the *P. knowlesi*-infected blood cell suspension on a Ficoll–Hypaque solution of density 1.076 g/ml. The leukocytes were removed at a second stage by centrifugation on a solution of density 1.08 g/ml. Eisen (1977) concentrated *P. chabaudi*-parasitized erythrocytes by centrifugation on a discontinuous bovine serum albumin (BSA) gradient at 40,000 *g* for 20 minutes. Most of the parasitized erythrocytes were concentrated at the boundary between the 15 and 25% layers. Siddiqui *et al.* (1978b) showed that a preparation containing 93% segmenters of cultured *P. falciparum* could be obtained from cultured blood cells containing only 6% segmenters by centrifugation of the cultured red cells on a discontinuous BSA gradient at 1500 *g* for 60 minutes. The yield was 83%. The segmenters accumulated at the interface between the bands of densities 1.07 and 1.08 g/ml.

Eling (1977) obtained pure preparations of *P. berghei*-infected mouse erythrocytes by centrifugation on a cushion of 28% Ficoll at 9000 *g* for 15 minutes. Higher yields were obtained after crisis when the majority of parasites are in reticulocytes. Similar conditions were used to obtain pure preparations of *P. berghei*-parasitized erythrocytes from the blood of infected rats and hamsters. With infected gerbil blood the Ficol concentration was reduced to 24 or 22% for obtaining parasitized erythrocytes with a purity of 80–95%. Separation of *P. vivax*-parasitized erythrocytes from *Aotus* blood was only partially successful.

Preparations considerably enriched in *P. falciparum* schizont-containing erythrocytes were obtained by sedimentation of the red cells in solutions which stimulate clumping of uninfected erythrocytes. Pasvol *et al.* (1978) used Plasmagel (a gelatin preparation), and Reese *et al.* (1978) used Physiogel (a chemically modified gelatin preparation) for this purpose.

For those working with a synchronized infection, parasites primarily in a given stage of development may be obtained by judicious choice of the time of blood collection. *Plasmodium lophurae* and *P. knowlesi* produce well-synchronized infections. Schizont-infected erythrocytes obtained by bleeding monkeys at the appropriate time were used for direct agglutination and antigenic variation studies of *P. knowlesi* parasites (Brown *et al.*, 1968; Brown and Brown, 1965). The synchronized development of *P. lophurae* made it possible for Trager *et al.* (1972) to obtain a preparation of almost pure trophozoites of this parasite for culture. If, however, the parasites are, like *P. berghei*, not naturally synchronized or lose their synchrony in culture, then one must either use procedures such as the gradient centrifugation just described to obtain parasites of a given stage or attempt to induce synchrony. Arnold and his associates (Arnold *et al.*, 1969; Shungu and Arnold, 1971) demonstrated that some degree of synchronization of *P. berghei* in mice could be induced by control of the photoperiod to which the host rats were exposed. An interesting approach for synchronization of *P. berghei* infection was taken with some success by Walter (1968) who brought about *in vivo* release of the parasites by injecting parasitized rat erythrocytes into mice previously immunized with normal rat erythrocytes. The infections which resulted were synchronized for several generations, presumably because the merozoites released by the hemolysis *in vivo* were infectious. Infection with *in vitro*-released parasites may also lead to synchronization (McAlliser, 1977). Successful synchronization of *P. berghei* infection would facilitate isolation of its specific stages from the blood and greatly simplify analysis of the developmental events in this otherwise most easily studied malaria parasite. Synchronized *P. falciparum* cultures have been obtained by Lambrose and Vanderberg (1979). The cultures were started with inocula treated with 5% sorbitol which destroyed mature forms of the parasite but young forms survived.

3. *Plasmodial Constituents from Parasitized Erythrocytes*

The present section will deal with procedures for preparing plasmodial constituents in which the erythrocyte–parasite complex is treated as a source of parasite material without first releasing the parasites from the host cell. Many early investigators simply disrupted the host-cell–parasite complex as the first step in preparing plasmodial antigens for serodiagnostic purposes. This approach was reevaluated many years later, when it was recognized that important constituents of the parasite may be located in the host cell outside the parasite's plasma membrane and thus be lost when the parasite is isolated.

The early procedures for preparing antigens from parasitized erythrocytes used hypotonic lysis, aqueous extraction, desiccation and reconstitution, extraction with alkali or alcohol, autolysis, or freezing and thawing. In many studies various combinations of these procedures were employed. Several representative procedures are described below. Gasbarrini (1913) was able to detect complement-fixing antibodies in sera of malarious patients with an antigen he prepared by washing parasitized erythrocytes with saline and hemolyzing the washed cells. Hemolysis was followed by desiccation, grinding, and extraction in saline. Pewny (1918) obtained precipitation reactions employing an antigen prepared by hypotonic lysis of infected blood followed by autolysis at body temperature for several days. Coggeshall and Eaton (1938) prepared a group-specific complement-fixing antigen from the blood of *P. knowlesi*-infected rhesus monkeys by treating the parasitized erythrocytes with three times their volume of distilled water for 48 hours (probably at 37°C). After centrifugation the supernatant containing hemoglobin was employed for the test. Another procedure they employed involved lyophilization of washed parasitized erythrocytes followed by grinding in a ball mill at $-70°C$, extraction in saline, and centrifugation to recover the supernatant for the test. Coggeshall and Eaton's (1938) use of the easily available heterologous plasmodia as a source of antigens for testing sera of human patients was a significant development which was followed by many other investigators who used various bird and animal plasmodia as sources of antigens for various serodiagnostic tests.

A nonsoluble plasmodial fraction was used in one of the early successful attempts to induce protection against *P. lophurae* (Jacobs, 1943). The antigen was prepared by treatment of washed parasitized blood with concentrated sucrose for 15–24 hours in the cold. The lysed product was then treated with protamine sulfate and sedimented. The sediment was washed and stored in phenol until used.

Soluble preparations of extracted parasitized erythrocytes commonly used by early investigators for serodiagnosis contained considerable amounts of hemoglobin. Removal of hemoglobin can be accomplished if the parasites are first released from the parasitized erythrocyte. If, however, a lysate is prepared directly from the parasitized erythrocyte, it will contain hemoglobin. The hemoglobin can be removed by a variety of fractionation methods. Davis (1948) separated antigen from hemoglobin by ammonium sulfate precipitation. By adding 36 g of ammonium sulfate to each 100 ml of lysate Davis obtained a precipitate which was largely free of hemoglobin and was useful for complement fixation (CF) testing after its resolution and dialysis.

In many recent studies the antigens were released from the parasitized erythrocytes by freezing and thawing. This treatment results in the lysis of 99% of the erythrocytes and releases plasmodial components, although many of the parasites may appear intact by Giemsa staining (McAlister, 1972). Some investigators combined freezing and thawing with various other physical procedures for disruption of parasitized erythrocytes. In some of these studies they fractionated the lysate to separate serologically or otherwise active components from unwanted constituents (e.g., hemoglobin). Kagan and his associates (Kagen, 1972) prepared *P. falciparum* antigens for use in passive hemagglutination tests by freezing and thawing parasitized *Aotus* erythrocytes and then further disintegrating them in a Ribe cell fractionator at 17,000 psi. The supernatant obtained following centrifugation of the lysate was employed for the test. Meuwissen *et al.* (1972) used a similarly prepared antigen for hemagglutination tests but subjected the frozen and thawed parasitized erythrocytes to a 10-second burst of sonic energy instead of passing them through a Ribe cell fractionator. Such antigens were also employed for the enzyme-linked immunosorbent assay (ELISA) of Voller *et al.* (1975) and in vaccination studies by Brown and Tanaka (1975).

Kortmann *et al.* (1971) used ultrasonic treatment to disrupt heavily parasitized (*P. falicparum*) placental blood. He then centrifuged the lysate and homogenized the pellet obtained to yield an antigen for capillary agglutination testing. The most extensive use of malarial antigens of placental origin was, however, in studies on precipitating antibodies to *P. falciparum* in West Africans (McGregor *et al.*, 1966). The use of the double immunodiffusion technique in these studies made it possible to identify separate plasmodial antigen–antibody systems, and the seroepidemiological studies that followed established the pattern of the response to the various antigens in different sections of the population (Wilson *et al.*, 1969; McGregor and Wilson, 1971). The studies also led to the demonstration of soluble plasmodial antigens in the plasma of infected and convalescing patients.

Initially unfractionated extracts from heavily infected placentas were employed for the double immunodiffusion tests by McGregor *et al.* (1966). The placental blood cells were collected after the placentas were minced, and the tissue debris was removed by filtration. After the blood cells were washed, the dark layer of heavily parasitized erythrocytes was collected and disintegrated in a Hughes press. The supernatant obtained following centrifugation at 18,000 *g* was employed for the tests. Antigens prepared from placentas heavily infected with mature forms of *P. falciparum* were more reactive than those prepared from peripheral blood or placental blood containing young parasites. A similar antigenic preparation was later fractionated by Turner and McGregor (1969). Two antigens, arbitrarily termed α and β, were identified by double immunodiffusion against hyperimmune human serum. Upon fractionation of the crude antigenic preparation by gel filtration on Sephadex G-200, three fractions of high absorbance were obtained of which the second contained a large proportion of hemoglobin. α-Antigen was associated chiefly with the first fraction, and its estimated molecular weight was between 300,000 and 900,000. When fractionated by polyacrylamide gel electrophoresis (PAGE) plasmodial antigens were found located at the top of the separation gel and stained with protein dyes as well as with periodic acid–schiff (PAS) and Feulgen reagents. β-Antigen was largely associated with the tail of the second fraction, and its estimated molecular weight was about 60,000. Several further attempts to separate α and β antigens on Sephadex G-200 gave inconsistent results (Wilson *et al.*, 1969). This led Wilson *et al.* (1969) to use a different "working nomenclature" based on the heat stability of the antigens. Antigens stable to heating at 100°C for 5 minutes were termed S (stable) antigens, and those destroyed or precipitated at 56°C for 30 minutes were termed L (labile) antigens. Another antigen termed R (resistant) antigen, was stable at 50°C but was destroyed at 100°C. This approach of discriminative inactivation can be regarded as fractionation in a broad functional sense. S, L, and R antigens were later identified in extracts of *Aotus* erythrocytes parasitized with *P. falciparum* (Wilson and Voller, 1972). They were also present in lysates prepared by sonication of placental blood (Williams, 1973).

S antigens cloesly correspond to the α antigens described by Turner and McGregor (1969) as they are contained in the first high-absorbance fraction and its trail upon fractionation on Sephadex G-200. The molecular weight of S antigens as estimated by gel filtration is about 400,000, however, ultracentrifugation of S antigens on sucrose gradients gives an s_{20} value of 4.4 which corresponds to a molecular weight of 60,000 for a globular protein. Such discrepancies suggest that S antigens are asymetric. They may be glycoproteins, as suggested by their heat stability and by their incomplete precipitation in 0.5 M trichloroacetic acid (TCA). Their antigenicity, however, is most likely associated with the protein moiety of the molecule, as it can be destroyed by the action of proteolytic enzymes. S antigens also appear in the serum. There is a wide range of these antigens, only a few of which are found in the serum of a patient during any one parasitemic episode.

L antigens, which are destroyed by heating at 56°C for 30 minutes, have been subdivided on the basis of other properties into La and Lb classes. At least three antigens of the La class can be extracted from parasitized placental blood (Wilson et al., 1969). Their molecular weights as estimated by gel filtration on Sephadex G-200 are about 250,000 for La-1 and 400,000 for La-2. La-1 antigens are more heat-labile than other L antigens and can be destroyed by heating to 55°C for 2 minutes. They also appear to aggregate when attempts are made to filter them in gels (Wilson et al., 1973). The pattern of appearance of antibodies to La antigens parallels the development of protective immunity. It is not inconceivable, therefore, that these antigens are important in stimulating the development of protective immunity (McGregor and Wilson, 1971). The Lb class of antigens constitutes a complex of at least three antigens. Gil filtration studies suggest that their molecular weight is about 32,000 (Wilson, et al., 1973). In this aspect they are similar to the β antigens described by Turner and McGregor (1969). Antibodies to these antigens appear in a small fraction of Gambian villagers (Wilson et al., 1969).

R antigen has been found in all extracts of parasitized placental blood. The molecular weight of this antigen is about 150,000 as determined by thin-layer chromatography on Sephadex G-200 (Wilson et al., 1969). R antigen can be separated from the other antigens of P. falciparum by elution from an ion-exchange column using a 0.05 M Tris–hydrochloric acid buffer of pH 8.0 (Wilson et al., 1973).

Recently Wilson and Ling (1978) fractionated lysates of infected placental blood on CM-cellulose. The first peak, eluted by 0.01 M phosphate buffer pH 6.5, was well separated from most of the hemoglobin and contained S, L, and R antigens.

Gel filtration, ion-exchange chromatography, and precipitation with ammonium sulfate were employed by various other investigators in obtaining plasmodial antigens from lysates of parasitized erythrocytes, primarily for serodiagnostic purposes. Sadun and his associates (Sadun and Gore, 1968; Sadun et al., 1969) obtained P. falciparum antigen for indirect hemagglutination (IHA) and soluble antigen fluorescent antibody (SAFA) tests by ion-exchange chromatography. Lysates were obtained by freezing and thawing parasitized chimpanzee erythrocytes, and the lysates were fractionated on DEAE-Sephadex A-25 columns. Most of the hemoglobin was eluted in the first fraction with 0.01 *M* buffer at pH 7.5. A fraction which was eluted with 0.1 *M* buffer at pH 6.5 contained the most reactive antigen for the SAFA test.

Wellde *et al.* (1969) compared several fractionation procedures while searching for antigens suitable for use in IHA tests. *Plasmodium berghei*-infected mouse and *P. falciparum*-infected chimpanzee erythrocytes were lysed by freezing and thawing, and the lysates were fractionated by ion-exchange chromatography using procedures previously described by Sadun and Gore (1968). The fraction eluted by passage through the column of 0.1 *M* phosphate buffer at pH 6.5 contained strongly reactive antigens. Fractionation was also done by initial precipitation of the lysate with 60% ammonium sulfate, followed by successive washings of the precipitate with decreasing concentrations of ammonium sulfate (50, 45, 37, 33, 24, and 5%). The supernatant of each wash was dialyzed and tested as an antigen for the IHA test. Strong antigenic activity was associated with the supernatants resulting from washing the initial precipitate with 50 and 33% ammonium sulfate. The supernatant fluid recovered following the initial precipitation step was treated with 70 and 76% ammonium sulfate, and the resulting precipitates were dissolved in phosphate-buffered saline (PBS) and dialyzed. The products of this step had the highest protein content among all fractions; they were, however, inactive in the IHA test. Gel filtration of the lysate on Sephadex G-200 yielded an active fraction which eluted before the hemoglobin. McAlister (1972) prepared lysates from *Aotus* erythrocytes parasitized with *P. falciparum* by the freezing and thawing procedure employed by Sadun and Gore (1968) and by Wellde *et al.* (1969). This procedure resulted in lysis of 99% of the erythrocytes, but many parasites appeared intact on microscopic examination of thin films of the lysate stained by the Giemsa technique. By comparison, treatment with a French pressure cell at 1000 psi resulted in complete lysis of the erythrocytes and in somewhat more damage to the parasites than resulted from freezing and thawing. The soluble components of both preparations were subjected to various fractionation procedures in a search for antigens reactive in the SAFA and IHA tests. Treatment with ammonium sulfate at 50% or higher saturation resulted in the precipitation of serologically active material. Most of the hemoglobin remained soluble after treatment with 62% saturated ammonium sulfate. Precipitates obtained by precipitation of lysates in which enough ammonium sulfate was dissolved to yield a 62% solution were further fractionated by gel filtration. The reactive antigens were eluted at or near the exclusion limit of Sephadex G-200 or in the void volume of Sepharose 4B columns. These results indicate that the molecular weight of the antigen involved is at least 800,000. The antigen purified on Sephadex G-200 columns reacted more strongly in IHA tests than the antigen prepared by ammonium sulfate precipitation only.

Todorovic *et al.* (1968a,b,c) used antigens they obtained from *P. gal-*

linaceum-infected blood cells in latex agglutination tests (Todorovic *et al.*, 1968d). Parasitized erythrocytes were disintegrated by sonication, and the supernatant obtained following centrifugation was fractionated by chromatography through 8% granulated agar. Protein-containing fractions were ultracentrifuged (190,000 *g* for 15 hours), and the pellets obtained were used for the tests after suspension in saline.

4. Release of Parasites from Parasitized Erythrocytes

a. Physical Procedures

i. Release by Osmotic Lysis. Osmotic lysis of infected erythrocytes usually combined with desiccation and further extraction by various means was employed by many early investigators to produce antigens for serodiagnostic purposes. Many of these procedures were described in the previous section. The preparations obtained were grossly contaminated with host cell constituents, notably hemoglobin. The most common use of hypotonic lysis for the release of malaria parasites is in preparing thick-drop preparations for microscopical diagnosis. While such treatment leaves the parasite in close association with the erythrocyte ghost, the removal of hemoglobin results in a considerable reduction in the sample volume and consequently in the concentration of parasites. That the parasites themselves are lysed along with the erythrocytes is apparent from their appearance in electron micrographs (Fig. 1).

Dulaney and Stratman-Thomas (1940) prepared a complement-fixing antigen by laking parasitized erythrocytes with distilled water. The hemoglobin was washed out, and the solid material, containing a mixture of erythrocytic stromata and parasites in various stages of disruption, was collected. This material was then dried under vacuum and stored until needed. When it was to be used, it was ground, reconstituted with saline, and frozen and thawed three times. After centrifugation, the clear supernatant fluid was used as antigen for CF tests. This antigen had the same type of group specificity as the lysate used by Coggeshall and Eaton (1938) but had the advantage of being relatively free of hemoglobin. Antigens prepared by procedures very similar to those of Dulaney and Stratman-Thomas (1940) have been used by Mayer and Heidelberger (1946) in studies on the use of the CF test in diagnosis of malaria, by Stein and Desowitz (1964) to sensitize erythrocytes for use in passive hemagglutination tests, and by Chavin (1966) for antigenic analysis of plasmodia by double immunodiffusion and immunoelectrophoresis techniques.

ii. Release by Ultrasound. It was shown by Verain and Verain (1956) that ultrasound disrupted red cells and released plasmodia. Later it was shown that parasite yield increased only to a limited degree with increases in the intensity of

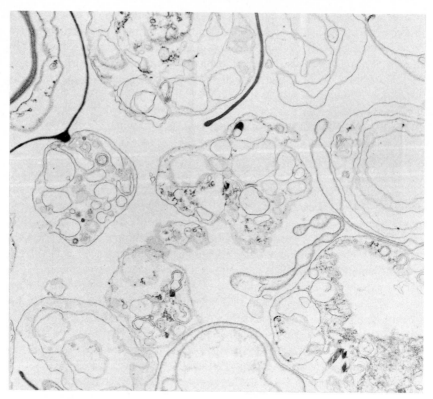

FIG. 1.   Electron micrograph of a thin section of *P. knowlesi* parasites freed by osmotic lysis of parasitized blood cells. The parasites are swollen and vacuolated. Many membranes of ruptured parasites are also present. (Photograph courtesy of Dr. M. Aikawa; from Cook *et al.*, 1969.)

the sonic energy used and the duration of the exposure (Rutledge and Ward, 1967) and that, while low-frequency ultrasound waves appeared to disrupt red cells more efficiently than high-frequency waves, no frequency existed which would break red cells but not plasmodia (Prior and Kreier, 1977). It is thus apparent that, in batch sonication systems, no combination of time, intensity, or frequency can be selected which will break red cells without also subsequently breaking the released parasites. The problem in the use of sonic energy for the release of plasmodia thus is one of developing a system permitting red cell disruption and then achieving prompt removal of the freed parasites from the sound field. This problem was resolved by the development of a continuous-flow system (Prior and Kreier, 1972a,b). The crucial technical aspect of the system is the design of the chamber. It must have a small void volume. The washed, parasitized red cells must pass through the ultrasound field in an ordered fashion, and there must be no eddies in which parasitized erythrocytes and parasites may

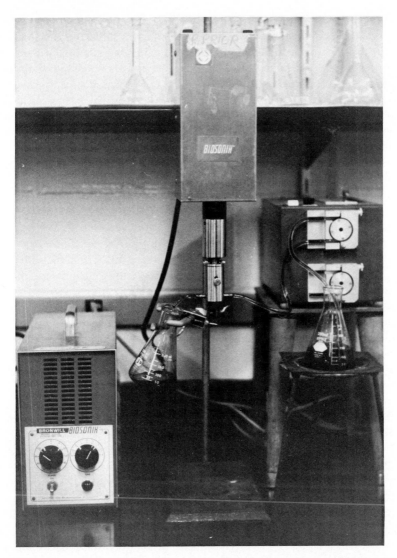

FIG. 2. The complete setup for CFS release of plasmodia from infected erythrocytes. A 10% suspension of washed parasitized erythrocytes is in the erlenmeyer flask on the right. The suspension of erythrocytes is pumped through the tube by the peristaltic pump just above and behind the flask. The suspension of erythrocytes is then passed through the flow chamber (center) attached to the probe of the sonic oscillator (top center). The mixture of broken and unbroken erythrocytes and freed parasites is collected in the flask just to the left of the chamber. The suspension of erythrocytes should be kept cold. This may be done by placing the flasks in a crushed ice bath. The disrupted material is strained through a pad of glass wool, and the parasites may be isolated by centrifugation or some other procedure.

be trapped and subjected to prolonged exposure to the disruptive forces of the ultrasound. The optimum rate of flow for maximum yield of parasites must be selected by experimentation for each continuous-flow system. Almost any reasonably powerful commercial sonicator may be used if fitted with a chamber which permits the ordered passage of a thin layer of suspended parasitized cells through the sound field (Fig. 2). A satisfactory system has been described in detail (Prior and Kreier, 1972b). Leukocytes and platelets must be removed from the blood cells by a suitable procedure before sonication, for sonication will cause release of nucleic acids which entrap the parasites and prevent their subsequent separation from erythrocyte debris. Prior and Krier (1972a,b) separated freed parasites from unbroken erythrocytes and erythrocyte debris by differential centrifugation. Short, low-force centrifugation was selected to remove the unbroken red cells, and then longer higher-force centrifugation was used to pellet the parasites; finely divided debris remained in the supernatant fluid. A practical procedure for selecting the conditions of centrifugation required to obtain parasites is to prepare a series of identical tubes of the effluent from the sonciation chamber, measure the height of the effluent column, and then choose an arbitrary gravity force, for example 300 g, and centrifuge for 5, 10, 15, 20, 25, and 30 minutes. Examination of the pellets will permit choice of appropriate centrifugation times at the selected gravity force to pellet all the unbroken red cells. Once appropriate centrifugation conditions for pelleting all the unbroken red cells are determined, supernatant fluids obtained by appropriate centrifugation of additional effluent may be placed in a series of tubes and after the column height is measured centrifuged at a standard gravity force, for example 600 g, for various times to determine the minimum time required to pellet the parasites. Centrifugation times at a given gravity are determined per centimeter of column height.

Thin-section electron micrographs have been published which show that relatively undamaged parasites free of entrapping erythrocyte membranes may be prepared by the sonication technique (Prior and Kreier, 1972a,b). The plasmodia obtained by sonic oscillation are in whatever stage of development they had obtained at the time of release (Kreier et al., 1976). Figure 3 shows a fairly typical preparation of sonically freed parasites. Parasites prepared by continuous-flow sonication (CFS) have been shown to be suitable as sources of antigen for CF tests (Prior and Kreier, 1972a), for studies on the mode of action of the host against the parasite (Hamburger and Kreier, 1975, 1976a,b; Green and Kreier, 1978), for study of the parasite's means of defense against the host

---

FIG. 3. Electron micrograph of a thin section of free *P. berghei* parasites prepared by differential centrifugation of a suspension of parasitized erythrocytes which has been disrupted by CFS. Parasites are in a variety of intraerythrocytic development stages. The majority are small trophozoites and merozoites or parasites transforming into or from merozoites. (Photograph courtesy of Drs. Prior and Kreier.)

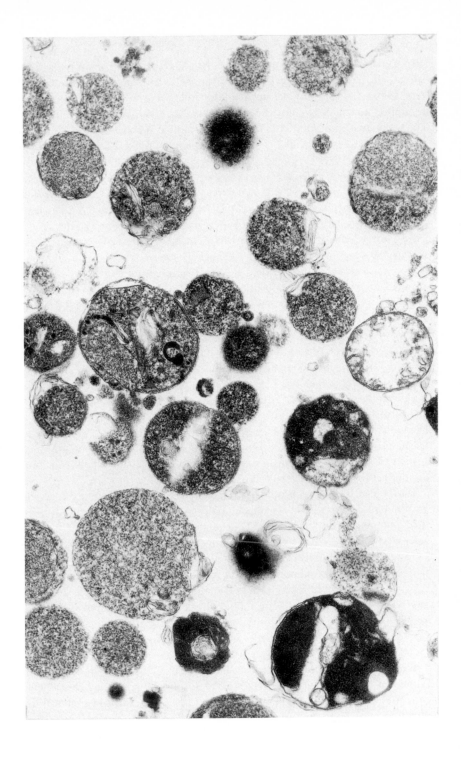

(Brooks and Kreier, 1978), and in vaccination studies (Saul and Kreier, 1977). The excellent state of preservation of the sonically freed parasites has made them very useful for study of the surface properties of free parasites, an area not previously amenable to study (Seed et al., 1973b, 1974; Seed and Kreier, 1976). The technique is not limited to use with plasmodia; *Babesia* have been freed by essentially the same procedures (Gravely and Kreier, 1974; Kreier et al., 1975).

iii. Release by Sudden Decreases in Pressure. The technique for release of plasmodia from erythrocytes by decompression under controlled conditions in a French pressure cell was developed by D'Antonio et al. (1966b). A 20% suspension of washed parasitized erythrocytes is prepared in buffered saline solution. This is extruded from the orifice of the French pressure cell at an appropriate pressure, usually between 800 and 1000 psi. The pressure chosen depends on the host–parasite system being studied and must be selected on the basis of trial and error (D'Antonio, 1972). The effluent from the cell is centrifuged at 500 g for 10 minutes to remove the unbroken red cells and gross debris, and then the parasites are collected by centrifugation of the supernatant at 3500 g for 5 minutes.

Such preparations were used for studies on the cytochrome oxidase of *P. knowlesi* (Scheibel and Miller, 1969a). Extracts of the released parasites were subjected to various fractionation procedures to separate antigens (D'Antonio et al., 1966b), a lytic factor (Fife et al., 1972), and components capable of inducing protective immunity (D'Antonio et al., 1970; D'Antonio, 1974; D'Antonio and Silverman, 1971; Schenkel et al., 1973, 1975). Micrographs showing isolated intact parasites obtained by French pressure cell treatment have been published (Kilby and Silverman 1969). Treatment of parasitized erythrocytes by this system yields some free parasites and much amorphous material which is probably derived in part from ruptured parasites (Fig. 4).

Most recently the bubble nucleation technique, commonly referred to as nitrogen cavitation was used by Wallach and his associates for the release of plasmodia (Wallach and Conley, 1977). The method involves the use of a pressure cell or "bomb" (e.g., an expanding nitrogen gas pressure homogenizer, Artisan Industries, Inc., Waltham, Massachusetts). The cell suspension is introduced into the bomb and equilibrated with nitrogen under pressure. Then the pressure is released. Bubbles of nitrogen form as the pressure decreases, and the shear forces associated with their growth and rupture break the erythrocyte membranes. The pressure conditions and the equilibrium time should be determined for each cell system by trial and error. The procedure described for the release of *P. knowlesi* (Wallach and Conley, 1977) is as follows.

Blood containing 20–30% schizont-infected cells is washed in PBS. The proportion of parasitized erythrocytes is increased to about 99% by centrifugation over a Ficoll–Hypaque gradient followed by a second centrifugation on Ficoll–Hypaque to remove leukocytes and platelets. Forty milliliters of washed cells

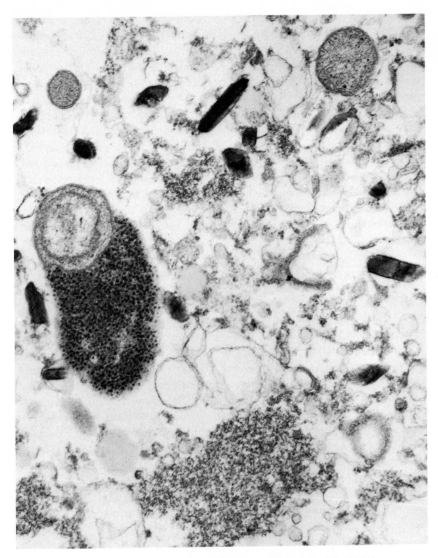

FIG. 4. Electron micrograph of a thin section of amorphous material which is a common contaminant of plasmodia obtained by the French pressure cell technique. Some intact parasites (not shown in this micrograph) are present in the preparations. (Photograph courtesy of Dr. M. Aikawa; from Cook *et al.*, 1969.)

(ca. 2×10^8 cells/ml) is equilibrated at 280 psi in the nitrogen bomb, and then the pressure is released. This procedure results in lysis of 50–80% of the parasitized red blood cells and damages no more than 35% of the parasites. The effluent is centrifuged to sediment the parasites differentially, and the unbroken erythrocytes and the released parasites are further separated from membranous debris by centrifugation at 9×10^3 g/min (sic) on a Ficoll–Hypaque gradient, density 1.08 g/ml. The sediment contains 35–50% of the total number of parasites and about 10% of the total erythrocyte membranes present in the starting materials. Further centrifugation steps are required to collect the bulk of the membrane material for further analysis. For accurate monitoring of the fate of the membrane material throughout the isolation procedure, a small number of parasitized erythrocytes initially labeled with ^{125}I may be added as a tracer to the bulk of the parasitized erythrocytes before introduction into the nitrogen bomb. At the time of writing of this chapter no micrographs of free parasites obtained by this technique were available.

iv. Release by Mechanical Shearing.   Erythrocytes from mice infected with *P. vinckei* were agglutinated with concanavalin. The agglutinated erythrocytes were washed by centrifugation and then suspended in Ringer's solution. The suspended erythrocytes were then forced through two membrane filters, first a 100-mesh nylon filter and then a 20-mesh one. The membranes of the cross-linked erythrocytes were torn, and the parasites released. The parasites were separated from the mixture by free-flow electrophoresis. The free parasites had a more rapid anodal mobility than uninfected or infected erythrocytes (Heidrich *et al.*, 1979). It is probable that this system of shearing cross-linked infected erythrocytes by forcing them through nylon sieves may be of general applicability. A great advantage of the system is its simplicity. The equipment needed is available to almost anyone; syringes, syringe filters, nylon screens, and lectins can be readily obtained at little cost. The use of free-flow electrophoresis to separate parasites from erythrocytes is quite complex and probably will be used only in well-equipped laboratories, but the parasites liberated by shearing probably could be collected by centrifugation also. The use of free-flow electrophoresis to separate parasites from erythrocytes is an example of the application of information obtained from a basic study (Seed and Kreier, 1976) to a useful separation technique and is thus a justification for support of basic research.

Very simple procedures for the release of malaria parasites have been described by Chow and Kreier (1972) and by McAlister and Gordon (1977). These procedures involve the extrusion by hand pressure of a 10% suspension of parasitized erythrocytes through a syringe fitted with a 27-gauge needle (Chow and Kreier, 1972) or extrusion through a filter membrane of 3.5-μm pore size (McAlister and Gordon, 1977).

b. Chemical and Immunological Procedures

i. Release by Treatment with Saponin. The use of saponin in lysing erythrocytes for the release of malaria parasites was introduced by Christopher and Fulton (1939). The procedure has been changed little by subsequent workers, who have used it as the first step in reducing the proportion of host material in their parasite preparations.

A. Zuckerman, working with her associates at the Hebrew University, was a major force in the reintroduction and establishment of the saponin lysis technique (Spira and Zuckerman, 1962). Zuckerman's adaptation of the original procedure has been described in detail (Zuckerman *et al.*, 1967) and in brief is as follows. The infected blood is collected in a sodium citrate solution to prevent coagulation, the plasma is removed, and the cells are washed in PBS by a series of centrifugations. Leukocytes and platelets may be partially removed by removing the buffy coat or by sedimentation of the cells through a 3.6% dextran solution. The erythrocytes are then mixed with 50 times their volume of a saponin solution containing 1 part saponin in 7500 parts PBS. The mixture is incubated at 37°C for 15 minutes with occasional stirring. The suspension is then centrifuged in the cold at 10,000 rpm (12,000 g) for 30–60 seconds. The supernatant fluid containing hemoglobin and much of the fluffy sediment containing erythrocyte stromata are discarded, and the procedure is repeated with half the original volume of saponin solution and with only a 10-minute incubation time. The suspension is centrifuged, and the pellet washed repeatedly with PBS to remove saponin and hemoglobin. The parasite preparation is lyophilized and stored under vacuum in the cold. Disruption of the parasites, if required, can be done prior to lyophilization or after reconstitution of the lyophilized material. Under these conditions of storage, antigenicity of the parasites, as determined by double immunodiffusion and immunoelectrophoresis techniques, is preserved for several years. Electron microscopy of thin sections of parasites prepared by saponin lysis of infected red cells reveals that the plasmodia are contained in the erythrocyte membranes (Fig. 5).

Since the recognition that the parasites collected following saponin lysis are contained in the erythrocyte membrane, attempts have been made to remove the membrane. Stauber and Walker (1946) used enzymatic digestion for this purpose. Digestion caused the parasites to become agglutinable by immune serum, but they were not free of membranes (Trager *et al.*, 1950). Kreier *et al.* (1965) fixed saponin-prepared *P. gallinaceum* parasites with Formalin and then broke the membranes which bound the parasites to the erythrocyte nuclei by sonication. These free parasites were morphologically intact, and could be agglutinated by serum from chickens which had recovered from malaria, but were not suitable for solubilization and further analysis because of the fixation. Cook *et al.* (1969)

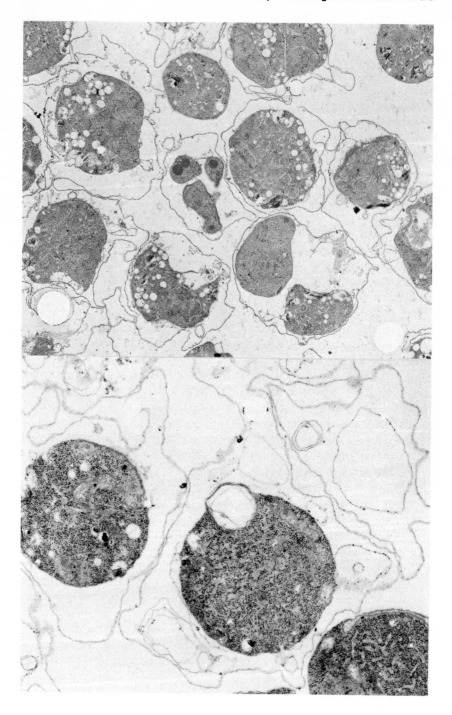

attempted removal of the erythrocyte membranes from saponin-released *P. knowlesi* by a variety of techniques. They observed that fixation with glutaraldehyde followed by mechanical agitation in a Waring blender yielded morphologically intact free parasites (Fig. 6), but they noted that these fixed parasites were of little use for metabolic studies. They also found that mechanical agitation without prior fixation disrupted the parasites and that treatment with sodium dodecyl sulfate lysed the parasites. Attempts by Cook and his associates (1969) to separate parasites from membrane debris by centrifugation on a sucrose gradient were unsuccessful.

A fairly complete separation of freed parasites from contaminating membrane material was recently reported by Siddiqui *et al.* (1978a,b) who employed a three-step gradient constructed of 37, 23, and 10% sucrose solutions and low-speed centrifugation to obtain free *P. falciparum* parasites. The parasites were concentrated within the 10% sucrose layer of the gradient. Eisen (1977) employed a four-step gradient constructed of 35, 25, 15, and 10% BSA solutions and high-speed centrifugation for the collection of *P. berghei* parasites. The free parasites accumulated at the boundary between the 10 and 15% BSA layers.

In attempts to ensure preservation of the parasites during saponin lysis various workers have introduced modifications of the original procedure. These have included decreasing the incubation time and temperature (Jerusalem, 1969; Jerusalem and Eiling, 1969; Van Dyke *et al.*, 1977), the use of balanced salt solutions for solution of the saponin (Siddiqui *et al.*, 1978b; Jerusalem *et al.*, 1969; Van Dyke *et al.*, 1977), and the addition of glucose to the lytic solution (Siddiqui *et al.*, 1978b; Van Dyke *et al.*, 1977).

In a recent study on the effects of various detergents and enzymes on erythrocytes, Siddiqui *et al.* (1978b) showed that saponin was the most efficient substance for hemolysis, for removal of membrane protein, and for removal of sialic acid from red cell membranes. They also showed that parasitized erythrocytes required higher concentrations of saponin for hemolysis than normal ones and emphasized the importance of specifying, when describing a saponin release procedure, the saponin/cell concentration ratio.

ii. Release by Treatment with Ammonium Chloride. Plasmodia may be released from their host cells by treatment of the parasitized erythrocytes with a 0.83% ammonium chloride solution buffered to pH 7.4 with 0.17 M Tris buffer (Martin *et al.*, 1971). One volume of a 50% erythrocyte suspension is added to 9

FIG. 5. Electron micrographs of thin sections of *P. knowlesi* prepared by saponin lysis of infected erythrocytes. (Top) Low-magnification micrograph showing a typical field. (Bottom) Higher-magnification micrograph showing several parasites. Many uninucleate trophozoites in a fairly good state of preservation can be seen, however, some vacuolation has occurred and the parasites are surrounded by host cell membranes. (Photographs courtesy of Dr. M. Aikawa; from Cook *et al.*, 1969.)

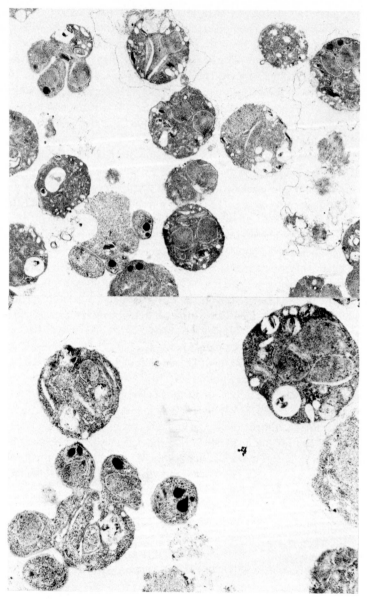

FIG. 6. Electron micrographs of thin sections of *P. knowlesi* prepared by saponin lysis of infected erythrocytes. Lysis was followed by fixation and shearing in a Waring blender. Many intact free parasites are present, however, some are still in membranous sacs, and vacuolation of the cytoplasm of some parasites is present. (Above) Low-magnification micrograph showing a field of parasites. (Below) Higher-magnification micrograph showing several free parasites including a schizont. (Photograph courtesy of Dr. M. Aikawa, from Cook *et al.*, 1969.)

volumes of the prewarmed (37°C) ammonium chloride solution, and the mixture is incubated at 37°C for 3 minutes. Subsequently, the mixture is centrifuged at 500 g for 12 minutes at room temperature and the sediment is washed twice in culture medium (minimal essential medium) supplemented with 10% fetal calf serum. The parasites in this sediment are reported to be free of red cell membrane, morphologically intact, and suitable for antigenic studies. An electron micrograph of free parasites produced by this technique is shown in Fig. 7. The crucial importance of controlling the time of exposure of the parasites to the lytic solution, to minimize their lysis, was emphasized in a later study of the technique (Prior *et al.*, 1973).

iii. Release by Lysis with Antiserum and Complement. The technique of release of plasmodia from host erythrocytes by treatment with specific anti-host erythrocyte antiserum and complement has been used most commonly for obtaining free parasites for culture (Trager, 1950, 1954) and for studies on plasmodial metabolism and enzyme activity (Langer *et al.*, 1967; Bowman *et al.*, 1960; Trigg *et al.*, 1975). A fairly typical procedure is that described by Trager *et al.* (1972) for releasing *P. lophurae*. Washed infected duck erythrocytes are sus-

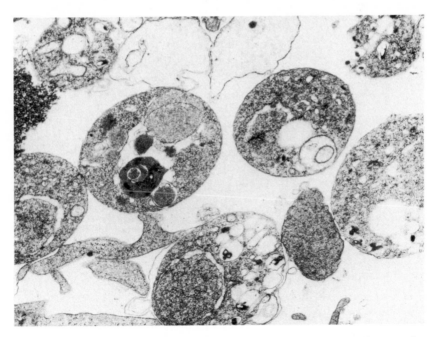

FIG. 7. Electron micrograph of a thin section of *P. berghei* parasites prepared by ammonium chloride lysis. A number of morphologically intact parasites and a moderate amount of debris are visible in the field. (Micrograph courtesy of Dr. John Finerty.)

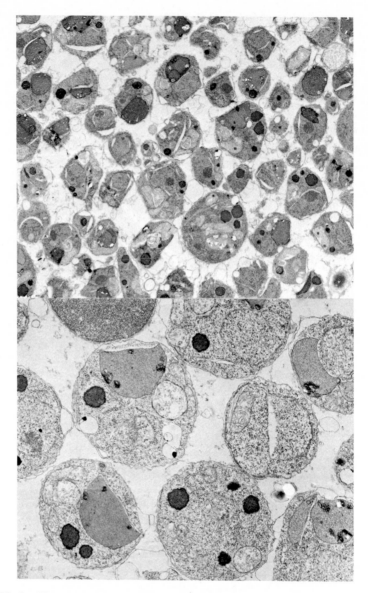

FIG. 8. Electron micrographs of thin sections of *P. lophurae* parasites prepared by immune lysis. (Above) Low-power view of a field showing large numbers of intact parasites and small amounts of membranous materials. (Below) Higher-power view of parasites showing the excellent morphological preservation of the parasites. (Micrographs courtesy of Drs. W. Trager and S. Langreth.)

pended in four times their volume of a balanced salt solution containing a lysed erythrocyte extract. To 6.3 ml of the suspension, 0.13 ml of guinea pig serum and 0.7 ml of antierythrocyte rabbit serum are added. The mixture is incubated for ½ hour at 40°C on a rocking platform and is swirled vigorously after 15 minutes and again at the end of the incubation period. A mild mechanical shear is effected by vigorous pipetting, and the material is centrifuged just long enough to obtain clearing of the fluid. The released parasites (Fig. 8) are then collected with the supernatant fluid. Earlier versions of the immune lysis procedure (Trager, 1950) included enzyme digestion with trypsin and DNase for removal of host cell membrane and nuclear material, but these treatments lowered the viability of the product (Trager *et al.*, 1972). This procedure was recently employed for releasing *P. lophurae* from which a histidine-rich protein was obtained (Kilejian, 1974).

   c. Natural Release.   All the procedures for obtaining erythrocytic stages of plasmodia described so far in this chapter have involved the use of chemical or physical means for disrupting the host erythrocyte membrane in order to release the contained parasites or to release components of the parasites. The parasites obtained by these procedures are in whatever stage of development they were at the time of the artifically induced erythrocyte rupture. In constrast, natural rupture of the parasitized erythrocyte results in preferential release of parasites in the final stages of development of the erythrocytic cycle, i.e., the merozoites. Natural release of the parasites depends on their development to maturity under suitable culture conditions. The description of these conditions is given in Volume 2, Chapter 6. Under proper culture conditions the parasites and their constituents are released into the culture medium without being exposed to the potentially harmful chemicals and physical conditions used for artifical lysis.

   Short-term cultures of *P. knowlesi* were used by Mitchell *et al.* (1973) for the production of merozoites. The merozoites obtained were later used for vaccination (Mitchell *et al.*, 1974, 1975). The procedure involves the culture of erythrocytes, a high proportion of which (75–95%) contain schizonts. The scarcity of uninfected cells minimizes reinvasion and allows progressive accumulation of the released merozoites. Maximal numbers of free merozoites are obtained after 2–7 hours in culture. Subsequent low-speed centrifugation of the cell suspension provides a supernatant containing 90% merozoites which are still considerably contaminated with intracellular schizonts. Separation of merozoites from schizont-containing erythrocytes is accomplished by agglutinating the latter using schizont-agglutinating serum (Mitchell *et al.*, 1973) or phytohemagglutinin (Mitchell *et al.*, 1975). The antiserum or lectin is added 30 minutes prior to the harvesting of merozoites. Forty percent of the merozoites are recovered, and the final product contains less than 1% normal or parasitized erythrocytes (Fig. 9, above) (Mitchell *et al.*, 1973). These merozoite preparations are mostly nonvi-

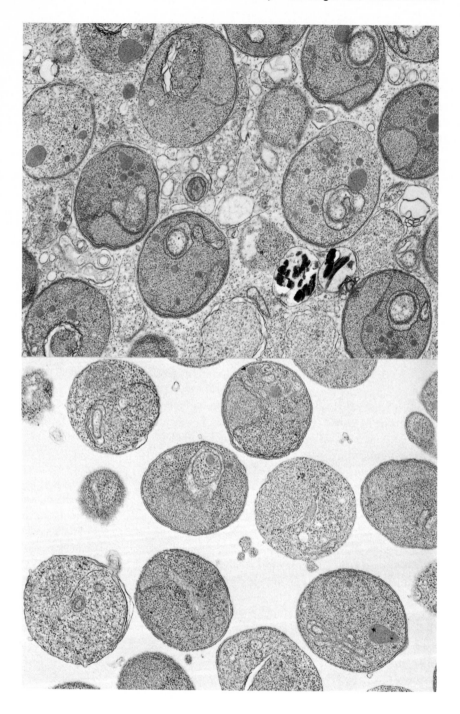

able by the time they have been prepared. To obtain viable merozoites a method has been devised by Dennis *et al.* (1975) for isolating merozoites as they are released from schizonts. The procedure involves the culturing of schizonts in a chamber with a floor consisting of a polycarbonate sieve of 2.0-μm pore size through which the merozoites are continuously drawn as they are released. The yield of merozoites is 50% of the expected total, and contaminating parasitized erythrocytes do not exceed 0.5% (Fig. 9, below).

The procedures now available for short-term culture of *P. falciparum* at high parasitemia (Siddiqui *et al.*, 1974) and the more recently developed techniques for continuous culture of this parasite (Trager and Jensen, 1976; Haynes *et al.*, 1976; Brackett *et al.*, 1978) will provide extremely important sources of *P. falciparum* merozoites.

Infected blood from a continuous culture served for the isolation of a histidine-rich protein from *P. falciparum* merozoites. The procedure for harvesting the parasites in this case involved culturing the parasitized erythrocytes under conditions which do not favor reinvasion and then collecting the merozoites by differential centrifugation (Kilejian and Jensen, 1977). A system for the continuous culture of *P. knowlesi* which has been recently reported (Butcher, 1978) should be useful for harvesting merozoites of this parasite.

Culture techniques for other plasmodia, *P. berghei* (Smalley and Butcher, 1975), for example, are less advanced. Despite the newness of the natural release techniques for obtaining erythrocytic merozoites, the usefulness of the culture procedures for obtaining merozoites for the study of host–parasite interactions (Cohen *et al.*, 1972; Miller *et al.*, 1975) has been proved. The most significant use of the merozoites obtained by natural release has been in vaccination studies (Cox, 1974; Mitchell *et al.*, 1974, 1975).

5. *Comparison of Release Procedures*

The value of a given procedure for releasing plasmodia from host cells is largely determined by the objectives of the specific study involved. Nevertheless, some general criteria can be used for evaluating the efficiency of a given release procedure. Basically, these are yield and quality. The quality of freed parasites can be evaluated in terms of viability, morphological integrity, and purity with regard to host cell contamination and antigenic activity.

The yield of released parasites has been specified in some of the studies on the release of plasmodia, but there is no uniform approach to such an evaluation.

FIG. 9. Electron micrographs of thin sections of *P. knowlesi* parasites released following maturation in culture. (Top) Parasites prepared by lectin agglutination of contaminating erythrocytes. (Bottom) Parasites prepared by the cell sieving procedure. The parasites are a fairly pure merozoite population. Less contaminating material is present in the preparation made by cell sieving than in the one made by lectin agglutination and centrifugation. (Micrographs courtesy of Drs. Cohen and Banister.)

Thus, for example, release by immune lysis has been reported to yield 2 ml of packed parasites per 100 ml of infected blood with 100% parasitemia (Kilejian, 1976). The blood harvested from 20 mice with 50% parasitemia when treated with saponin yielded parasites which when disrupted yielded about 30 mg parasite protein (*P. berghei*).(Spira, 1965). In another study on saponin release of parasites, blood from 200 infected mice yielded 1.5–2 ml packed material (Mannweiler and Oelerich, 1969). Continuous collection of naturally released *P. knowlesi* parasites yielded 50% of the expected total (Dennis *et al.*, 1975).

Viability of the released parasites is essential for studies on infectivity, invasion *in vitro*, metabolic activity, and *in vitro* growth. The stage of development of the released parasites should be considered in viability testing. Thus, while released trophozoites and schizonts may continue to develop *in vitro* (Langreth and Trager, 1973; Trager *et al.*, 1972), merozoites quickly lose their ability to invade host cells (Dennis *et al.*, 1975; Dvorak *et al.*, 1975). Those using infectivity tests should consider the possibility that among free blood stage parasites only the fully developed merozoites are potentially infective (Walter, 1968). Thus when viability is inferred from metabolic activity, one has to take into account that most free parasite preparations contain viable but noninfectious forms of parasites (Kreier *et al.*, 1976), host cell membranes (Cook *et al.*, 1969; Seed *et al.*, 1973a; Kilby and Silverman, 1969), and soluble enzymes (Tsukamoto, 1974). These contaminants plus contaminating leukocytes, platelets, and possibly host cell organelles may affect the results of metabolic experiments with free parasites. Thus, metabolic activities such as respiration, which are carried out by parasites in immature stages of development and which may continue in disrupted parasites (Scheibel and Miller, 1969a,b), cannot be regarded as completely satisfactory criteria for viability, as they only reflect certain aspects of viability.

The infectivity of saponin-released parasites was initially demonstrated by Christophers and Fulton (1939). This finding was later confirmed (Zuckerman and Ristic, 1968). Saponin-released parasites may develop *in vitro* (Trager *et al.*, 1972), maintaining their ability to incorporate amino acids (reviewed by Sherman, 1977b) and nucleic acid precursors (Van Dyke *et al.*, 1977; reviewed in Sherman, 1977a) into the corresponding macromolecules. Similarly, parasites released by immune lysis are infective (Walter, 1968; McAlister and Gordon, 1977; Bowman *et al.*, 1960) and capable of extracellular growth while maintaining the metabolic activities essential for growth (Trager *et al.*, 1972; Sherman, 1977a,b).

Naturally released *P. knowlesi* merozoites are capable of invading erythrocytes *in vitro*, although invasiveness is quickly lost (Dennis *et al.*, 1975; Dvorak *et al.*, 1975). Naturally released merozoites do not incorporate amino acids, for example, isoleucine, until after reinvasion (Cohen *et al.*, 1969, 1972).

Release by continuous flow sonication (CFS) yields infective parasites (Prior and Kreier, 1972a,b; Kreier et al., 1976). The CFS-released parasites, unlike parasites in red cells, interact directly with protective antibody as demonstrated in comparative infectivity tests (Hamburger and Kreier, 1975). As a relatively small fraction of CFS preparations of P. berghei contain fully developed, potentially infective merozoites, metabolic studies combined with infectivity studies should add important quantitative information on the viability of parasites prepared by this procedure. It should be noted that increasing the void volume of the sonication chamber and decreasing the flow rate may account for loss of viability of parasites released by CFS (McAlister and Gordon, 1977).

Electron microscopical examinations of naturally released parasites (see Fig. 9) (Dennis et al., 1975), as well as of parasites released by CFS (see Fig. 3) (Kreier et al., 1976; Prior and Kreier, 1972a,b; Prior et al., 1973), saponin lysis (see Fig. 5) (Aikawa and Cook, 1972; Cook et al., 1969; Trager et al., 1972; Kilby and Silverman, 1969), and immune lysis (see Fig. 8) (Trager et al., 1972; Cook et al., 1969) show that the morphological integrity of the released parasites is largely preserved, an observation compatible with the demonstration of viability and infectivity of at least some of the parasites released by these techniques.

The viability of parasites obtained by other release procedures is, at best, doubtful. Parasites released by hypotonic lysis, for example, are nonviable (Christophers and Fulton, 1939). It was noted by Cook et al. (1969) that most parasites were more sensitive to osmotic shock than some of the erythrocytes. Seed et al. (1976) observed that merozoites were the most sensitive to osmotic stress of any of the blood forms of plasmodia. Osmotically released parasite preparations were incapable of incorporating [^{3}H]adenosine into parasite nucleic acids (Van Dyke et al., 1977). Electron microscopical examination showed complete disruption of osmotically released parasites (see Fig. 1) (Cook et al., 1969; Kilby and Silverman, 1969; Aikawa and Cook, 1972). French pressure cell-released parasites were initially reported to be viable (D'Antonio et al., 1966b), but other studies showed that parasites prepared by this technique were severely damaged (see Fig. 4) (Trager et al., 1972; Cook et al., 1969; Kilby and Silverman, 1969; Aikawa and Cook, 1972) (see Fig. 4) and failed to develop in vitro (Trager et al., 1972). Plasmodia released by treatment with ammonium chloride have been shown to possess some degree of morphological preservation (see Fig. 7) (Martin et al., 1971; Prior et al., 1973). These parasite preparations were initially found to be infective (Martin et al., 1971), however, more recently it has been noted that free parasites prepared by this method are quiescent and lack typical merozoite movement (McAlister and Gordon, 1977) and are unable to incorporate [^{3}H]adenosine (Van Dyke et al., 1977). Information on the viability and morphology of parasites released by nitrogen cavitation (Wallach and Conley, 1977) is not yet available.

The degree of freedom of released parasites from host cell contamination has been given much attention because of the implications of such contamination in metabolic and immunological studies. As effective removal of leukocytes and platelets is now possible, the chief difficulty remains complete removal of the erythrocyte envelope from the individual parasites and the quantitative assessment of membrane contamination in the parasite preparations. Naturally released parasites, being mostly fully developed merozoites, are free of the outer membrane of the erythrocyte as well as of the membrane of the parasitophorous vacuole (Dennis *et al.*, 1975; Ladda, 1969). Some of the parasites, especially the merozoites, released by CFS are also free of the membrane of the parasitophorous vacuole, and essentially all are free of the outer membrane of the erythrocyte (kreier *et al.*, 1976). *Plasmodium lophurae* released by immune lysis are essentially free of the erythrocyte outer membrane but are still within the parasitophorous vacuole (Langreth and Trager, 1973). In general, removal of the parasitophorous vacuole membrane is not achieved by most artificial release procedures (Trager *et al.*, 1972; Cook *et al.*, 1969; Langreth and Trager, 1973; Kilby and Silverman, 1969; Aikawa and Cook, 1972). Furthermore, saponin treatment (Trager *et al.*, 1972; Stauber and Walker, 1946; Cook *et al.*, 1969; Aikawa and Cook, 1972), treatment with a French pressure cell (Trager *et al.*, 1972; Cook *et al.*, 1969), and hypotonic lysis (Cook *et al.*, 1969) leave many of the parasites still enveloped by the outer membrane of the erythrocyte as well as the membrane of the parasitophorous vacuole.

The identification of erythrocyte membrane material in preparations of released parasites has been a problem. Even if the individual parasites are released from the membrane, it is impossible to quantitate, by microscopy, the amount of membrane contamination left in the preparation. It has recently been shown that erythrocyte membranes can be differentiated from parasite membranes by their affinity for colloidal iron stains (Seed *et al.*, 1973a; Miller *et al.*, 1973) or by their affinity for a variety of lectins (Seed and Kreier, 1976). Stains which differentiate the erythrocyte membrane from the parasite are potentially useful for quantitative determination of host cell contamination in preparations of released parasites. Most recently Wallach and Conley (1977) have partially solved the problem of monitoring erythrocyte membrane contamination by adding erythrocytes, whose outer membranes are labeled, to the parasitized erythrocytes prior to lysis. They then monitor the amount of radioactive label present as a measure of membrane contamination throughout the isolation procedure. This technique cannot be used to detect contamination with the membrane of the parasitophorous vacuole, as this membrane cannot be labeled prior to cell lysis by presently available techniques.

There are various implications for immunological studies of the viability, morphological integrity, and degree of host cell contamination of parasite preparations. Viability is indeed important when released parasites are to be used for culture. Where antigenic analysis is concerned, viability and morphological integrity can serve as general criteria for evaluating the state of the starting material (Zuckerman and Ristic, 1968). Some serological tests require viable parasites, e.g., penetration inhibition tests (Cohen *et al.*, 1969), and some such as direct agglutination (Kreier *et al.*, 1965) and the indirect fluorescent antibody test (Hamburger and Kreier, 1976b) require intact parasites, but many serological tests (CF, SAFA, IHA, ELISA, and Immunoprecipitation) require only extracts or fractions of parasites (Brown, 1969; Fife, 1972; Mathews *et al.*, 1975; Meuwissen *et al.*, 1972; Voller *et al.*, 1975; Sadun and Gore, 1968; Wellde *et al.*, 1969; Spira, 1965). It should be emphasized that the release of parasites from the parasitized erythrocyte may by itself result in a loss of serologically active antigens. Thus Lund and Powers (1976) found that, for a passive hemagglutination test, the antigen obtained by freezing and thawing schizont-infected cells was as good as the antigen obtained from saponin-released parasites but that the yield from the free parasites was smaller.

Less severe problems may result from the use of contaminated antigen in serological tests than from the use of contaminated antigen for immunization. Individuals immunized with vaccine contaminated with erythrocyte membranes may develop antierythrocyte antibodies (Diggs, 1966; Hamburger and Zuckerman, 1976a). Such antibodies may cause erythroblastosis fetalis in infants born to immunized women. This condition has occurred in calves born to cows immunized against anaplasmosis with a blood origin parasite preparation (Dennis *et al.*, 1970).

Erythrocyte membranes will fix complement with sera of individuals with malaria (Heidelberger and Mayer, 1944), and the active components, which are at least in part lipid, will sensitize erythrocytes for hemagglutination and will precipitate in gel with serum from infected subjects (Seed and Kreier, 1969). Antibodies to erythrocyte membranes develop in individuals with many diseases, and erythrocyte membrane contamination in antigen to be used for serodiagnosis of malaria may cause false positive reactions. In general, host cell contamination if present in large quantities may reduce the sensitivity and the specificity of serological tests employing extracts of parasite preparations.

Comparative evaluation of antigen preparations used for immunization is an undeveloped field. Jerusalem and Eling (1969) made a comparison of the induction of protective immunity in mice by saponin-released, hemolytic antiserum and complement-released and dilute formol-released *P. berghei*. They concluded that the method of release of the parasite was irrelevant to the antigenicity. Desowitz (1975) compared the immunogenicity for rats of several subfractions of saponin-prepared *P. berghei* parasites in what was basically a study of adjuvants. He reported that alum-precipitated components of the soluble portions of saponin-prepared *P. berghei* parasites were not immunogenic. Saul and Kreier (1977) compared the immunogenicity in rats of various fractions of sonically released *P. berghei*. They found protective antigen in both soluble and insoluble portions of the parasites. The techniques they describe could be applied to a comparison of the various antigens currently being used. These workers emphasize the importance of careful quantitative analysis of the immunogens if valid comparisons are to be made.

6. Plasmodial Constituents from Freed Parasites

For most studies the collection of released parasites is only part of the preparation process. The subsequent steps generally are disruption of the collected parasites and separation of the soluble from the insoluble material by centrifugation. In some studies this initial separatory step is followed by fractionation of the parasites' constitutents. A great variety of techniques have been applied for the disruption of released malaria parasites. These include lysis by distilled water (Cook *et al.*, 1971), by Triton X-100 (Sherman *et al.*, 1975), by freezing and thawing (Sherman and Hull, 1960; Sherman, 1964), by sonication (Todorovic *et al.*, 1968a; Diggs, 1966; Sodeman and Meuwissen, 1966; Ward and Conran, 1966), by treatment with a French pressure cell (D'Antonio *et al.*, 1966b; D'Antonio, 1972; Scheibel and Miller, 1969a) or a Hughes press (Spira and Zuckerman, 1962), and by homogenization in a Potter homogenizer (Jerusalem, 1969; Jerusalem *et al.*, 1971), a Ten Broek homogenizer (Rock *et al.*, 1971), or a Virtis homogenizer (Corradetti *et al.*, 1966).

a. Serological Studies on Constituents of Freed Parasites. A variety of serological techniques use plasmodial extracts and fractions prepared from released parasites. Complement-fixing antigens were initially prepared from lysates of parasitized erythrocytes. The use of extracts from parasites released by hypotonic lysis was introduced in the 1940s (Dulaney and Stratman-Thomas, 1940; Mayer and Heidelberger, 1946). More recently complement-fixing antigens were prepared from parasites released by CFS (Prior and Kreier, 1972a), saponin lysis (Ward and Conran, 1966; Mahoney *et al.*, 1966), and French pressure cell treatment (D'Antonio *et al.*, 1966a,b; Mohoney *et al.*, 1966). Efforts to purify complement-fixing antigens and to reduce the anticomplementary activity led to fractionation of the crude extracts. D'Antonio *et al.* (1966b) used a French pressure cell to release and disintegrate *P. knowlesi* parasites and fractionated the soluble extract on Sephadex G-200 to obtain a complement-fixing antigen of high molecular weight. Mahoney *et al.* (1966) prepared extracts from saponin-released parasites by subjecting them to extrusion at high pressure from a French pressure cell. Both these groups then separated soluble from insoluble fractions by a series of centrifugations and extractions and tested the various fractions in CF, IHA, SAFA, double immunodiffusion, and slide flocculation tests. Mahoney reported that complement-fixing activity was associated with the insoluble fractions and was eliminated by treatment with *n*-butanol. The particulate nature of soluble complement-fixing antigens was noted by Mayer and Heidelberger (1946). That immunogenic fractions could be particulate was observed by D'Antonio et al. (1970) and by Saul and Kreier (1977). The latter workers detected immunogenicity in soluble as well as particulate materials. It should be noted that the term ''soluble plasmodial antigen'' is frequently used in the literature to describe the supernatant obtained by centrifugation of disintegrated parasites at speeds which will remove pigment and other visible debris, but only ultracentrifugation of disintegrated parasites will sediment small particulate or aggregated material and yield truly soluble preparations (Mahoney et al., 1966).

Unlike early complement-fixing antigens, IHA antigens were initially prepared from released parasites, and the use of erythrocyte lysates was a later development. The original procedure described by Stein and Desowitz (1964) involved hypotonic lysis of the erythrocytes and grinding of the released parasites. Release by hypotonic lysis followed by freezing and thawing of the parasites or disintegration by extrusion from a French pressure cell was later employed by Rogers et al. (1968). Bray and El-Nahal (1966) and Mahoney et al. (1966) released the parasites by saponin treatment and disintegrated them by freezing and thawing (Bray and El-Nahal, 1966) or by extrusion from a French pressure cell (Mahoney et al., 1966). The soluble fraction of the various extracts was employed as antigen. Ultracentrifugation of such supernatants yielded a true soluble antigen which was active in IHA and a sediment capable on inhibiting the reaction (Mahoney et al., 1966). In a comparative study, Kagan (1972) employed various release procedures, disintegration, and fractionation methods for preparing IHA antigens. He concluded that treatment with distilled water containing 0.01% Triton X-100 gave a better recovery of parasites than saponin lysis, pressure lysis, or hypontonic lysis without additives. Kagan (1972) also found disintegration of parasites by a Ribe cell fractionator to give a better antigen than various other disintegration procedures including freezing and thawing, grinding in a tissue grinder, sonication, and lyophilization followed by pressure and pressure release disruption. Kagan (1972) also fractionated the soluble extracts he obtained by various techniques previously described by others including gel filtration, ion-exchange chromatography, ammonium sulfate precipitation, and Rivanol precipitation. He found Rivanol precipitation to be the most satisfactory procedure of those he tested.

Mahoney et al. (1966) showed that soluble as well as insoluble fractions of P. knowlesi, including residues left after extraction with n-butanol, gave precipitation lines in double immunodiffusion tests with sera from artificially immunized monkeys but not with sera from individuals which had recovered from infection.

b. Antigenic Analysis of Constituents of Freed Parasites. The use of the techniques of precipitation in agar, e.g., double immunodiffusion (Ouchterlony) and immunoelectrophoresis, have contributed substantially to the antigenic analysis of plasmodia. These techniques are capable of revealing separate antigen–antibody systems, thus making it possible to identify species-specific antigens in mixtures of antigens (Hamburger and Zuckerman, 1978). Recently, crossed immunoelectrophoresis (CIE), another technique of precipitation in agar, has been used to identify stage-specific antigens (Deans *et al.*, 1978). The use of these techniques makes possible a modern approach to the study of malarial antigens and antibodies. With these approaches attempts are made to fractionate plasmodial extracts and identify and characterize separate antigens.

The use of PAGE with primate, avian, and rodent plasmodia has indicated that extracts of plasmodia consist of complex mixtures of potentially antigenic components (Chavin, 1966; Sodeman and Meuwissen, 1966; Ward and Conran, 1966; Zuckerman, 1964, 1969; Spira *et al.*, 1965; Kreier *et al.*, 1976; Grothaus and Kreier, 1980). Extracts have been resolved into more than 10 protein fractions. The most extensive studies on antigens of human plasmodia were done on *P. falciparum* antigens prepared by direct lysis of parasitized erythrocytes from placental blood. In these studies antisera from human patients were used. Important information on the antigenic composition of plasmodia has also been obtained from studies on the more easily manageable animal plasmodia. Such studies were done on simian (Mahoney *et al.*, 1966; Deans *et al.*, 1978; Williamson, 1967; Banki and Bucci, 1964a,b; Brown *et al.*, 1970), rodent (Spira and Zuckerman, 1962; Diggs, 1966; Zuckerman and Spira, 1963; Zuckerman, 1964), and avian (Sherman, 1964; Spira and Zuckerman, 1964) plasmodia and employed extracts of released parasites (usually released by saponin lysis) and antisera from artifically immunized animals. Such antisera, particularly those prepared in rabbits, contain precipitins against more antigenic components than sera from recovered animals (Williamson, 1967; Banki and Bucci, 1964a,b; Brown *et al.*, 1970; Zuckerman, 1964; Zuckerman *et al.*, 1969) and are thus capable of providing a more complete antigenic profile of the extracts. Such antisera, however, may contain antibodies against host cell components (Diggs, 1966; Hamburger and Zuckerman, 1976a; Spira and Zuckerman, 1966). The advantage of the use of sera from recovered subjects over that of sera from artificially immunized animals is that recovered animal sera contain antibodies induced by the viable parasite in the susceptible host. The possibility that such sera may contain induced protective antibodies as well as a proportion of antibodies irrelevant to immunity may make them suitable for the identification of antigens stimulating protective responses (Hamburger and Zuckerman, 1976b).

A variety of fractionation procedures followed by double immunodiffusion and immunoelectrophorsis have been used to identify antigens in various plasmodial extracts. Chavin (1966) used several procedures to fractionate *P. berghei* extracts obtained by the homogenization of parasites released from erythrocytes by hypotonic lysis. Rivanol precipitation of the extract almost completely separated parasite materials from host hemoglobin and provided plasmodial antigens serologically active in double immunodiffusion tests. In Chavin's agar plates 8–10 precipitation lines developed. The various procedures Chavin (1966) used in attempting fractionation of the antigens were analytical ultracentrifugation, sucrose density gradient ultracentrifugation, gel filtration on Sephadex G-100 and G-200, ion-exhange chromatophraphy on DEAE-cellulose or on CM-cellulose, and block electrophoresis with starch or with Pevikon–Gehon. Ion-exchange chromatography yielded up to three fractions, and the other procedures yielded only one fraction or protein peak. None of the procedures provided useful fractionation of the plasmodial antigens. Mannweiler and Oelerich (1969) fractionated extracts obtained by freezing and thawing saponin-released *P. berghei*. He used gel filtration and preparative PAGE for the fractionation and determined the antigenic activity of the fractions obtained by double immunodiffusion tests. The antigenically active fractions eluted in one peak upon filtration of the extracts through Sephadex G-75, G-100, and G-200 columns. Photoabsorbance monitoring of continuously collected eluates from preparative PAGE columns revealed a single absorbance peak and two trailing shoulders. Separation of the serologically active components into individual fractions did not occur. Hamburger and Zuckerman (1976a,b) successfully fractionated a rather similar extract by another preparative PAGE approach. In their study the gels were cut into 12 slices following electrophoresis, and the components in each were eluted. Slices were also used directly for immunization. The extract was resolved into about 10 protein fractions, seen as bands on PAGE, and gave 10 precipitation lines with serum from artifically immunized rabbits in double diffusion tests. Each of the protein bands in the PAGE columns could in turn be resolved into one or two bands by gel diffusion techniques. The molecular weights of the various components of the extract ranged between 8000 and 130,000. Some of the fractions contained glycoproteins and RNA. Of the 12 slices into which the PAGE gels were cut, slices 4 and 5 and 7 and 8 contained species-specific antigens capable of inducing a degree of protection against or enhancement of infection in animals into which they were injected. Of all the slices, 4 and 5 and 7 and 8 gave the strongest precipitation lines with sera from recovered hyperimmune rats. Most of the protein of *P. berghei* was in slices 4 and 5. The protein appearing in slices 4 and 5 of the PAGE gels could also be separated from most other *P. berghei* components in the mixtures by ion-exchange chromatography of the extract on DEAE-Sephadex (Hamburger and Zuckerman, 1978).

c. Immunization with Constituents of Freed Parasites. Partial characterization of protective antigens used for vaccination was accomplished with the rodent plasmodium *P. berghei* by Hamburger and Zuckerman (1976b) and Grothaus and Kreier (1980). Most other vaccination studies did not, however, attempt antigenic characterization of the fractions used for immunization. Extensive vaccination studies with fractions of French pressure cell-released parasites were conducted in Silverman's laboratory. In the initial studies by D'Antonio *et al.* (1970) the parasites (*P. berghei*) were fractionated by gel filtration on Sephadex G-200. In later studies with *P. knowlesi*, fractionation on Sephadex G-200 (D'Antonio, 1972; Schenkel *et al.*, 1973), or BioGel A 1.5 (Simpson *et al.*, 1974) was used. All the columns tested yielded a void volume fraction capable of inducing protection. Further fractionation by centrifugation on sucrose density gradients gave fractions with increased immunogenicity (Simpson *et al.*, 1974).

Kilejian (1974) isolated a histidine-rich polypeptide from *P. lophurae*. After release from the host erythrocytes by immune lysis the parasites were disintegrated by sonication and the extract centrifuged on a sucrose cushion. The pellet was extracted with 0.1 *N* sodium hydroxide to remove hemozoin, and the resulting pellet was dissolved in 0.9 *N* acetic acid. Alternatively the sucrose pellet was directly extracted with acetic acid. Amino acid analysis of the polypeptide obtained by these treatments showed it to have a very high histidine content. The purity of the product was monitored by PAGE, and a single band was obtained. This polypeptide may be involved in the penetration of erythrocytes by merozoites (Kilejian, 1976) and has been demonstrated to induce protection against *P. lophurae* (Kilejian, 1978).

Saul and Kreier (1977) obtained a soluble antigen by gently washing sonically freed *P. berghei* in cold saline. This antigen stimulated as strong a protective response as the free parasites from which it was washed. On analysis by PAGE this antigen was shown to be a protein and to represent a small subset of the soluble antigens which could be released from the parasites by freezing and thawing. Brooks and Kreier (1978) have shown that the merozoite capsule is antiphagocytic and suggest that the antigen of Saul and Kreier (1977) may be this capsular material. Grothaus and Kreier (1980) confirmed the observations of Saul and Kreier (1977) that a soluble immunogen could be obtained by gentle washing of sonically freed *P. berghei*. They further demonstrated that this material is approximately 20-fold more potent as an immunogen than are the free parasites. The relationship of the soluble material isolated by Saul and Kreier to the various soluble and membrane fractions shown by others to stimulate protection is at present under investigation.

d. Biochemical Characteristics of Plasmodia. Plasmodial proteins are antigenic, and some are also enzymatically active. Nevertheless, it appears that combined antigenic and enzymatic analyses of plasmodial constituents are largely lacking. Such combined studies may provide important information on the biological activity of antigens, as well as on the specific identity of enzymes. Furthermore, ligand activities may serve as markers in the molecular characterization of plasmodial proteins. Another area in plasmodial biochemistry and molecular biology yet to benefit from advances in the characterization and purification of plasmodial antigens is that of cell-free protein-synthesizing systems. An extensive account of the biochemical and metabolic activities of plasmodia is available in Chapter 5, Volume 1. Here we will only discuss those aspects of fractionation and electrophoretic characterization of plasmodial enzymes which may aid the immunologist attempting similar fractionation and characterization of plasmodial constituents for immunological studies. We will also mention briefly the use of plasmodial components in cell-free protein-synthesizing systems.

Several plasmodial enzymes participating in carbohydrate metabolism including enzymes involved in glycolysis, the pentose phosphate pathway, and the tricarboxylic acid cycle have been identified electrophoretically. Purification of plasmodial enzymes, in general, is a relatively undeveloped field, but even in cases where a high degree of purity was accomplished no antigenic characterization of the product was undertaken. Langer et al. (1967) used electrophoresis to identify 6-phosphogluconate dehydrogenase (6-PGD), glucose-6-phosphate dehydrogenase (G-6-PD), and transketolase in soluble extracts obtained by homogenization of P. berghei parasites released from erythrocytes by immune lysis. These studies were later extended to include lactic dehydrogenase (LDH) (Phisphumvidhi and Langer, 1969). Sherman et al. (1971) detected NADP-glutamate dehydrogenase in extracts of saponin-released P. lophurae. Extensive electrophoretic studies on plasmodial enzymes and isozymes were carried out by Carter and his colleagues. They defined the electrophoretic profiles of various enzymes, mainly those involved in carbohydrate metabolism, which exist among plasmodial species and subspecies. In the initial studies (Carter, 1970, 1972) glucose phosphate isomerase (GPI), malate dehydrogenase (MDH), 6-PGD, and adenylate kinase were identified in extracts of P. berghei released by immune lysis and disintegrated with a solution of Triton X-100. In further studies these enzymes, as well as LDH (Carter, 1973; Carter and McGregor, 1973; Carter and Voller, 1973a,b, 1975) and glutamate dehydrogenase (Carter, 1974), were identified in lysates of parasitized erythrocytes. The studies were extended to include human and simian plasmodia (Carter and McGregor, 1973; Carter and Voller, 1973a,b, 1975). In a recent study pyruvate kinase was identified electrophoretically by Oelschlegel et al. (1975). NADP-glutamate dehydrogenase of P. chabaudi was purified 1400-fold by Walter et al. (1974). For this purpose soluble extracts of saponin-released, sonically disintegrated parasites were subjected to stepwise fractionation involving precipitation with ammonium sulfate followed by column chromatography on DEAE-cellulose, hydroxyapatite, CM-cellulose and Sepharose, and by isoelectrofocusing. The isoelectric point of the NADP-glutamate dehydrogenase of P. chabaudi was 4.55, and its molecular weight was 200,000 as determined by gel filtration and 245,000 as determined by centrifugation in a sucrose gradient.

Studies on carbon dioxide fixation by plasmodia also involved attempts at enzyme purification. Phosphoenolpyruvate carboxylase of *P. berghei* was concentrated 14- to 20-fold by ammonium sulfate precipitation and gel filtration on a column of agarose beads (Siu, 1967; Forrester and Siu, 1971). This enzyme was purified 400-fold by ammonium sulfate precipitation followed by ion-exchange chromatography on DEAE-cellulose and cellulose phosphate columns (McDaniel and Siu, 1972).

The enzymes hydroxymethyldihydropteridine pyrophosphokinase and dihydropteroate synthetase, involved in folate metabolism, were identified in soluble extracts of *P. berghei*. They were eluted together in the void volume or close to it upon gel filtration on Sephadex G-100 or G-200 columns but could be separated from each other by ion-exchange chromatography on DEAE-Sephadex A-50 columns (Ferone, 1973). Walter and Königk (1974) were not able to separate materials bearing these two enzymes of folate metabolism in extracts of *P. chabaudi* but succeeded in concentrating them so that enzymatic activity of the concentrate was 950-fold greater than in the starting material. This was accomplished by subjecting the soluble extracts of the parasites to a series of fractionation steps. These involved ammonium sulfate precipitation of the material obtained by a series of chromatographic treatments of the extract on CM-cellulose, hydroxyapatite, DEAE-cellulose, Sephadex G-200, and DEAE-Sephadex A-50. Other enzymes involved in folate metabolism have also been subjected to fractionation and purification. Dihydrofolate reductase of *P. berghei* was eluted from Sephadex G-100 columns close to the void volume (Ferone *et al.*, 1968). The enzyme was precipitated from the soluble parasite extract by the addition of 35–75% ammonium sulfate, and its molecular weight, as determined by gel filtration on Sephadex G-200 columns, was $190,000 \pm 10\%$. The dihydrofolate reductase of *P. knowlesi* has a similar molecular weight, i.e., 200,000 (Gutteridge and Trigg, 1971). The dihydrofolate reductase of *P. lophurae* was shown by similar methods to have a molecular weight of only 103,000 (Platzer, 1974). Thymidylate synthetase of *P. berghei* was concentrated 50-fold by ion-exchange chromatography of parasitized erythrocyte lysates. A molecular weight of 100,000 was determined for this enzyme by gel filtration on Sephadex G-100 (Reid and Friedkin, 1973).

The presence of proteolytic enzymes in plasmodia is obvious from their ability to utilize host cell hemoglobin. Both acid and alkaline proteases have been detected in plasmodia (reviewed by Sherman, 1977b). An acid, membrane-bound proteinase of *P. berghei* was partially purified (Levy and Chow, 1973) by treatment of *P. berghei* membranes with Triton X-100 followed by ammonium sulfate precipitation and gel filtration on Sephadex G-100. This enzyme had a molecular weight of less than 68,000. The breakdown product of hemoglobin within the parasite, hemozoin, was the subject of numerous studies, some involving its purification (reviewed by Sherman, 1977b).

Cell-free protein-synthesizing systems using plasmodial components have been described, but until very recently no attempts had been made to identify the antigenic properties of the products. Cook *et al.* (1969) described a method for obtaining *P. knowlesi* ribosomes and other subcellular particles. Saponin-released parasites were disintegrated by treatment with water containing 0.005 *M* magnesium chloride, and the lysates were centrifuged on a continuous sucrose gradient. Free ribosomes and rough microsomal membranes were contained in a band with a density of 1.22 g/ml. *In vitro* protein synthesis, as measured by the incorporation of ^{14}C-labeled amino acids into TCA-insoluble material, was demonstrated using this microsomal fraction supplemented with a soluble part of *P. knowlesi*. In a later study, Cook *et al.* (1971) harvested ribosomes from a *P. knowlesi* extract by a series of centrifugations and homogenizations of the pellets, followed by treatment with sodium deoxycholate and filtration on a 0.45-μm filter. The mode of activation of amino acids for protein synthesis was studied by Ilan and his associates (Ilan and Ilan, 1969; Ilan *et al.*, 1969). They used a soluble *P. berghei* extract as a source of amino acid tRNA synthetase and tRNA from *Escherichia coli* or rabbit liver. In a series of studies by Sherman and his associates (Sherman *et al.*, 1975; Sherman, 1976; Sherman and Jones, 1976) ribosomes of *P. knowlesi* and *P. lophurae* were harvested by centrifugation from parasites released by immune lysis and disintegrated by a lytic solution containing Triton X-100. The ribosomes were utilizied for *in vitro* protein synthesis with endogenous RNA or synthetic polyuridylic acid and a rabbit or duck reticulocyte fraction. Protein synthesis was monitored by the incorporation of radioactively labeled amino acids. Recently Egitt *et al.* (1978) demonstrated translation of mRNA of *P. knowlesi* in a cell-free system. The resulting polypeptides were examined by sodium dodecyl sulfate (SDS) PAGE before and after precipitation with immune serum. It was shown that *P. knowlesi*-specific polypeptides were synthesized. Attempts were made to identify variant-specific antigens by comparing the SDS PAGE profiles of precipitates obtained with homologous and heterologous antisera. The results of these attempts were inconclusive. Similar studies by the same authors using RNA isolated from *Trypanosoma brucei* and a monospecific antivariant serum indeed demonstrated the *in vitro* synthesis of variant-specific *T. brucei* polypeptides (Egitt *et al.*, 1977).

It can be readily seen from this brief discussion of the biochemistry of plasmodia that many of the techniques used by biochemists can be used by immunologists for isolating antigens. It is also apparent that the use of biochemical and enzymatic markers by immunologists or of immunological markers by biochemists would improve the work of both groups.

While there is no reason to believe that at present *in vitro* synthesizing systems constructed by mixing components isolated from plasmodia and host cells are likely to have any advantage in providing antigens for immunization or serology over direct isolation of the desired antigens, the approach should not be abandoned. Technologies which at inception may be very cumbersome frequently when developed become very advantageous. One may hope that such will be the case with *in vitro* systems for the synthesis of cellular products. Even if these technologies do not become of practical use, the knowledge of the biological processes gained in developing them is of value in itself.

7. Parasite-Associated Materials from Erythrocytic Stages of the Parasite in the Erythrocyte Membrane, Plasma, and Culture Fluids

During the intraerythrocytic development of the malaria parasite changes may develop in the erythrocyte membrane, and plasmodial constituents may be found in the erythrocyte membrane. Under certain conditions plasmodial constituents may be released into the plasma or into culture fluids. Once released in the host, the fate of these materials, including hemozoin, residual bodies, and soluble material from the parasitophorous vacuole depends on the efficiency of phagocytosis and the immune state of the animal; if they are released in *in vitro* cultures, they may simply accumulate.

a. Parasite-Associated Material in the Erythrocyte Membrane. Eaton (1938) observed that immune serum from monkeys infected with *P. knowlesi* agglutinated schizont-containing red cells. Uninfected erythrocytes from the blood were not agglutinated, nor were erythrocytes containing rings or more advanced trophozoites. Thus, these parasite materials must make their way into the red cell membrane from the inside through the erythrocyte cytoplasm as the parasites mature. The parasite materials in the membranes of erythrocytes containing *P. knowlesi* schizonts are variant antigens (Brown *et al.*, 1968). Erythrocytes containing various other plasmodia have parasite-associated materials in their cytoplasm also (Aikawa *et al.*, 1975) but, as specific antiplasmodial antiserum will not usually agglutinate these erythrocytes (Brown, 1974), these materials probably do not extend through the membrane. Todorovic *et al.* (1968a) reported that fluorescein-labeled antibody specific for soluble antigens in the serum caused fluorescence and stimulated phagocytosis of erythrocytes of chickens with *P. gallinaceum* infection and caused fluorescence of free merozoites. These results suggest that the parasite-associated materials in or on the erythrocytes and on the merozoites, and the soluble materials in the serum, are antigenically at least similar. Unfortunately, this work was done with outbred chickens, and it is not possible to exclude the possibility that the results reported were caused by antibodies to blood group antigens rather than parasite antigens.

Morphological changes in the parasitized erythrocyte have been demonstrated by light and electron microscopy (reviewed by Aikawa, 1977), but only very recently have attempts been made to isolate the parasite-associated constituents in the membrane of the parasitized erythrocyte and characterize them. Bannister *et al.* (1975) showed that labeled immunoglobulin from monkeys infected with *P. vivax* bound to membranes of vesicles in the parasitized erythrocyte. Poels *et al.* (1978) similarly showed that *P. berghei*-parasitized reticulocytes, but not oxyphilic cells, had plasmodial antigens exposed on their membranes. Kilejian *et al.* (1977) prepared antisera against *P. falciparum*- and *P. coatneyi*-parasitized erythrocytes having "knob-like protrusions." After absorption with normal erythrocytes this antiserum bound to the protrusions but not to the normal parts of the membranes, demonstrating the immunological distinctness of the knobs. In a later study, Kilejian and Olson (1978) obtained membrane-rich fractions of lysed, parasitized erythrocytes by centrifugation on a discontinuous sucrose gradient. With SDS PAGE knob-rich membranes from erythrocytes parasitized with mature schizonts showed a band not present in membranes of normal erythrocytes or parasitized erythrocytes not showing knobs. The protein of this band had a molecular weight of 70,000–80,000. This component bound concanavalin A. It could be labeled metabolically with radioactive methionine by *in vitro* cultivation of parasitized erythrocytes with radioactively labeled amino acids.

Wallach and Conley (1977) used nitrogen cavitation to prepare membrane vesicles from radioiodinated *P. knowlesi*-parasitized erythrocytes and from normal rhesus erythrocytes and compared the SDS PAGE profiles of both preparations. Membranes from parasitized erythrocytes contained a glycoprotein component, not present in uninfected erythrocytes, which had a molecular weight between 125,000 and 130,000. Other proteins of normal erythrocyte membranes appeared to be degraded or to be deleted from parasitized erythrocytes. Schmidt-Ulrich *et al.* (1978) extended the study of Wallach and Conley (1977) by immunochemically and metabolically characterizing the protein and glycoprotein components of membranes of parasitized erythrocytes. They isolated schizonts by centrifugation on a discontinuous dextran gradient. From these schizonts they prepared membrane vesicles. Membranes of parasites and erythrocytes were solubilized with Triton X-100 and subjected to immunochemical analysis. By CIE with antisera against parasites and against erythrocytes they detected four parasite-specific antigens in the membranes of the parasitized erythrocytes. In addition at least three proteins, not present in uninfected erythrocyte membranes, were detected in the membranes of parasitized erythrocytes by bidimensional isoelectrofocusing and SDS PAGE. These proteins could be metabolically labeled with ^{14}C-labeled amino acids and glucosamine and had isoelectric points of 4.5, 4–5, and 5.2 and molecular weights of 55,000, 65,000, and 50,000, respectively. Deans *et al.* (1978) also detected parasite-specific antigens on membranes of *P. knowlesi*-parasitized erythrocytes by CIE.

b. Materials of Parasite Origin in the Plasma. Antigenic proteins of parasite origin have been detected in the plasma or serum of monkeys, ducks, rodents, chickens, and man with acute malaria (reviewed by Smith *et al.*, 1972).

Eaton (1939) was the first to demonstrate parasite antigens in the plasma of infected animals. He found them in the sera of monkeys infected with *P. knowlesi*. These antigens were reactive in CF tests but did not induce protective immunity. Soluble plasmodial antigens in the plasma of mice infected with *P. berghei* (Jerusalem, 1968), ducklings infected with *P. lophurae* (Corwin and Cox, 1969), and chickens infected with *P. gallinaceum* (Smith *et al.*, 1969) did induce protective immunity on injection into uninfected hosts. Circulating plasmodial antigens of *P. lophurae* (Sherman, 1964), *P. gallinaceum* (Todorovic *et al.*, 1967, 1968a; Smith *et al.*, 1969), *P. berghei*, and *P. vinckei*, (Seitz, 1972, 1975), as well as of human plasmodia (McGregor *et al.*, 1966, 1968; McGregor and Wilson, 1971), have been characterized by double immunodiffusion, immunoelectrophoresis, and counter current immunoelectrophoresis techniques. Malaria-associated antigens in the serum of chickens infected with *P. gallinaceum* were the subject of several fractionation and immunochemical studies as well as biophysical analyses. Todorovic *et al.* (1968a) fractionated sera containing soluble antigen on a column of granular agar and then ultracentrifuged the effluent to obtain plasmodial antigens. These antigens reacted in the slide precipitation test with homologous and heterologous immune sera. Todorovic *et al.* (1968a) further analyzed the biophysical and biochemical properties as well as the serological activity of the antigens they obtained from the serum by ultracentrifugation and by column chromatopraphy on agar, Sephadex, and BioGel columns (Todorovic *et al.*, 1967, 1968a,b). The antigens had sedimentation coefficients of 3 and 5 S and were rendered serologically inactive in gel precipitation (Todorovic *et al.*, 1968a) and tube latex agglutination (Todorovic *et al.*, 1968d) by treatment with trypsin, pepsin, and papain. Heating to 56°C did not affect their antigenicity, but heating to 65°C caused partial destruction of their serological activity. Exposure to temperatures above 65°C completely destroyed their serological activity, as did treatment with phenol (1:100), dialysis against distilled water, treatment with sodium chloride solutions with concentrations in excess of 4%, exposure to a pH above 9.0, and treatment with lipase. The last-mentioned finding suggests that the antigens had a lipid component. Smith *et al.* (1969) isolated a soluble antigen (SA1) for which a molecular weight of 500,000–700,000 was determined by gel filtration, ultracentrifugation, and disc electrophoresis. The antigen was precipitated from the serum with 12.5% sodium sulfate. Lykins *et al.* (1971) demonstrated three antigens, termed SA1, SA2, and SA3, which had molecular weights of 500,000–1,000,000; 150,000–250,000; and less than 70,000, respectively, as determined by gel filtration. These antigens could be separated by precipitation with sodium sulfate and by batch fractionation with DEAE-cellulose. SA2 was also precipitated by dextran sulfate. It was not clear whether these antigens arose from the parasites alone or whether they were produced as a result of action of the parasites on the erythrocyte. Fluorescent-labeled antibody to the soluble antigens stained the whole erythrocyte–parasite complex if the contained parasites were mature, but stained only the parasites if they were young forms (Todorovic et al., 1968a).

McGregor et al. (1968) were the first to study soluble plasmodial antigens in the serum of humans. There studies were done on Gambian children acutely infected with P. falciparum. Wilson et al. (1969) found that most of the antigens in the serum of the Gambian children with acute P. falciparum malaria, as well as serologically identical antigens in extracts of parasitized erythrocytes from infected placentas from women with P. falciparum infection, were stable at 100°C for 5 minutes. These antigens were termed S (stable) antigens. Other antigens found in lysates of parasitized erythrocytes which were named La (labile-a), Lb (labile-b), and R (resistant) antigens were not usually detected in the serum. In two individuals R antigens were found in the serum (Wilson et al., 1969). S antigens were also identified in the serum of infected Aotus monkeys (Wilson and Voller, 1970) and in sera of Nigerian children (Williams and Houba, 1972). S antigens were originally reported to have molecular weights of about 400,000 and 60,000 as determined by gel filtration and sucrose gradient centrifugation, respectively (Wilson et al., 1969). More recently (Wilson and Ling, 1978) molecular weights of S antigens from plasma of infected Aotus and infected children were determined by SDS PAGE. From these studies values of 130,000–148,000 and 150,000–210,000, respectively, were estimated. The origin of S antigens is not yet clear. The S antigens are not found in extracts of normal erythrocytes, thus they must be of plasmodial origin. They cannot be labeled metabolically in vitro by ^{14}C-labeled amino acids by treatment under the same conditions which permitted labeled amino acids to be incorporated into La, Lb, and R antigens (Wilson, 1974). S antigens generally disappear from the serum within days, or at most several weeks, following cessation of parasitemia (Wilson et al., 1975; Williams and Houba, 1972). They appear to be weakly immunogenic, and antibodies to them are rarely found in young children (McGregor et al., 1968; Wilson et al., 1969). Antibodies against La antigens in contrast are readily demonstrable in individuals of all age groups. It has been suggested that the absence of La antigens from the serum is a result of rapid complexing with antibodies, followed by removal from the serum (Wilson et al., 1969). Soluble antigen–antibody complexes in the serum of individuals with acute P. falciparum infection have been demonstrated by Houba and Williams (1972). To isolate and identify antigen–antibody complexes in serum Houba and Williams used column chromatography on Sephadex G-200, absorption with antisera to human globulins, treatment of complex-containing sera with mercaptoethanol and citric acid, and double immunodiffusion in gel. In a later study Houba et al. (1976) used sensitive radioimmunoassay techniques to detect antigen–antibody complexes in infected human serum. The sensitive methods used by Houba and Williams made it possible to detect antigen–antibody complexes even in individuals with quartan malaria. Such complexes are suspected of being the cause of renal immunopathology in malaria (Ward and Conran, 1966; Soothhill and Hendrickse, 1967; Allison *et al.*, 1969).

c. Soluble Plasmodial Constituents in Culture Fluids.   The occurrence of malaria-associated antigens in the plasma suggests that such antigens may be released from the parasitized erythrocytes. Indeed the release of acid- and antibody-precipitable material has been observed in cultures of erythrocytes parasitized with *P. knowlesi* (Cohen *et al.*, 1969; McColm *et al.*, 1977), *P. falciparum* (Wilson and Bartholomew, 1975), and *P. berghei* (Weissberger *et al.*, 1978). The release appears to occur primarily during late schizogony.

Wilson and Bartholemew (1975) detected antigens belonging to the L, R, and S classes in supernatants of cultured *P. falciparum*-parasitized erythrocytes. McColm *et al.* (1977), extending earlier observations by Cohen *et al.* (1969), investigated the release of proteins by erythrocytic stages of *P. knowlesi* during the cultivation of parasitized erythrocytes labeled with [^{3}H]isoleucine *in vitro*. They found that maximal amounts of TCA-insoluble radioactive material were present in the culture fluids at the time of merozoite release and reinvasion. Ultrafiltration studies indicated that the TCA-soluble fraction contained small peptide chains as well as free [^{3}H]isoleucine. That some of the released components were particulate in nature was shown by membrane filtration, gel filtration, and ultracentrifugation studies. With SDS PAGE the culture fluids revealed two major labeled polypeptide species, one of 45,000 and the other of 49,000 molecular weight. In a recent study Weissberger *et al.* (1978) found that supernatants from cultured *P. berghei*-parasitized erythrocytes contained serologically identifiable plasmodial constituents. Such supernatants also caused lymphoblast transformation *in vitro* and induced protective immunity in rats.

The possibility of the release of plasmodial antigens from cultured free parasites has not been investigated, although some such preparations are capable of incorporating amino acids and are largely free of soluble erythrocytic constituents which may add complexity to the analysis of plasmodial constituents in culture fluids. It should be mentioned in this context that parasites released by CFS even when only stirred in the cold for 2 hours liberate into the suspension fluid a major protein component (Saul and Kreier, 1977; Grothaus and Kreier, 1980), while other components, detectable in extracts of the parasite (Spira and Zuckerman, 1966; Kreier *et al.*, 1976), are present in a relatively small proportion. Furthermore, such ''wash-off'' material was about 20-fold more potent in inducing protective immunity than were the parasites themselves (Grothaus and Kreier, 1980).

C. Isolation of Exoerythrocytic Parasites

Mass *in vitro* cultivation of exoerythrocytic stages of avian plasmodia in cell cultures is technically feasible (Pipkin and Jensen, 1958; Davis *et al.*, 1966;

Huff, 1969). Exoerythrocytic merozoites may be obtained by centrifugation of the cell culture medium overlay (Holbrook *et al.*, 1974). Exoerythrocytic merozoites of *P. lophurae* and *P. fallax* can be obtained thus in quantity. In contrast, the *in vitro* cultivation of exoerythrocytic stages of mammalian plasmodia is very difficult. This difficulty is partly because the exoerythrocytic stages of mammalian plasmodia, unlike those of avian plasmodia, undergo only a limited number of generations of reproduction and must, therefore, always be produced from sporozoites, and partly because their host cell, the liver parenchyma cell, is difficult to cultivate. It is difficult to obtain germ-free sporozoites from conventionally reared mosquitoes, and this also complicates the culture procedure (Huff, 1964). Fowley *et al.* (1978a,b) have cultured liver cells from rats infected with *P. berghei* sporozoites. The exoerythrocytic schizonts in the liver cells mature in the cultures. The advantage of this procedure over direct infection of liver cultures with sporozoites is that the rat's reticuloendothelial system removes contaminating microorganisms, and sterile cultures are obtained. Avian exoerythrocytic parasites will grow radily in embryonic mouse liver cells (Beaudoin *et al.*, 1974), but only sparse growth of mammalian parasites in cultured liver cells have been reported (Doby and Barker, 1976). Beaudoin recently (Beaudoin, 1977) reemphasized that the host cell specificity of exoerythrocytic malarial parasites may not be a useful guide in choosing cells for *in vitro* cultures.

Immunization of turkeys with Formalin-killed *P. fallax* exoerythrocytic merozoites conferred some stage-specific protection against exoerythrocytic forms of the parasite but did not protect against infection by blood forms (Holbrook *et al.*, 1974). Some evidence exists that injection of avian erythrocytic merozoites will confer protection against infection with *P. berghei* sporozoites (Holbrook *et al.*, 1976). Beaudoin (1977) has recently questioned whether cultivated exoerythrocytic parasites will be a useful source of antigen for a malaria vaccine. A more complete discussion of the use of exoerythrocytic merozoites for immunization is presented in this volume, Chapter 5.

D. Isolation of Plasmodial Parasites in Sexual Stages of Development

1. General Considerations

The sexual forms of malaria parasites start their existence as intracellular gametocytes in the blood of the infected vertebrate but become sexually mature, undergo fertilization, and complete the sexual cycle in the invertebrate as extracellular parasites. The early sexual forms, the gametocytes, gametes, and ookinetes, can be grouped together with regard to isolation problems. The source of gametocytes, like that of asexual blood forms, is the blood of infected vertebrates. Continuous *in vitro* cultures of *P. falciparum* may be a source of gametocytes (Trager and Jensen, 1976; Carter and Miller, 1978). Isolation from cultured blood cells should not be much more difficult than isolation from blood cells of infected hosts. Gamete formation followed by fertilization and ookinete formation, which under natural conditions take place in the lumen of the mosquito's midgut, can take place *in vitro* under suitable culture conditions. These processes occur quickly and thus require only short-term *in vitro* culture. The low rates of gamete formation and fertilization under *in vitro* conditions are factors which limit the usefulness of the system. The mere possibility of obtaining sexual forms of malaria parasites from a source other than the mosquito encourages continuing work on *in vitro* systems.

The isolation of oocysts and sporozoites presents a much more complicated problem than the isolation of gametocytes, gametes, and ookinetes. Oocysts and sporozoites can be obtained from infected mosquitoes, but the isolation procedures are tedious and the quantities harvested are relatively small. *In vitro* cultures are not, as yet, a practical source of the sporogonic stages of the parasite. The long-term culture conditions required are complex and are far from being fully understood. These culture conditions have been recently reviewed and their prospects evaluated by Vanderberg *et al.* (1977) (see also Volume 2, Chapter 5).

2. Gametocytes, Gametes, and Ookinetes

The isolation of *P. falciparum* gametocytes was described by Kass *et al.* (1971a). The procedure involves sedimentation of parasitized erythrocytes in a salt solution containing 3% gelatin, followed by the separation of gametocytes on a Sepharose 4B column. The gametocytes collected in the first few effluent tubes are leukocyte-free and contain only minute numbers of trophozoites. Extracts of the gametocytes contain a stage-specific protein which appears as a unique band on PAGE. The extracts stimulated blast transformation of lymphocytes from *P. falciparum* patients (Kass *et al.*, 1971a).

Gwadz (1976) recently reported that immunization of chickens with Formalin-treated or x-irradiated *P. gallinaceum*-infected red cells, including those containing gametocytes, inhibited oocyte formation in mosquitoes fed on the challenged chickens, while barely affecting the sexual infections (see also this volume, Chapter 7). These findings suggested a possible new approach for malaria control and raised new interest in the immunogenic properties of gametocytes. It was suggested that antibodies taken into the mosquito's gut with the blood meal acted upon the gametes. Carter and Chen (1976) obtained a high degree of inhibition of oocyte formation by immunization with gametes. To obtain gametes they collected infected blood containing gametocytes, washed the blood cells in a medium which inhibited gamete release, and then suspended the gametocytes in a solution which stimulated gamete formation. The gametes were collected by a series of centrifugations. The gametes were irradiated before use as vaccine to suppress infectivity of contaminating asexual parasites. More recently Gwadz *et al.* (1978) reported that antibodies in the vaccinated birds inhibited microgametocyte motility and prevented *in vitro* ookinete formation. Gwadz *et al.* also showed that removal of the immune serum from the parasitized cell suspension and its replacement with normal serum rendered them infective to mosquitoes fed the cells through a membrane. Similar findings were reported with *P. knowlesi* malaria, but effective transmission-blocking immunity in this case required vaccination with antigen incorporated into Freund's complete adjuvant (FCA). As gametocytes of *P. falciparum* can now be produced *in vitro* (Trager and Jensen, 1976; Carter and Miller, 1978), isolation of these gametocytes by centrifugation or column procedures (Kass *et al.*, 1971a,b) and their testing in transmission-blocking vaccines should be possible. *Plasmodium berghei* ookinetes may be isolated from mosquito midguts in large numbers (Weiss and Vanderberg, 1976). Midguts are dissected from mosquitoes 9–12 or 18–24 hours after engorgement. A variety of antibiotics are added to the medium in which the midguts are suspended. The guts are ground in a Ten Broeck tissue grinder, and the homogenate digested with collagenase and hyaluronidase at 20°–21°C for 45–60 minutes while being gently stirred. The digest is then centrifuged at 50 g for 5 minutes to sediment the ookinetes. The ookinetes in the pellet are then further cleaned by gradient centrifugation. These preparations, although containing viable ookinetes, are heavily contaminated with microorganisms. Mosquito cell culture systems have been described for the development of ookinetes from gametocytes (Alger, 1968; Rosales-Ronquillo and Silverman, 1974). Ookinetes will also develop from gametocytes in cultures of fathead minnow epithelial cells (Rosales-Ronquillo *et al.*, 1974), but ookinete yields in cell culture systems are small and further development does not occur (Shapiro *et al.*, 1975). A simple *in vitro* technique that produces ookinetes of *P. berghei* reproducibly and in relatively large numbers was recently described by Weiss and Vandenberg (1977). The procedure involved the culturing of blood taken aseptically from an infected hamster in commerically available culture media. Eagle's minimal medium with Earle's salts and added fetal calf serum were found to be satisfactory. It was calculated that under these conditions about 1% of the observed macrogametocytes became fertilized and formed ookinetes.

3. Oocysts and Sporozoites

As it is not at present possible to obtain masses of sterile sporozoites from cultures inoculated with gametocyte-containing blood, the common source of sporozoites for study is the salivary glands or whole bodies of infected mosquitoes. It is possible to obtain relatively small numbers of clean sporozoites by dissecting the salivary glands from the mosquito, placing the freed glands on a microscope slide under a coverslip in saline solution, and causing a current of fluid to pass under the coverslip by dropping saline on one side and withdrawing it from the other with a capillary tube. The sporozoites leave the glands, enter the saline, and are collected with it. Simple centrifugation permits concentration of the sporozoites in the saline (Corradetti *et al.*, 1964). It is possible to obtain relatively large numbers of sporozoites by grinding whole mosquitoes with a loose-fitting Teflon tissue grinder, or mosquito thoraxes or abdomens suspended in tissue culture medium 199. After grinding, the heavier fragments are sedimented by centrifugation and the sporozoites are subsequently separated from most of the remaining debris by centrifugation on a bovine serum albumin–Renografin gradient. The sporozoites are concentrated in the region of the gradient with a specific gravity of about 1.10 (Krettli *et al.*, 1973). Bosworth *et al.* (1975) described a procedure for mass isolation of *Anopheles stephensi* salivary glands infected with sporozoites. Decapitated mosquitoes are washed on a 22-gauge mesh plastic screen and then spread as a monolayer on a glass plate between tracks formed by feeler gauges of specific thicknesses which serve as spacers. A roller is passed over the tracks. The salivary glands are expelled from the bodies, but the bodies are not crushed because the spacers maintain an appropriate distance between the roller and the glass plate. The expelled glands may be washed from the bodies by screening and collected for further processing to obtain sporozoites. Large numbers of relatively clean *P. berghei* sporozoites were recently separated from mosquito debris on a DEAE-cellulose column (Whatman, DE 52) (Mack *et al.*, 1978). Infected mosquitoes or their thoraxes were homogenized in an all-glass homogenizer with medium 199, and gross debris was removed by centrifugation. The sporozoite-containing material was preincubated in a medium containing equal parts medium 199 and 35% BSA. The sporozoite-containing medium was then diluted in the column buffer (containing Trizma base, sodium phosphate, sodium chloride, and 1.8% glucose at pH 8.2 and ionic strength 0.121) and passed through the column. A yield of 42.0% of the available sporozoites and about a 90% reduction in bacterial and fungal contaminations were obtained. The sporozoites were mobile, infective, and reactive in the circumsporozoite precipitation test (Vanderberg *et al.*, 1969) and capable of inducing protective immunity (Nussenzweig *et al.*, 1972). Another procedure for isolating *P. berghei* sporozoites involves filtration of homogenized infected mosquitoes through a set of four filters made up of Whatman no. 2, Nucleopore 8-μm, Whatman no. 2, and Nucleopore 3-μm filters. Filtration is followed by two centrifugations on a gradient made of Renografin 60 mixed with medium 199 and normal mouse serum. By this method 24,000–200,000 sporozoites were obtained from 50 infected mosquitoes (Wood *et al.*, 1978).

Nussenzweig *et al.* (1972) demonstrated that x-irradiated sporozoites induced protective immunity against sporozoite-induced infections, but attempts to isolate an immunogenic subfraction of the sporozoites have not succeeded. In order to avoid the problem of bacterial contamination of sporozoites obtained from mosquitoes, the human immunizations attempted to date have used direct feeding by irradiated mosquitoes (see this volume, Chapter 4). As germ-free mosquitoes can now be grown under sterile conditions (Rosales-Ronquillo *et al.*, 1973), the harvesting of sterile sporozoites may be possible from sterile mosquitoes if not from culture.

III. CONCLUSIONS

A variety of procedures for the release of erythrocytic stages of plasmodia have been described. All have their uses and limitations. Recent application of isotope labeling techniques has allowed a quantitative approach to the assessment of erythrocyte membrane contamination in preparations of released plasmodia. A large volume of information has accumulated on techniques for the isolation of plasmodia, their constituents, and their products. The information available is often but not always sufficient to permit quantitative and qualitative evaluation of the various isolation procedures. The criteria of purity plus criteria of simplicity of production can serve as guidelines for the choice of a release procedure most suitable for any specific purpose.

Culture techniques have made it possible to obtain relatively large numbers of erythrocytic merozoites from *P. knowlesi* and *P. falciparum*. They have also provided a source of soluble plasmodial constituents released to the culture fluid materials, which if released *in vivo* may be promptly destroyed by the host's defense systems. The metabolic labeling of plasmodial proteins *in vitro* is an important tool for the study of plasmodial polypeptides, whether they are in the parasite, in the parasitized erythrocyte, or in the culture fluid. The development of continuous culture of *P. falciparum* thus opens up many new research possibilities. The simple continuous-culture techniques for *P. falciparum* parasites which are within the reach of scientists who, because of limited facilities, have so far concentrated their research on the convenient and relatively inexpensive small animal parasites will permit them to expand their activities. The experimentation in antigenic analysis, fractionation, and molecular biology these scientists have done with rodent plasmodia can now be done with falciparum plasmodia also. The only serious impediment to a shift to study of cultured falciparum parasites remains the scarcity and cost of the primate hosts needed for studies on host–parasite interaction.

A variety of plasmodial fractions have been prepared for serological purposes, and the application of sensitive electrophoretic and immunoelectrophoretic techniques to antigenic analysis of plasmodial extracts and fractions has yielded important information. However, studies combining purification with characterization of immunobiologically active plasmodial constituents are still in the future, although a few promising developments in this area have been reported. It is probable that such studies will still have to be done with rodent plasmodia, because they will require large numbers of test animals for evaluation of the biological characteristics of the isolated plasmodial fractions.

Procedures are available for obtaining quantities of exoerythrocytic merozoites of avian plasmodia, but we do not have satisfactory procedures for obtaining exoerythrocytic merozoites of mammalian plasmodia.

A few techniques have been described for obtaining relatively large numbers of gametocytes, gametes, and ookinetes. The use of gametocytes and gametes in the induction of transmission-inhibiting immunity has opened an interesting approach to vaccination. The *in vitro* production of ookinetes from gametes has made it possible to devise an *in vitro* system for monitoring transmission-inhibiting antibodies. Fertilization, if possible under controlled *in vitro* conditions, may open the possibility of genetic studies if suitable culture systems for inducing sporogony or if effecient membrane feeding methods for mosquitoes became available.

While procedures are now available for obtaining preparations of parasites in most of the asexual intraerythrocytic forms as well as for obtaining gametocyto-cytes, gametes, oocysts, and sporozoites, our inability to induce the complete sporogonic development of the plasmodia *in vitro* remains a problem.

REFERENCES

Agency for International Development (1976). "Proposed Strategy for Expediting Research and Development for a Malaria Vaccine." US Department of State, Office of Health, Washington, D.C.

Aikawa, M. (1977). Variations in structure and function during the life cycle of malarial parasites. *Bull. W.H.O.* **55**, 139–155.

Aikawa, M., and Cook, R. T. (1972). *Plasmodium*: Electron microscopy of antigen preparations. *Exp. Parasitol.* **31**, 67–74.

Aikawa, M., Miller, L. H., and Rabbage, J. (1975). Caveola-vesicle complexes in the plasmalemma of erythrocytes infected by *Plasmodium vivax* and *P. cynomolgi*. *Am. J. Pathol.* **79**, 285–294.

Alger, N. E. (1968). *In vitro* development of *Plasmodium berghei* ookinetes. *Nature (London)* **218**, 774.

Allison, A. C., Houba, V., Hendrikse, R. G., de Petris, S., Edington, G. H., and Adeniyi, A. (1969). Immune complexes in the nephrotic syndrome of Africian children. *Lancet* **1**, 1232–1237.

Arnold, J.D., Lallis, F., and Martin, D. C. (1969). Augmentation of growth and division synchrony and of vascular sequestration of *Plasmodium berghei* by the photoperiodic rhythm. *J. Parasitol.* **55**, 597–608.

Baggaley, V. C., and Atkinson, E. M. (1972). Use of CF 12 columns for preparation of DNA from rodent malarias. *Trans. R. Soc. Trop. Med. Hyg.* **66**, 4.

Banki, G., and Bucci, A. (1964a). Research on antigenic structure of *Plasmodium berghei*. *Parasitologia* **6**, 251–257.

Banki, G., and Bucci, A. (1964b). Antigenic structure of *Plasmodium cynomolgi* and its relationship with the antigenic structure of *Plasmodium berghei*. *Parasitologia* **6**, 269–274.

Bannister, L. H., Butcher, G. A., Dennis, E. D., and Mitchell, G. H. (1975). Structure and invasive behavior of *Plasmodium knowlesi* merozoites *in vitro*. *Parasitology* **71**, 483-491.

Beaudoin, R. L. (1977). Should cultivated exoerythrocytic parasites be considered as a source of antigen for a malaria vaccine? *Bull. W.H.O.* **55**, 373-376.

Beaudoin, R. L., Strome, C. P. A., and Clutter, W. G. (1974). Cultivation of avian malaria parasites in mammalian liver cells. *Exp. Parasitol.* **36**, 355-359.

Bosworth, A. B., Schindler, I., and Frier, J. E. (1975). Mass isolation of *Anopheles stephensi* salivary glands infected with malaria sporozoites. *J. Parasitol.* **61**, 769-772.

Bowman, I. B. R., Grand, P. T., and Kermack, W. O. (1960). The metabolism of *Plasmodium berghei*, the malaria parasite of rodents. I. The preparation of the erythrocytic form of *P. berghei* separated from the host cell. *Exp. Parasitol.* **9**, 131-136.

Brackett, R. G., Cole, G. C., Greene, T. J., and Jacobs, R. L. (1978). "*In Vitro* Propagation of *P. falciparum* for Merozoite Antigen," NMRI/USAID/WHO Workshop on the Immunology of Malaria. NMRI, Bethesda, Maryland. *Bull. W.H.O.* **57** (Suppl. 1), 33-36 (1979).

Bray, R. S. (1957). Studies on malaria in chimpanzees. II. *Plasmodium vivax. Am. J. Trop. Med. Hyg.* **6**, 514-520.

Bray, R. S. (1960). Studies on malaria in chimpanzees. VIII. The experimental transmission and the pre-erythrocytic phase of *Plasmodium malariae* with a note on the host-range of the parasite. *Am. J. Trop. Med. Hyg.* **9**, 455-465.

Bray, R. S., and El-Nahal, H. M. S. (1966). Indirect haemagglutination test for malaria antibody, *Nature (London)* **212**, 83.

Brooks, C., and Kreier, J. P. (1978). Role of surface coat in *in vitro* attachment and phagocytosis of *Plasmodium berghei* by peritoneal macrophages. *Infect. Immun.* **20**, 827-835.

Brown, I. N. (1969). Immunological aspects of malaria infection. *Adv. Immunol.* **11**, 267-349.

Brown, I. N., Brown, K. N., and Hills, L. A. (1966). The separation of *Plasmodium knowlesi* from host cells. *Trans. R. Soc. Trop. Med. Hyg.* **60**, 3.

Brown, I. N., Brown, K. N., and Hills, L. A. (1968). Immunity to malaria: The antibody response to antigenic variation by *Plasmodium knowlesi. Immunology* **14**, 127-138.

Brown, K. N. (1974). "Antigenic Variation and Immunity to Malaria," Ciba Found. Symp. No. 25 (New Ser.). Elsevier, Amsterdam.

Brown, K. N., and Brown, I. N. (1965). Immunity to malaria: Antigenic variation in chronic infections of *Plasmodium knowlesi. Nature (London)* **208**, 1286-1288.

Brown, K. N., and Tanaka, A. (1975). Vaccination against *Plasmodium knowlesi* malaria. *Trans. R. Soc. Trop. Med. Hyg.* **69**, 350-353.

Brown, K. N., Brown, I. N., Trigg, P. I., Phillips, R. S., and Hills, L. A. (1970). Immunity to malaria. II. Serological response of monkeys sensitized by drug-suppressed infection or by dead parasitized cells in Freund's complete adjuvant. *Exp. Parasitol.* **28**, 318-338.

Butcher, G. A. (1978). "Factors Affecting the *in Vitro* Culture of *Plasmodium falciparum* and *Plasmodium knowlesi*," NMRI/USAID/WHO Workshop on the Immunology of Malaria. NMRI, Bethesda, Maryland.

Carter, R. (1970). Enzyme variation in *Plasmodium berghei. Trans. R. Soc. Trop. Med. Hyg.* **64**, 401-406.

Carter, R. (1972). Electrophoretic forms of glucose phosphate isomerase in oocysts and blood parasites of *P. berghei. Trans. R. Soc. Trop. Med. Hyg.* **66**, 542.

Carter, R. (1973). Enzyme variation in *Plasmodium berghei* and *Plasmodium vinckei. Parasitology* **66**, 297-307.

Carter, R. (1974). Variation in glutamate dehydrogenase in subspecies of *Plasmodium berghei. Trans. R. Soc. Trop. Med. Hyg.* **68**, 274.

Carter, R., and Chen, D. H. (1976). Malaria transmission blocked by immunization with gametes of the malaria parasite. *Nature (London)* **263**, 57-60.

Carter, R., and McGregor, I. A. (1973). Enzyme variation in *Plasmodium falciparum* in the Gambia. *Trans. R. Soc. Trop. Med. Hyg.* **67**, 830–837.

Carter, R., and Miller, L. H. (1978). "A Method for the Study of Gametogenesis by *Plasmodium falciparum* in Culture: Evidence for Environmental Modulation of Gametogenesis," NMRI/USAID/WHO Workshop on the Immunology of Malaria. NMRI, Bethesda, Maryland.

Carter, R., and Voller, A. (1973a). Enzyme typing of malaria parasites. *Br. Med. J.* **1**, 149–150.

Carter, R., and Voller, A. (1973b). Enzyme variants in primate malaria parasites. *Trans. R. Soc. Trop. Med. Hyg.* **67**, 14–15.

Carter, R., and Voller, A. (1975). The distribution of enzyme variation in populations of *Plasmodium falciparum* in Africa. *Trans. R. Soc. Trop. Med. Hyg.* **69**, 371–376.

Chavin, S. I. (1966). Studies on the antigenic constituents of *Plasmodium berghei*. I. Immunologic analysis of the parasite constituents. II. Fractionation of the parasite constituents. *Mil. Med.* **13**, Suppl., 1124–1136.

Chow, J. S., and Kreier, J. P. (1972). *Plasmodium berghei*: Adherence and phagocytosis by rat macrophages *in vitro*. *Exp. Parasitol.* **31**, 13–18.

Christophers, S. R., and Fulton, J. D. (1939). Experiments with isolated malaria parasites (*Plasmodium knowlesi*) free from red cells. *Ann. Trop. Med. Parasitol.* **33**, 161–170.

Coatney, G. R., Collins, W. E., and Contacos, P. G. (1971). "The Primate Malaria." US Dept. of Health, Education and Welfare, Bethesda, Maryland.

Coggeshall, L. T., and Eaton, M. D. (1938). The complement fixation reaction in monkey malaria. *J. Exp. Med.* **67**, 871–882.

Cohen, S., Butcher, G. A., and Crandall, R. B. (1969). Action of malaria antibody *in vitro*. *Nature (London)* **223**, 368–371.

Cohen, S., Butcher, G. A., and Mitchell, G. H. (1972). *In vitro* studies of malaria antibody. *Proc. Helminthol. Soc. Wash.* **39**, Sepc. Issue, 231–237.

Cook, R. T., Aikawa, M., Rock, R. C., Little, W., and Sprinz, H. (1969). The isolation and fractionation of *Plasmodium knowlesi*. *Mil. Med.* **134**, Suppl., 866–884.

Cook, R. T., Rock, R. C., Aikawa, M., and Fournier, M. J. (1971). Ribosomes of the malarial parasite, *Plasmodium knowlesi*. I. Isolation, activity and sedimentation velocity. *Comp. Biochem. Physiol. B* **39**, 897–911.

Corradetti, A., Verolini, F., Sebastiani, A., Proietti, A. M., and Amati, L. (1964). Fluorescent antibody testing with sporozoites of plasmodia. *Bull. W.H.O.* **30**, 747–750.

Corradetti, A., Verolini, F., Ilardi, A., and Bucci, A. (1966). Immunoelectrophoretic analysis of water soluble antigens extracted from parasitic bodies of *Plasmodium berghei* separated from the blood. *Bull. W.H.O.* **35**, 802–805.

Corwin, R. M., and Cox, H. W. (1969). The immunogenic activity of the nonspecific serum antigens of acute hemosporidian infections. *Mil. Med.* **134**, Suppl., 1258–1265.

Cox, F. E. G. (1974). Vaccination against malaria. *Nature (London)* **252**, 268.

D'Antonio, L. E. (1972). *Plasmodium*: A resume of the isolation of a vaccine fraction by the French pressure cell technique. *Exp. Parasitol.* **31**, 75–81.

D'Antonio, L. E. (1974). Vaccination against malaria: Evaluation of a plasmodial vaccine fraction and a preliminary study of some immunologic adjuvants in a primate model system: A brief report. *J. Am. Osteopathol. Assoc.* **74**, 649–652.

D'Antonio, L. E., and Silverman, P. H. (1971). Malaria resistance: Artificial induction with a partially purified plasmodial fraction. *Science* **121**, 1176.

D'Antonio, L. E., von Doenhoff, A. E., Jr., and Fife, E. H., Jr. (1966a). Serological evaluation of the specificity and sensitivity of purified malaria antigens prepared by a new method. *Mil. Med.* **131**, Suppl.,1152–1156.

D'Antonio, L. E., von Doenhoff, A. E., Jr., and Fife, E. M., Jr. (1966b). A new method for isolation and fractionation of complement fixing antigens from *Plasmodium knowlesi*. *Proc. Soc. Exp. Biol. Med.* **123**, 30–34.

D'Antonio, L. E., Spira, D. T., Fu, R. C., Dagnillo, D. M., and Silverman, P. H. (1970). Malaria resistance: Artificial induction with a partially purified plasmodial fraction. *Science* **168**, 1117–1118.

Davis, A. G., Huff, C. G., and Palmer, T. T. (1966). Procedures for maximum production of exoerythrocytic stages of *Plasmodium fallax* in tissue culture. *Exp. Parasitol.* **19**, 1–8.

Davis, B. D. (1948). Complement fixation with soluble antigens of *Plasmodium knowlesi* and *Plasmodium lophurae*. *J. Immunol.* **58**, 269–281.

Deans, J. A., Dennis, E. D., and Cohen, S. (1978). Antigenic analysis of sequential erythrocytic stages of *Plasmodium*. *Parasitology* **77**, 333–344.

Dennis, E. D., Mitchell, G. H., Butcher, G. A., and Cohen, S. (1975). *In vitro* isolation of *Plasmodium knowlesi* merozoites using polycarbonate sieves. *Parasitology* **71**, 475–481.

Dennis, R. A., O'Hara, P. J., Young, M. F., and Dorris, K. D. (1970). Neonatal immunohaemolytic anemia and icterus of calves. *J. Am. Vet. Med. Assoc.* **156**, 1861–1869.

Desowitz, R. S. (1975). *Plasmodium berghei*: Immunologic enhancement of antigens by adjuvant addition. *Exp. Parasitol.* **38**, 6–13.

Diggs, C. L. (1966). Immunodiffusion studies of *Plasmodium berghei*: Interactions of an extract of the erythrocytic forms with rabbit antisera. *Exp. Parasitol.* **19**, 237–248.

Doby, J. M., and Barker, R. (1976). Essais d'obtention *in vitro* des formes préerythrocytaires de *Plasmodium vivax* en cultures de cellules hépatiques humaines inoculées par sporozoites. *C. R. Seances Soc. Biol. Ses Fil.* **170**, 661–665.

Dulaney, A. D., and Stratman-Thomas, W. K. (1940). Complement fixation in human malaria. I. Results obtained with various antigens. *Immunology* **39**, 247–255.

Dvorak, J. A., Miller, L. H., Whitehouse, W. C., and Shiroshi, T. (1975). Invasion of erythrocytes by malaria merozoites. *Science* **187**, 748–750.

Eaton, M. D. (1938). The agglutination of *Plasmodium knowlesi* by immune serum. *J. Exp. Med.* **67**, 857–870.

Eaton, M. D. (1939). The soluble malarial antigen in the serum of monkeys infected with *Plasmodium knowlesi*. *J. Exp. Med.* **69**, 517–553.

Egitt, M. J., Tappenden, L., and Brown, K. N. (1977). Translation in a reticulocyte cell-free system of RNA isolated from blood and culture forms of *Trypanosoma brucei*. *Parasitology* **75**, 133–141.

Egitt, M. J., Tappenden, L., and Brown, K. N. (1978). "Synthesis of *Plasmodium knowlesi* Polypeptides in a Cell-free System," NMRI/USAID/WHO Workshop on the Immunology of Malaria. NMRI, Bethesda, Maryland. *Bull. W.H.O.* **57** (Suppl. 1), 109–113 (1979).

Eisen, H. (1977). Purification of intracellular forms of *Plasmodium chabaudi* and their interactions with the erythrocyte membrane and with serum albumen. *Bull. W.H.O.* **55**, 333–338.

Eling, W. (1977). Ficoll fractionation for the separation of parasitized erythrocytes from malaria infected blood. *Bull. W.H.O.* **55**, 105–114.

Eling, W., Van Zon, A. and Jerusalem, C. (1977). The course of a *Plasmodium berghei* infection in six different mouse strains. *Z. Parasitenkd.* **54**, 29–45.

Ferone, R. (1973). The enzymatic synthesis of dihydropteroate and dihydrofolate by *Plasmodium berghei*. *J. Protozool.* **20**, 459–464.

Ferone, R., Burchall, J. J., and Hitchings, G. H. (1968). *Plasmodium berghei* dihydrofolate reductase: Isolation, properties and inhibition by antifolates. *Mol. Pharmacol.* **5**, 49–59.

Ferrebee, J. W., and Geiman, Q. M. (1946). Studies on malarial parasites. III. A procedure for preparing concentrates of *Plasmodium vivax*. *J. Infect. Dis.* **78**, 173–179.

Fife, E. H., Jr. (1971). Advances in methodology for immunodiagnosis of parasitic diseases. *Exp. Parasitol.* **30**, 132–163.

Fife, E. H., Jr. (1972). Current state of serological tests used to detect blood parasite infections. *Exp. Parasitol.* **31**, 136–152.

Fife, E. H., Jr., von Doenhoff, A. E., Jr., and D'Antonio, L. E. (1972). *In vitro* and *in vivo* studies on a lytic factor isolated from *Plasmodium knowlesi*. *Proc. Helminthol. Soc. Wash.* **39**, Spec. Issue, 373–382.

Foley, D. A., Kennard, J., and Vanderberg, J. P. (1978a). *Plasmodium berghei*: Infective exoerythrocytic schizonts in primary monolayer cultures of rat liver cells. *Exp. Parasitol.* **46**, 166–178.

Foley, D. A., Kennard, J., and Vanderberg, J. P. (1978b). Preparation of rat hepatic cell suspensions that include infective exoerythrocytic schizonts. *Exp. Parasitol.* **46**, 179–188.

Forrester, L. J., and Siu, P. M. L. (1971). Phosphoenolpyruvate carboxylase from *Plasmodium berghei*. *Comp. Biochem. Physiol. B* **38**, 73–85.

Fulton, J. D., and Grant, P. T. (1956). The sulfur requirements of the erythrocytic forms of *Plasmodium knowlesi*. *Biochem. J.* **63**, 274–282.

Gasbarrini, A. (1913). Das Bordet-Gengousche phenomen (Kemplement ablenkung) bei Malaria. *Z. Immunitaetsforsch. Exp. Ther., I* **20**, 178–197.

Gravely, S. M., and Kreier, J. P. (1974). *Babesia microti* (Gray strain): Removal from infected hamster erythrocytes by continuous flow ultrasonication. *Z. Tropenmed. Parasitol.* **25**, 198–206.

Green, T., and Kreier, J. P. (1978). Demonstration of a role of cytophilic antibody in resistance to the malaria parasite (*Plasmodium berghei*) in rats. *Infect. Immun.* **18**, 138–145.

Grothaus, G. D., and Kreier, J. P. (1980). Isolation of a soluble component of *Plasmodium berghei* which induces immunity in rats. *Infect. Immun.* **28**, 245–253.

Gutteridge, B. W., and Trigg, P. I. (1971). Action of pyrimethamine and related drugs against *Plasmodium knowlesi in vitro*. *Parasitology* **62**, 431–444.

Gwadz, R. W. (1976). Malaria: Successful immunization against the sexual stages of *Plasmodium gallinaceum*. *Science* **193**, 1150–1151.

Gwadz, R. W., Carter, R., and Green, I. (1978). "Gamete Vaccines and Transmission-Blocking Immunity in Malaria," NMRI/USAID/WHO Workshop on the Immunology of Malaria. NMRI, Bethesda, Maryland.

Hamburger, J., and Kreier, J. P. (1975). Antibody mediated elimination of malaria parasites (*Plasmodium berghei*) *in vivo*. *Infect. Immun.* **12**, 339–345.

Hamburger, J., and Kreier, J. P. (1976a). Interaction between protective antibodies and malaria parasites (*Plasmodium berghei*): Involvement of low avidity antibodies. *Z. Tropenmed. Parasitol.* **27**, 385–390.

Hamburger, J., and Kreier, J. P. (1976b). *Plasmodium berghei*: Use of free blood stage parasites to demonstrate protective humoral activity in the serum of recovered rats. *Exp. Parasitol.* **40**, 158–167.

Hamburger, J., and Zuckerman, A. (1976a). *Plasmodium berghei*. I. Immunochemical properties of fractions of a soluble extract. *Exp. Parasitol.* **39**, 460–478.

Hamburger, J., and Zuckerman, A. (1976b). *Plasmodium berghei*. II. Immunobiological properties of fractions of a soluble extract. *Exp. Parasitol.* **39**, 479–495.

Hamburger, J., and Zuckerman, A. (1978). *Plasmodium berghei*. III. The partial separation of a putative species-specific antigen from a soluble extract. *Isr. J. Med. Sci.* **14**, 557–562.

Haynes, J. D., Diggs, C. L., Hines, F. A., and Desjardin, R. E. (1976). Culture of human malaria parasites, *Plasmodium falciparum*. *Nature (London)* **263**, 767–769.

Heidelberger, M., and Mayer, M. M. (1944). Normal human stromata as antigens for complement fixation in the sera of patients with relapsing vivax malaria. *Science* **100**, 359–360.

Heidelberger, M., Mayer, M. M., and Demarest, C. R. (1946). Studies in human malaria. I. The preparation of vaccines and suspensions containing plasmodia. *J. Immunol.* **52**, 325–330.

Heidrich, H. G., Rüssmann, L., Bayer, B., and Jung, A. (1979). Free flow electrophoresis for the separation of malaria infected and uninfected mouse erythrocytes and for the isolation of free parasites (*Plasmodium vinkei*): A new rapid technique for the liberation of malaria parasites from host cells. *Z. Parasitenkd.* **58**, 151–159.

Hickman, R. L. (1969). The use of subhuman primates for experimental studies of human malaria. *Mil. Med.* **134**, Suppl., 741-756.

Holbrook, T. W., Palczak, N. C., and Stauber, L. A. (1974). Immunity to exoerythrocytic forms of malaria. III. Stage specific immunization against exoerythrocytic forms of *Plasmodium fallax*. *J. Parasitol.* **60**, 348-354.

Holbrook, T. W., Spitalny, G. L., and Palczak, N. C. (1976). Stimulation of resistance in mice to sporozoite induced *Plasmodium berghei* malaria by injections of avian exoerythrocytic forms. *J. Parasitol.* **62**, 670-675.

Homewood, C. A., and Neame, K. D. (1976). A comparison of methods used for the removal of white cells from malaria-infected blood. *Ann. Trop. Med. Parasitol.* **70**, 249-251.

Houba, V., and Williams, A. I. O. (1972). Soluble serum antigens of *P. falciparum* in Nigerians. II. Immunochemical study. *Afr. J. Med. Sci.* **3**, 309-317.

Houba, V., Lambert, P. H., Voller, A., and Soyanwo, H. A. O. (1976). Clinical and experimental investigation of immune complexes in malaria. *Clin. Immunol. Immunopathol.* **6**, 1-12.

Huff, C. G. (1964). Cultivation of exoerythrocytic stages of malaria parasites. *Am. J. Trop. Med. Hyg.* **13**, 171-177.

Huff, C. G. (1969). Exoerythrocytic stages of avian and reptilian malarial parasites. *Exp. Parasitol.* **24**, 383-421.

Ilan, J., and Ilan, J. (1969). Aminoacyl transfer ribonucleic acid and synthetases from a cell-free extract of *Plasmodium berghei*. *Science* **164**, 560-562.

Ilan, J., Ilan, J., and Tokuyasu, K. (1969). Amino acid activation for protein synthesis in *Plasmodium berghei*. *Mil. Med.* **134**, Suppl., 1026-1031.

Jacobs, H. R. (1943). Immunization against malaria: Increased protection by vaccination of ducklings with saline-insoluble residues of *Plasmodium lophurae* mixed with bacterial toxin. *Am. J. Trop. Med.* **23**, 597-606.

Jerusalem, C. (1968). Active immunization against malaria (*Plasmodium berghei*). I. Definition of antimalaria immunity. *Z. Tropenmed. Parasitol.* **19**, 171-180.

Jerusalem, C. (1969). Active immunization against malaria (*P. berghei*). IV. Immunization with non-viable antigen. *Z. Tropenmed. Parasitol.* **20**, 430-439.

Jerusalem, C., and Eling, W. (1969). Active immunization against *Plasmodium berghei* malaria in mice using different preparations of plasmodial antigens and different pathways of administration. *Bull. W.H.O.* **40**, 807-818.

Jerusalem, C., Weiss, M. L., and Poels, L. (1971). Immunological enhancement in malaria infection (*Plasmodium berghei*). *J. Immunol.* **107**, 260-268.

Kagan, I. G. (1972). Malaria: Seroepidemiology and serologic diagnosis. *Exp. Parasitol.* **31**, 126-135.

Kass, L., Willerson, D., Jr., Rieckmann, K. H., Carson, P. E., and Becker, R. P. (1971a). *Plasmodium falciparum* gametocytes: Electron microscopic observations on material obtained by a new method. *Am. J. Trop. Med. Hyg.* **20**, 187-194.

Kass, L., Willerson, D., Jr., Rieckmann, K. H., and Carson, P. E. (1971b). Blastoid transformation of lymphocytes in falciparum malaria. *Am. J. Trop. Med. Hyg.* **20**, 195-198.

Kilby, V. A. A., and Silverman, P. H. (1969). Isolated erythrocytic forms of *Plasmodium berghei*—An electron microscopical study. *Am. J. Trop. Med. Hyg.* **18**, 836-859.

Kilejian, A. (1974). A unique histidine-rich polypeptide from the malaria parasite *Plasmodium lophurae*. *J. Biol. Chem.* **249**, 4050-4655.

Kilejian, A. (1976). Does a histidine-rich protein from *Plasmodium lophurae* have a function in merozoite penetration. *J. Protozool.* **23**, 272-277.

Kilejian, A. (1978). A purified antigen as a possible model for a malaria vaccine. *Proc. Int. Congt. Parasitol., 4th, 1978* Sect. E, p. 6.

Kilejian, A., and Jensen, J. B. (1977). A histidine-rich protein from *Plasmodium falciparum* and its interaction with membranes. *Bull. W.H.O.* **55**, 191-197.

Kilejian, A., and Olson, J. (1978). "Proteins and Glycoproteins from Human Erythrocytes Infected with *Plasmodium falciparum*," NMRI/USAID/WHO Workshop on the Immunology of Malaria. NMRI, Bethesda, Maryland. *Bull. W.H.O.* **57** (Suppl. 1), 101–107 (1979).

Kilejian, A., Abati, A., and Trager, W. (1977). *Plasmodium falciparum* and *Plasmodium coatneyi*: Immunogenicity of "knob like protrusions" on infected erythrocyte membranes. *Exp. Parasitol* **42**, 157–164.

Kortmann, H. F., Lelijveld, J., Ross, J. P. J., and Lohr, K. F. (1971). A capillary agglutination test for malaria. *Bull. W.H.O.* **45**, 839–844.

Kreier, J. P. (1977). The isolation and fractionation of malaria-infected cells. *Bull. W.H.O.* **55**, 317–331.

Kreier, J. P., Pearson, G. L., and Sillwill, D. (1965). A capillary agglutination test using *Plasmodium gallinaceum* parasites freed from erythrocytes: A preliminary report. *Am. J. Trop. Med. Hyg.* **14**, 529–532.

Kreier, J. P., Gravely, S. M., Seed, T. M., Smucker, R., and Pfister, R. M. (1975). *Babesia* sp.: The relationship of stage of development to structure of intracellular and extracellular parasites. *Z. Tropenmed. Parasitol.* **26**, 9–18.

Kreier, J. P., Hamburger, J., Seed, T. M., Saul, K., and Green, T. (1976). *Plasmodium berghei*: Characteristics of a selected population of small free blood stage parasites. *Z. Tropenmed. Parasitol.* **27**, 82–88.

Krettli, A., Chen, D. R., and Nussenzweig, R. S. (1973). Immunogenicity and infectivity of sporozoites of mammalian malaria isolated by density gradient centrifugation. *J. Parasitol.* **20**, 662–665.

Ladda, R. L. (1969). New insights into the fine structure of rodent malarial parasites. *Mil. Med.* **134**, Suppl., 825–865.

Lambros, C., and Vanderberg, J. P. (1979). Synchronization of *Plasmodium falciparum* erythrocytic stages in culture. *J. Parasitol.* **63**, 418–420.

Langer, B. W., Phisphumvidhi, P., and Friedlander, Y. (1967). Malaria parasite metabolism: The pentose cycle in *Plasmodium berghei*. *Exp. Parasitol.* **20**, 68–76.

Langreth, S. G., and Trager, W. (1973). Fine structure of the malaria parasite *Plasmodium lophurae* developing extracellularly *in vitro*. *J. Protozool.* **20**, 606–613.

Levy, M. R., and Chow, S. C. (1973). Activity and some properties of an acid proteinase from normal and *Plasmodium berghei*-infected red cells. *J. Parasitol.* **59**, 1064–1070.

Lund, M. N., and Powers, K. G. (1976). The preparation of malaria haemagglutination antigen. *Ann. Trop. Med. Parasitol.* **70**, 284–291.

Lykins, J. D., Smith, A. R., Voss, E. W., and Ristic, M. (1971). Physical separation of three soluble malarial antigens from the serum of chickens infected with *Plasmodium gallinaceum*. *Am J. Trop. Med. Hyg.* **20**, 394–402.

McAlister, R. O. (1972). Fractionation of the serologically reactive antigens of *Plasmodium falciparum*. *Proc. Helminthol. Soc. Wash.* **39**, Spec. Issue, 554–562.

McAlister, R. O. (1977). Time-dependent loss of viability of *Plasmodium berghei* merozoites *in vitro*. *J. Parasitol.* **63**, 455–463.

McAlister, R. O., and Gordon, D. M. (1976). Schizont-infected cell enrichment in rodent malaria. *J. Parasitol.* **62**, 664–669.

McAlister, R. O., and Gordon, D. M. (1977). Studies on the invasive ability of malarial merozoites (*Plasmodium berghei*). *J. Parasitol.* **63**, 448–454.

McColm, A. A., Shakespeare, P. G., and Trigg, P. I. (1977). Release of protein by erythrocytic stages of *Plasmodium knowlesi* during cultivation *in vitro*. *Bull. W.H.O.* **55**, 277–283.

McDaniel, H. G., and Siu, P. M. L. (1972). Purification and characterization of phosphoenopyruvate carboxylase from *Plasmodium berghei*. *J. Bacteriol.* **109**, 385–390.

McGregor, I. A. (1971). Immunity to plasmodial infections: Considerations of factors relevant to malaria in man. *Int. Rev. Trop. Med.* **4**, 1-52.

McGregor, I. A., and Wilson, R. J. M. (1971). Precipitating antibodies and immunoglobulins in *P. falciparum* infections in the Gambia, West Africa. *Trans. R. Soc. Trop. Med. Hyg.* **65**, 136-145.

McGregor, I. A., Hall, P. J., Williams, K., and Hardy, C. L. S. (1966). Demonstration of circulating antibodies to *Plasmodium falciparum* by gel-diffusion techniques. *Nature (London)* **210**, 1384-1386.

McGregor, I. A., Turner, M. W., Williams, K., and Hall, P. (1968). Soluble antigens in the blood of African patients with severe *Plasmodium falciparum* malaria. *Lancet* **1**, 881-884.

Mack, S. R., Vanderberg, J. P., and Nawrot, R. (1978). Column separation of *Plasmodium berghei* sporozoites. *J. Parasitol.* **64**, 166-168.

Mahoney, D. F., Redington, B. C., and Schoenbechler, M. J. (1966). The preparation and serologic activity of plasmodial fractions. *Mil. Med.* **131**, Suppl., 1141-1151.

Mannweiler, E., and Oelerich, S. (1969). Untersuchungen über die antigenen eigenschaften von *Plasmodium berghei*. *Z. Tropenmed. Parasitol.* **20**, 265-279.

Martin, W. J., Finerty, J., and Rosenthal, A. (1971). Isolation of *Plasmodium berghei* (malaria) parasites by ammonium chloride lysis of infected erythrocytes. *Nature (London)* **233**, 260-261.

Mathews, H. M., Fried, J. A., and Kagan, I. G. (1975). The indirect haemagglutination test for malaria: Evaluation of antigens prepared from *Plasmodium falciparum* and *Plasmodium vivax*. *Am. J. Trop. Med. Hyg.* **24**, 417-422.

Mayer, M. M., and Heidelberger, M. (1946). Studies in human malaria. V. Complement fixation reactions. *J. Immunol.* **54**, 89-102.

Meuwissen, J. H. E. T., Leeuwenberg, D. E. M. and Molenkamp, G. E. (1972). Studies on various aspects of the indirect haemagglutination test for malaria. *Bull. W.H.O.* **46**, 771-782.

Miller, L. H. (1976). Innate resistance in malaria. *Exp. Parasitol.* **40**, 132-146.

Miller, L. H., and Chien, S. (1971). Density distribution of red cells infected by *Plasmodium knowlesi* and *Plasmodium coatneyi*. *Exp. Parasitol.* **29**, 451-456.

Miller, L. H., Powers, K. G., Finerty, J., and Vandenberg, J. P. (1973). Difference in surface change between host cells and malarial parasites. *J. Parasitol.* **59**, 925-927.

Miller, L. H., Aikawa, M., and Dvorak, J. A. (1975). Malaria (*Plasmodium knowlesi*) merozoites: Immunity and the surface coat. *J. Immunol.* **114**, 1237-1242.

Mitchell, G. H., Butcher, G. A., and Cohen, S. (1973). Isolation of blood stage merozoites from *Plasmodium knowlesi* malaria. *Int. J. Parasitol.* **3**, 443-445.

Mitchell, G. H., Butcher, G. A., and Cohen, S. (1974). A merozoite vaccine effective against *Plasmodium knowlesi* malaria. *Nature (London)* **252**, 311-313.

Mitchell, G. H., Butcher, G. A., and Cohen, S. (1975). Merozoite vaccination against *Plasmodium knowlesi* malaria. *Immunology* **29**, 397-407.

Nussenzweig, R. S., Vanderberg, J., Spitalny, G. L., Rivera, C. I. O., Orton, C., and Most, H. (1972). Sporozoite induced immunity in mammalian malaria: A review. *Am. J. Trop. Med. Hyg.* **21**, 722-728.

Oelschlegel, F. J., Jr., Sander, B. J., and Brewer, G. J. (1975). Pyruvate kinase in malaria host-parasite interaction. *Nature (London)* **255**, 345-347.

Pasvol, G., Wilson, R. J. M., Smalley, M. E., and Brown, J. (1978). Separation of viable schizont-infected red cells of *Plasmodium falciparum* from human blood. *Ann. Trop. Med. Parasitol.* **72**, 87-88.

Pewny, W. (1978). Präzipitinversuche bei Malaria. *Wien. Klin. Wochenschr.* **31**, 205-206.

Phisphumvidhi, P., and Langer, B. W., Jr. (1969). The lactic acid dehydrogenase of *Plasmodium berghei*. *Exp. Parasitol.* **24**, 37-41.

Pipkin, A. C., and Jensen, D. V. (1958). Avian embryos and tissue culture in the study of parasitic protozoa. I. Malarial parasites. *Exp. Parasitol.* **7**, 491–530.

Platzer, E. G. (1974). Dihydrofolate reductase in *Plasmodium lophurae* and duckling erythrocytes. *J. Protozool.* **21**, 400–405.

Poels, L. G., Van Niekerk, C., and Franken, M. A. M. (1978). Plasmodial antigens exposed on the surface of infected reticulocytes: Their role in induction of protective immunity in mice. *Isr. J. Med. Sci.* **14**, 575–581.

Prior, R. B., and Kreier, J. P. (1972a). Isolation of *Plasmodium berghei* by use of a continuous-flow ultrasonic system: A morphological and immunological evaluation. *Proc. Helminthol. Soc. Wash.* **39**, Spec. Issue, 563–574.

Prior, R. B., and Kreier, J. P. (1972b). *Plasmodium berghei* freed from host erythrocytes by a continuous-flow ultrasonic system. *Exp. Parasitol.* **32**, 239–243.

Prior, R. B., and Kreier, J. P. (1977). The effects of ultrasound on erythrocytes of chickens with *Plasmodium gallinaceum* infection. *Ohio J. Sci.* **77**, 91–96.

Prior, R. B., Smucker, R. A., Kreier, J. P., and Pfister, R. M. (1973). A comparison by electron microscopy of *Plasmodium berghei* freed by ammonium chloride lysis to *P. berghei* freed by ultrasound in a continuous flow system. *J. Parasitol.* **59**, 200–201.

Reese, R. T., Langreth, S. G., and Trager, W. (1978). "Isolation of Stages of the Human Parasite *Plasmodium falciparum* from Culture and from Animal Blood," NMRI/USAID/WHO Workshop on the Immunology of Malaria. NMRI, Bethesda, Maryland. *Bull. W.H.O.* **57** (Suppl. 1), 53–61 (1979).

Reid, V. E., and Friedkin, M. (1973). Thymidylate synthetase in mouse erythrocytes infected with *Plasmodium berghei*. *Mol. Pharmacol.* **9**, 74–80.

Richards, W. H. G., and Voller, A. (1969). The normal course of *Plasmodium falciparum* in owl monkeys. *Trans. R. Soc. Trop. Med. Hyg.* **63**, 3.

Richards, W. H. G., and Williams, S. G. (1973). The removal of leukocytes from malaria infected blood. *Ann. Trop. Med. Parasitol.* **67**, 249–250.

Rock, R. C., Standefer, J. C., Cook, R. T., Little, W., and Sprinz, H. (1971). Lipid composition of *Plasmodium knowlesi* membranes: Comparison of parasites and microsomal subfractions with host rhesus erythrocyte membranes. *Comp. Biochem. Physiol. B* **33**, 425–437.

Rodhain, J., and Jadin, J. (1964). La transmission du *Plasmodium falciparum* au chimpanze splenectomise. *Ann. Soc. Belge Med. Trop.* **44**, 531–536.

Rogers, T. E. (1969). Analytical serology of protozoa. *In* "Analytical Serology of Microorganisms" (J. B. C. Kwapinski, ed.) Vol. 1, pp. 549–637. Wiley (Interscience), New York.

Rogers, W. A., Fried, J. A., and Kagan, I. G. (1968). A modified indirect microhemagglutination test for malaria. *Am. J. Trop. Med. Hyg.* **17**, 804–809.

Rosales-Ronquillo, M. C., and Silverman, P. H. (1974). *In vitro* ookinete development of the rodent malaria parasite, *Plasmodium berghei*. *J. Parasitol.* **60**, 819–824.

Rosales-Ronquillo, M. C., Simons, R. W., and Silverman, P. H. (1973). Aseptic rearing of *Anopheles stephensi (Diptera-Culicidae)*. *Ann. Entomol. Soc. Am.* **66**, 949–954.

Rosales-Ronquillo, M. C., Hienber, G., and Silverman, P. H. (1974). *Plasmodium berghei* ookinete formation in a nonvector cell line. *J. Parasitol.* **60**, 1039–1040.

Rowley, P. T., Siddiqui, W. A., and Geiman, Q. M. (1967). Separation of malaria parasites according to age by density gradient centrifugation. *J. Lab. Clin. Med.* **70**, 933–938.

Rutledge, L. C., and Ward, R. A. (1967). Effects of ultrasound on *Plasmodium gallinaceum* infected chick blood. *Exp. Parasitol.* **20**, 167–176.

Sadun, E. H., and Gore, R. W. (1968). Mass diagnostic test using *Plasmodium falciparum* and chimpanzee erythrocyte lysate. *Exp. Parasitol.* **23**, 277–285.

Sadun, E. H., Gore, R. W., Wellde, B. T., and Clyde, D. F. (1969). Malarial antibodies in human volunteers: A comparison of the soluble antigen fluorescent antibody (SAFA) and the indirect hemagglutination (IHA) tests using as antigen *Plasmodium falciparum* parasitized erythrocyte lysates. *Mil. Med.* **134**, Suppl., 1294–1299.

Saul, K., and Kreier, J. P. (1977). Immunization of rats with antigen from a population of free parasites rich in merozoites. *Z. Tropenmed. Parasitol.* **28**, 302–318.

Scheibel, L. W., and Miller, J. (1969a). Glycolytic and cytochrome oxidase activity in plasmodia. *Mil. Med.* **134**, Suppl., 1074–1080.

Scheibel, L. W., and Miller, J. (1969b). Cytochrome oxidase activity of platelet-free preparations of *Plasmodium knowlesi. J. Parasitol.* **55**, 825–829.

Schenkel, R. H., Simpson, G. L., and Silverman, P. H. (1973). Vaccination of rhesus monkeys (*Macaca mulatta*) against *Plasmodium knowlesi* by the use of nonviable antigens. *Bull. W.H.O.* **48**, 597–604.

Schenkel, R. H., Cabrera, E. J., Barr, M. L., and Silverman, P. H. (1975). A new adjuvant for use in vaccination against malaria. *J. Parasitol.* **61**, 549–550.

Schmidt-Ulrich, R., Wallach, D. H. F., and Lightholder, J. (1978). "Fractionation of *P. knowlesi*-Induced Antigens of Rhesus Monkey Erythrocyte Membranes," NMRI/USAID/WHO Workshop on the Immunology of Malaria. NMRI, Bethesda, Maryland. *Bull. W.H.O.* **57** (Suppl. 1), 115–121 (1979).

Seed, T. M., and Kreier, J. P. (1969). Autoimmune reactions in chickens with *Plasmodium gallinaceum* infection: The isolation and characterization of a lipid from trypsinized erythrocytes which reacts with serum from acutely infected chickens. *Mil. Med.* **134**, Suppl., 1220–1227.

Seed, T. M., and Kreier, J. P. (1976). Surface properties of extracellular malaria parasites: Electrophoretic and lectin binding characteristics. *Infect. Immun.* **14**, 1139–1347.

Seed, T. M., Aikawa, M., and Sterling, C. R. (1973a). An electron microscope-cytochemical method for differentiating membranes of host red cells and malaria parasites. *J. Protozool.* **20**, 603–605.

Seed, T. M., Aikawa, M., Prior, R. B., Kreier, J. P., and Pfister, R. M. (1973b). *Plasmodium* sp.: Topography of intra- and extracellular parasites. *Z. Tropenmed. Parasitol.* **24**, 525–535.

Seed, T. M., Aikawa, M., Sterling, C., and Rabbage, J. (1974). Surface properties of extracellular malaria parasites: Morphological and cytochemical study. *Infect. Immun.* **9**, 750–761.

Seed, T. M., Brindley, D., Aikawa, M., and Rabbage, J. (1976). *Plasmodium berghei*: Osmotic fragility of malaria parasites and mouse host erythrocytes. *Exp. Parasitol.* **40**, 380–390.

Seitz, H. M. J. (1972). Demonstration of malarial antigens in the sera of *Plasmodium berghei*-infected mice. *J. Parasitol.* **58**, 179–180.

Seitz, H. M. J. (1975). Counter-current immunoelectrophoresis for the demonstration of malarial antigens and antibodies in the sera of rats and mice. *Trans. R. Soc. Trop. Med. Hyg.* **69**, 88–90.

Shapiro, M., Espinal-Tejada, C., and Nussenzweig, R. (1975). Evaluation of a method for *in vitro* development of the rodent malaria parasite *Plasmodium berghei. J. Parasitol.* **61**, 1105–1106.

Sherman, I. W. (1964). Antigens of *Plasmodium lophurae. J. Protozool.* **11**, 409–417.

Sherman, I. W. (1976). The ribosomes of the simian malaria parasite *Plasmodium knowlesi*. II. A cell free protein synthesizing system. *Cimp. Biochem. Physiol. B* **53**, 447–450.

Sherman, I. W. (1977a). Transport of amino acids and nucleic acid precursors in malarial parasites. *Bull. W.H.O.* **55**, 211–225.

Sherman, I. W. (1977b). Amino acid metabolism and protein synthesis in malarial parasites. *Bull. W.H.O.* **55**, 265–276.

Sherman, I. W., and Hull, R. W. (1960). The pigment (hemozoin) and proteins of the avian malaria parasite *Plasmodium lophurae. J. Protozool.* **7**, 409–416.

Sherman, I. W., and Jones, L. A. (1976). Protein synthesis by a cell-free preparation from the bird malaria *Plasmodium lophurae. J. Protozool.* **23**, 277–281.

Sherman, I. W., Peterson, I., Tanigoshi, L., and Ting, I. P. (1971). The glutamate dehydrogenase of *Plasmodium lophurae* (avian malaria). *Exp. Parasitol.* **29**, 433–439.

Sherman, I. W., Cox, R. A., Higginson, B., McLaren, D. J., and Williamson, J. (1975). The ribosomes of the simian malaria parasite *Plasmodium knowlesi*. I. Isolation and characterization. *J. Protozool.* **22**, 568–572.

Shungu, D. M., and Arnold, J. D. (1971). Synchronization of growth and division of rat adapted *Plasmodium vinckei chabaudi* by photoperiodic rhythm. *Trans. R. Soc. Trop. Med. Hyg.* **65**, 684–685.

Siddiqui, W. A., Schnell, J. V., and Richmond-Crum, S. (1974). *In vitro* cultivation of *Plasmodium falciparum* at high parasitemia. *Am. J. Trop. Med. Hyg.* **23**, 1015–1018.

Siddiqui, W. A., Kromer, K. and Richmond-Crum, S. M. (1978a). *In vitro* cultivation and partial purification of *Plasmodium falciparum* antigen suitable for vaccination studies in *Aotus* monkeys. *J. Parasitol.* **64**, 168–169.

Siddiqui, W. A., Kan, S. C., Kramer, K., and Richmond-Crum, S. M. (1978b). "*In Vitro* Production and Partial Purification of *Plasmodium falciparum* Antigen," NMRI/USAID/WHO Workshop on the Immunology of Malaria. NMRI, Bethesda, Maryland. *Bull. W.H.O.* **57** (Suppl. 1), 75–82 (1979).

Simpson, G. L., Schenkel, R. H., and Silverman, P. H. (1974). Vaccination of rhesus monkeys against malaria by use of sucrose density fractions of *Plasmodium knowlesi* antigens. *Nature (London)* **247**, 304–306.

Siu, P. M. L. (1967). Carbon dioxide fixation in plasmodia and the effect of some antimalarial drugs on the enzyme. *Comp. Biochem. Physiol.* **23**, 785–795.

Smalley, M. E., and Butcher, G. A. (1975). The *in vitro* culture of the blood stages of *Plasmodium berghei*. *Int. J. Parasitol.* **5**, 131–132.

Smith, A. R., Lykins, J. D., Voss, E. W., and Ristić, M. (1969). Identification of an antigen and specific antibody in the sera of chickens infected with *Plasmodium gallinaceum*. *J. Immunol.* **103**, 6–14.

Smith, A. R., Karr, L. J., Lykins, J. D., and Ristic, M. (1972). Serum soluble antigens of malaria: A review. *Exp. Parasitol.* **31**, 120–125.

Sodeman, W. A., Jr., and Meuwissen, J. H. E. T. (1966). Disc Electrophoresis of *Plasmodium berghei*. *J. Parasitol.* **52**, 23–25.

Soothhill, J. F., and Hendrickse, R. G. (1967). Some immunological studies of the nephrotic syndrome of Nigerian children. *Lancet* **2**, 629–632.

Spira, D. (1965). Antigenic structure of some parasites of the family Plasmodiidae. Ph.D. Thesis, Hebrew University, Jerusalem, Israel.

Spira, D., and Zuckerman, A. (1962). Antigenic structure of *Plasmodium vinckei*. *Science* **137**, 536–537.

Spira, D., and Zuckerman, A. (1964). Antigenic analysis of the erythrocytic stages of *Plasmodium gallinaceum*. *J. Protozool.* **11**, Suppl., 43–44.

Spira, D., and Zuckerman, A. (1966). Recent advances in the antigenic analysis of plasmodia. *Mil. Med.* **131**, Suppl., 1117–1123.

Spira, D., Hamburger, J., and Zuckerman, A. (1965). Disc electrophoretic patterns of plasmodial extracts. *J. Protozool.* **13**, Suppl., 34–35.

Stauber, L. A., and Walker, H. A. (1946). Preparation and properties of erythrocyte-free avian plasmodia. *Proc. Soc. Exp. Biol. Med.* **63**, 223–227.

Stein, B., and Desowitz, R. S. (1964). The measurement of antibody in human malaria by a formolized tanned sheep cell haemagglutination test. *Bull. W.H.O.* **30**, 45–49.

Taliaferro, W. H. (1930). "The Immunology of Parasitic Infections." Johns, Bale Sons and Danielson Ltd., London.

Todorovic, R., Ferris, D., and Ristic, M. (1967). Immunogenic properties of serum antigens from chickens infected with *Plasmodium falciparum*. *Ann. Trop. Med. Parasitol.* **61**, 117–124.

Todorovic, R., Ferris, D. H., and Ristic, M. (1968a). Antigens of *Plasmodium gallinaceum*. I.

Biophysical and biochemical characterization of explasmodial antigens. *Am. J. Trop. Med. Hyg.* **17**, 685–694.

Todorovic, R., Ferris, D. H., and Ristic, M. (1968b). Antigens of *Plasmodium gallinaceum*. II. Immunoserologic characterization of explasmodial antigens and their antibodies. *Am. J. Trop. Med. Hyg.* **17**, 695–701.

Todorovic, R., Ristic, M., and Ferris, D. (1968c). Soluble antigens of *Plasmodium gallinaceum*. *Trans. R. Soc. Trop. Med. Hyg.* **62**, 51–57.

Todorovic, R., Ristic, M., and Ferris, D. (1968d). A tube latex agglutination test for the diagnosis of malaria. *Trans. R. Soc. Trop. Med. Hyg.* **62**, 58–68.

Trager, W. (1950). Studies on the extracellular cultivation of an intracellular parasite (avian malaria). I. Development of the organism in erythrocytic extracts and the favoring effect of adenosine triphosphate. *J. Exp. Med.* **92**, 349–366.

Trager, W. (1954). Co-enzyme A and the malaria parasite *Plasmodium lophurae*. *J. Protozool.* **1**, 231–237.

Trager, W., and Jensen, J. B. (1976). Human malaria parasites in continuous culture. *Science* **193**, 673–675.

Trager, W., Stauber, L. A., and Ben Harel, S. (1950). Innate and acquired agglutinins in ducks to the malaria parasite *Plasmodium lophurae*. *Proc. Soc. Exp. Biol. Med.* **75**, 766–771.

Trager, W., Langreth, S. E., and Platzer, E. G. (1972). Viability and fine structure of extracellular *Plasmodium lophurae* prepared by different methods. *Proc. Helminthol. Soc. Wash.* **39**, Spec. Issue, 220–230.

Trigg, P. I., Shakespeare, P. G., Burt, S. J., and Kyd, S. I. (1975). Ribonucleic acid synthesis in *Plasmodium knowlesi* maintained both *in vivo* and *in vitro*. *Parasitology* **71**, 199–209.

Tsukamoto, M. (1974). Differential detection of soluble enzymes specific to a rodent malaria parasite, *Plasmodium berghei*, by electrophoresis in polyacrylamide gels. *Trop. Med.* **16**, 55–69.

Turner, M. W., and McGregor, I. A. (1969). Studies on the immunology of human malaria. I. Preliminary characterization of antigens in *Plasmodium falciparum* infections. *Clin. Exp. Immunol.* **5**, 1–16.

Vanderberg, J. P., Nussenzweig, R., and Most, H. (1969). Protective immunity produced by the injection of x-irradiated sporozoites of *Plasmodium berghei*. V. *In vitro* effects of immune serum on sporozoites. *Mil. Med.* **134**, 1183–1190.

Vanderberg, J. P., Weiss, M. M., and Mack, S. R. (1977). *In vitro* cultivation of the sporogonic stages of *plasmodium*: A review. *Bull. W.H.O.* **55**, 377–392.

Van Dyke, K., Trush, M. A., Wilson, M. E., and Stealey, P. K. (1977). Isolation and analysis of nucleotides from erythrocyte-free malaria parasites (*Plasmodium berghei*) and potential relevance to malaria chemotherapy. *Bull. W.H.O.* **55**, 253–265.

Verain, A., and Verain, A. (1956). Influence de ultrason sur *Plasmodium berghei*. *C. R. Seances Soc. Biol. Ses Fil.* **150**, 1189–1190.

Voller, A., Huldt, G., Thors, C., and Engvall, E. (1975). New serological test for malaria antibodies. *Br. Med. J.* **1**, 659–661.

Wallach, D. F. H., and Conley, M. (1977). Altered membrane proteins of monkey erythrocytes infected with simian malaria. *J. Mol. Med.* **2**, 119–136.

Walter, R. D. (1968). Untersuchungen über die Entwicklung frier erythrozytärer Schizonten bei Infektionen mit *Plasmodium berghei* und *Plasmodium chabaudi*. *Z. Tropenmed. Parasitol.* **19**, 415–426.

Walter, R. D., and Königk, E. (1974). Purification and properties of the 7,8-dihydropterate synthesizing enzyme from *Plasmodium chabaudi*. *Hoppe-Seyler's Z. Physiol. Chem.* **355**, 431–437.

Walter, R. D., Nordmeyer, J. P., and Königk, E. (1974). NADP-specific glutamate dehydrogenase from *Plasmodium chabaudi*. *Hoppe-Seyler's Z. Physiol. Chem.* **355**, 495–500.

Ward, R. A., and Cadigan, F. C. (1966). The development of erythrocytic stages of *Plasmodium falciparum* in the gibbon *Hylobates lar*. *Mil. Med.* **131**, Suppl., 944–951.

Ward, P. A., and Conran, P. B. (1966). Immunopathologic studies of simian malaria. *Mil. Med.* **131**, Suppl., 1225–1232.

Ward, P. A., Morris, J. H., Gould, D. J., Bourke, A. T. C., and Cadigan, F. C., Jr. (1965). Susceptibility of the gibbon *Hylobates lar* to falciparum malaria. *Science* **150**, 1604–1605.

Weiss, M. M., and Vanderberg, J. P. (1976). Studies on *Plasmodium* ookinetes. I. Isolation and concentration from mosquito midguts. *J. Protozool.* **23**, 547.

Weiss, M. M., and Vanderberg, J. P. (1977). Studies on *Plasmodium* ookinetes. II. *In vitro* formation of *Plasmodium berghei* ookinetes. *J. Parasitol.* **63**, 932–934.

Weissberger, H., Golenser, J., and Spira, D. T. (1978). "Soluble Antigens Released *in vitro* from Erythrocytes Infected with *Plasmodium berghei*," NMRI/USAID/WHO Workshop on the Immunology of Malaria. NMRI, Bethesda, Maryland. *Bull. W.H.O.* **57** (Suppl. 1), 83–84 (1979).

Wellde, B. T., Stechschulte, D. J., Schoenbechler, M. J., and Colgate, W. A. (1969). An indirect hemagglutination test for malaria using an antigen from the lysate of parasitized erythrocytes. *Mil. Med.* **134**, Suppl., 1284–1293.

Williams, A. I. O. (1973). Preparation of malarial placenta antigen for immunodiffusion studies in a Nigerian population. *Trans. R. Soc. Trop. Med. Hyg.* **67**, 621–630.

Williams, A. I. O., and Houba, V. (1972). Soluble serum antigens of *P. falciparum* in Nigerians. I. Local incidence of malarial soluble serum antigens and antibodies. *Afr. J. Med. Sci.* **3**, 295–307.

Williamson, J. (1967). Antigens of *Plasmodium knowlesi*. *Protozoology* **11**(Suppl. to *J. Helminthol.*), 85–104.

Williamson, J., and Cover, B. (1966). Separation of blood cell free trypanosomes and malaria parasites on a sucrose gradient. *Trans. R. Soc. Trop. Med. Hyg.* **60**, 425–427.

Wilson, R. J. M. (1974). The production of antigens by *Plasmodium falciparum in vitro*. *Int. J. Parasitol.* **4**, 537–547.

Wilson, R. J. M., and Bartholomew, R. K. (1975). The release of antigens by *Plasmodium falciparum*. *Parasitology* **71**, 183–192.

Wilson, R. J. M., and Ling, I. (1978). "Fractionation and Characterization of *Plasmodium falciparum* Antigens," NMRI/USAID/WHO Workshop on the Immunology of Malaria. NMRI, Bethesda, Maryland.

Wilson, R. J. M., and Voller, A. (1970). Malarial S-antigens from man and owl monkey infected with *Plasmodium falciparum*. *Parasitology* **61**, 461–465.

Wilson, R. J. M., and Voller, A. (1972). A comparison of malarial antigens from human and *Aotus* monkey blood infected with *Plasmodium falciparum*. *Parasitology* **64**, 191–195.

Wilson, R. J. M., McGregor, I. A., Hall, P., Williams, K., and Bartholomew, R. (1969). Antigens associated with *Plasmodium falciparum* infections in man. *Lancet* **2**, 201–205.

Wilson, R. J. M., McGregor, I. A., and Wilson, M. E. (1973). The stability and fractionation of malarial antigens from the body of Africans infected with *Plasmodium falciparum*. *Int. J. Parasitol.* **3**, 511–520.

Wilson, R. J. M., McGregor, I. A., and Hall, P. I. (1975). Persistence and recurrence of S-antigens in *Plasmodium falciparum* infections in man. *Trans. R. Soc. Trop. Med. Hyg.* **69**, 460–467.

Wood, D. E., Smrkovski, L. L., McConnell, E., Pancheco, N. D., and Bawden, M. P. (1978). "The Use of Membrane Screen Filters in the Isolation of *Plasmodium berghei* Sporozoites from Mosquitoes," NMRI/USAID/WHO Workshop on the Immunology of Malaria. NMRI, Bethesda, Maryland. *Bull. W.H.O.* **57** (Suppl. 1), 69–74 (1979).

World Health Organization (1975). Developments in malaria immunology. *W.H.O., Tech. Rep. Ser.* 579.

Young, M. D., Porter, J. A., Jr., and Johnson, C. M. (1966). *Plasmodium vivax* transmitted from man to monkey to man. *Science* **153**, 1006–1007.

Zuckerman, A. (1964). The antigenic analysis of plasmodia. *Am. J. Trop. Med. Hyg.* **13**, Suppl., 209–213.

Zuckerman, A. (1969). Current status of the immunology of malaria and the antigenic analysis of plasmodia. *Bull. W.H.O.* **40**, 55–66.

Zuckerman, A. (1970). Malaria of lower mammals. *In* "Immunity to Parasitic Animals" (G. J. Jackson, R. Herman, and I. Singer, eds.), Vol. 2, pp. 793–829. Appleton, New York.

Zuckerman, A., and Ristic, M. (1968). Blood parasite antigens and antibodies. *In* "Infectious Blood Diseases of Man and Animals" (D. Weinman and M. Ristic, eds.), Vol. 1, pp. 79–122. Academic Press, New York.

Zuckerman, A., and Spira, D. (1963). Electrophoretic patterns of extracts of rodent plasmodia. *J. Protozool.* **10**, Suppl., 34.

Zuckerman, A., and Yoeli, M. (1954). Age and sex as factors influencing *P. berghei* infections in intact and splenectomized rats. *J. Infect. Dis.* **94**, 255–236.

Zuckerman, A., Spira, D., and Hamburger, J. (1967). A procedure for the harvesting of mammaliam plasmodia. *Bull. W.H.O.* **37**, 431–436.

Zuckerman, A., Goberman, V., Ron, N., Spira, D., Hamburger, J., and Burg, R. (1969). Antiplasmodial precipitins demonstrated by double diffusion in agar gel in the serum of rats infected with *Plasmodium berghei*. *Exp. Parasitol.* **24**, 299–312.

2

Methods for Measuring the Immunological Response to Plasmodia

A. Voller, J. H. E. Meuwissen, and J. P. Verhave

I. INTRODUCTION

In this chapter an attempt will be made to describe antibody responses which occur during plasmodial infections. The measurement of these responses has become important in recent years, as they can provide means of identifying infected persons as well as valuable epidemiological evidence. The theory and practice of the methods used for these purposes will be described in detail.

There is frequently confusion in the minds of nonimmunologists concerning the relationship of antibody presence and functional immunity. It should be stressed at the outset that detectable antibody does not necessarily indicate or act as a measure of protective immunity in an individual or in a population. In some instances antibody levels correlate with the degree of protection, but there are many exceptions to this. As yet there is no immunological test for malaria which can directly and invariably yield results reflecting the functional immune status against malaria.

Until recently it was thought that under natural conditions the initiation of a malaria infection by a mosquito's introduction of sporozoites did not lead to a marked serological response. During recent years, however, it has been found by experimental studies that normal sporozoites and those treated in various ways and presented to the host by natural bites or under various abnormal conditions can elicit antibody responses. These studies will be dealt with in Section II. Recently Nardin and Nussenzweig (1978) reported that the sporozoite-specific circulating antibodies can also be detected in people living in endemic malarious areas. Their role in functional antimalarial immunity still has to be established.

There is no evidence so far that the liver cell-inhabiting stage can also evoke a strong host reaction, although *in vitro* studies show that these exoerythrocytic forms (EEFs) of malaria parasites are antigenically reactive. However, when the blood is invaded by the malaria parasite, we can see the classic serological response develop, and it is a consideration of this response that constitutes the greater part of this chapter.

Because of the vast literature on this subject it is impossible to review and cite all the published work. Selected works will be taken to illustrate particular points, and the choice will inevitably reflect the authors' interests, prejudices, and personal involvement.

II. THE ANTIBODY RESPONSE AGAINST SPOROZOITES

In the past, several tests have been used for demonstrating antisporozoite antibodies. Mulligan *et al.* (1940) developed a direct agglutination test for sporozoites. Similar experiments were performed by Richards (1966), but this test has not been successfully used since then because of technical difficulties. Currently the following serological tests are in use.

A. Circumsporozoite Precipitation Test

Sporozoites develop a threadlike precipitate when incubated in serum from rodents immunized with radiation-attenuated sporozoites, and this test is specific for antibodies against sporozoites. Sera from animals with a blood-induced infection do not react in the circumsporozoite precipitation (CSP) test. The CSP test becomes positive slowly after one inoculation with sporozoites, depending on the administered dose. The titer increases after subsequent inoculations and levels off at a dilution of 1:80 (Nussenzweig *et al.*, 1972a,b). These reactions are best seen in animals immunized with mature sporozoites administered by the intravenous route (Spitalny and Nussenzweig, 1972). The CSP antibodies are also seen in sporozoite-immunized monkeys and in man exposed to infected irradiated mosquitoes (Nussenzweig, 1977; Clyde *et al.*, 1975), but individual variations are considerable as compared with the situation in rodents. Nonirradiated sporozoites injected into animals protected with chloroquine against parasitemia also induce CSP antibodies (Verhave, 1975). Nonirradiated sporozoites of primate plasmodia elicit CSP antibodies in insusceptible hosts (Nussenzweig *et al.*, 1973; Nussenzweig and Chen, 1974).

This CSP reaction seems to involve the binding of antibodies to the sporozoite, thus forming a thick surface coat. This coat, as seen with electron microscopy, is not evenly distributed but is thicker toward the posterior end, suggesting capping and shedding of the precipitate (Cochrane *et al.*, 1976).

Technical Details of the Circumsporozoite Precipitation Test.   The technique of the CSP test is based simply on the incubation of sporozoites in a drop of a serum dilution. The preparation is overlaid with a coverslip and incubated for 30 minutes at 37°C. The presence of antibodies is judged from the presence of a precipitate in at least 2 out of 20 sporozoites under phase-contrast.

B. Sporozoite Neutralization Test

Sporozoites need to be alive to produce a CSP coat, but they readily become noninfective upon *in vitro* incubation in immune sera or after inoculation into immune animals (Nussenzweig *et al.*, 1972a,b).

Another method for the detection of antibody activity, designated the sporozoite-neutralizing activity (SNA) tests, was based on this principle.

This activity is not detectable in sporozoite-primed animals, but after secondary exposure it is readily observed up to serum dilutions of 1:80. It can be observed in rodents as well as in primates, and it seems to play a major role in the protective mechanism against sporozoites. The exact nature of the action of antibodies in preventing sporozoites from infecting hepatocytes is still obscure.

Technical Details of the Sporozoite Neutralization Test.   Equal volumes of a serum dilution and a sporozoite suspension are incubated for 45 minutes at room temperature with vigorous shaking. Three thousand of the sporozoites are then injected intravenously into normal mice. Serum dilutions are considered to have SNA when more than one-half of the inoculated mice remain parasitologically negative.

C. Indirect Fluorescent Antibody Test

Sporozoites are very immunogenic and cause a detectable antibody response with the indirect fluorescent antibody (IFA) test shortly after their inoculation. These sporozoites can be irradiation-attenuated or nonattenuated, and they induce these antibodies when inoculated via the intravenous route or by biting mosquitoes. Sporozoites induce antibodies in susceptible as well as insusceptible hosts.

The work of Golenser *et al.* (1977) shows that the antibody response in rats after exposure to biting mosquitoes is already detectable with frozen sporozoite antigen after 3 days and quickly increases to high titers after 1 week. One booster inoculation of sporozoites forces the titers to an even higher level, where they level off despite further boosters. The number of inoculated sporozoites appears to influence the antibody reaction, since it was found that priming through bites of 2–4 mosquitoes did not reveal detectable titers, whereas 10–15 mosquitoes induced low titers and 30–40 mosquitoes gave the highest titer values. This effect is resolved after the second bite. Exposure to a few mosquitoes boosts the antibody response to the same height as exposure to many mosquitoes (Golenser *et al.*, 1978). Even the bite of a single infected mosquito may induce an increase in the IFA titer established by one previous intravenous inoculation of sporozoites (McConnell, 1978). Absorption of immune sera with sporozoites has indicated that the antibodies are sporozoite-specific. The passive transfer of antisporozoite immune serum into rats reduces the number of detectable EEFs, indicating that the antibodies have specifically neutralized most of the inoculated sporozoites (Golenser *et al.*, 1978). The specificity of antibodies against sporozoites was beautifully demonstrated by Nardin and Nussenzweig (1978), using both frozen sporozoites and viable sporozoites for the IFA test. Hansen *et al.* (1980) found both IgM and IgG antibodies against frozen sporozoites in sera from immunized mice. They also observed that in the process of immunization there was an initial drop in the titer after the first two boosters; the third booster inoculation did not affect the titer level, which might be attributable to the state of antibody excess achieved after completion of the immunization procedure. Also, Bawden *et al.* (1978) found high antisporozoite titers in mice and rabbits immunized with sporozoites. They developed an inhibition test for checking the specificity of the fluorescence agains sporozoites.

Technical Details of the Indirect Fluorescent Antibody Test with Sporozoites. The antigen used in the IFA technique consists of sporozoites applied to slides with a 12-pronged applicator (Voller and O'Neill, 1971); the slides are subsequently stored at −70°C. Sporozoites are collected from homogenized infected mosquitoes with the use of a biphasic gradient as described by Beaudoin *et al.* (1977) or as modified by J. P. Verhave and R. E.

Vermeulen (personal communication) using 60% Urografin (Schering Ag., West Berlin) instead of diatrozoate, and 15% calf serum instead of 15% bovine serum albumin. The suspensions are not completly pure, and some mosquito debris is present on the antigen slides as well. This debris fluoresces in serum from animals immunized intravenously with sporozoite suspensions contaminated with debris but not in serum from animals immunized by bites of infected mosquitoes. However, this factor does not interfere with the proper reading of fluorescing sporozoites. Another point to be made is that frozen sporozoites tend to have cracks in their surface membrane through which intracellular contents may escape (Vanderberg *et al.*, 1969). Antigen preparations treated with anti-sporozoite immune serum often show the fluorescing sporozoite in the midst of a little pool of fluorescing material. These technical inconveniences can be circumvented by using sporozoites obtained from a DEAE-cellulose column (Moser *et al.*, 1978; Mack *et al.*, 1978), resulting in a less contaminated preparation in which the surface membranes of sporozoites remain intact. Vermeulen (in preparation) applies a gradient centrifugation method using a discontinuous Urografin gradient, followed by further purification of the sporozoite-containing layer on a continuous gradient of Percoll.

D. Interstage Cross-Reactivity

One of the first reports dealing with serological reactions between different stages was by Sodeman and Jeffery (1964) who used a direct fluorescent antibody test with *Plasmodium gallinaceum* sporozoites and serum from blood-induced infections in chickens. Much later Golenser *et al.* (1977) investigated with the IFA technique whether blood forms cross-reacted with antibodies against frozen sporozoites of *P. berghei*. One exposure to sporozoites under chloroquine cover induces antibodies that are detectable in the IFA test only with sporozoite antigen and not with blood schizonts. However, after repeated exposure to sporozoites, blood schizonts fluoresce with such sera. It is highly unlikely that a chloroquine-aborted parasitemia accounts solely for this cross-reactivity, since irradiated sporozoites and sporozoites inoculated into rabbits, or into rats under pyrimethamine cover, induce some reactivity as well (Meuwissen *et al.*, 1978). This has been confirmed by Nardin and Nussenzweig (1978), Hansen (1980), and Bawden *et al.* (1978).

These titers against blood schizonts are greatly reduced after the absorption of such sera with frozen and thawed infected blood. But after absorption with sporozoites only the antisporozoite titers are reduced and not the anti-blood form titers. The reverse situation has also been tested. Rats infected with and immune to blood forms were checked for antibodies. Sera from these animals showed anti-blood form antibodies, but sporozoite antigen also reacted shortly after infection. Absorption with frozen and thawed infected blood reduced the anti-blood form titers but not the antisporozoite titers (Golenser *et al.*, 1978), and absorption with sporozoites affected only the reactivity to sporozoite antigen (Verhave *et al.*, 1978).

These findings make it likely that both developmental stages share antigenic determinants. The stage-specific antigens cover or dominate those shared with the other stages, or the latter may only induce antibodies of lower avidity.

E. Intra- and Interspecies Cross-Reactivity

Using the CSP test Vanderberg *et al.* (1969) and Nussenzweig *et al.* (1972b) found cross-reactivity between *P. chabaudi* and *P. vinckei* and sera from mice immune to sporozoites of *P. berghei*. *Plasmodium chabaudi* immune sera also reacted with sporozoites of *P. berghei*. In a different model Verhave *et al.* (1980) failed to observe serological cross-reactivity between species of *P. berghei* and *P. yoelii* in rats with the IFA test. However, some cross-reactivity was observed between subspecies strains, i.e., *P. berghei berghei* strains ANKA and SP 1 i-RLL, and between *P. yoelii yoelii* and *P. yoelii nigeriensis*. Rodent sera with antibodies against *P. berghei* sporozoites do not react with sporozoites from primate plasmodia (Nussenzweig *et al.*, 1972b; Golenser *et al.*, 1977). Antibodies against sporozoites from primate malarias have not so far been demonstrated extensively with the CSP test. Such antibodies can be readily induced in incompatible hosts such as rats (Nussenzweig *et al.*, 1973; Nussenzweig and Chen, 1974). It was found that cross-reactivity was demonstrable between strains of *P. cynomolgi* or *P. falciparum* but not between these species. Sporozoites from one strain of *P. falciparum* induced CSP antibodies that readily cross-reacted with falciparum sporozoites of various geographic isolates. And the same was found for the *P. vivax* model (Clyde *et al.*, 1975; McCarthy and Clyde, 1977).

F. Antibodies and Protection

Protection against sporozoite infection is at least partly antibody-mediated. It has been shown that passive transfer of immune mouse sera prior to the administration of infective sporozoites rapidly neutralizes the greater part of the infected inoculum. Thereby the number of EEFs developing in the liver is reduced, but eventually all animals become patent and die of the infection (Nussenzweig *et al.*, 1969). Antisporozoite serum from rats had the same effect, but serum from rats immune to blood stages did not (Golenser *et al.*, 1978). The CSP antibodies are not believed to be the sole responsible factor in antisporozoite protection. The antibodies can be induced with disrupted and immature sporozoites, and their production can be induced via routes other than the intravenous one and yet induce no protection (Spitalny and Nussenzweig, 1973). The reverse situation is also possible: Established protection without detectable CSP antibodies was found in splenectomized and immunized mice (Spitalny and Nussenzweig, 1976).

A sporozoite immunization schedule covering several months is needed to render monkeys or humans immune, i.e., protected against primate malarias. This can be related to the technical difficulty of obtaining suitable amounts of primate sporozoites within a short period of time. This is probably also the cause of variability of the CSP antibody response in *P. cynomolgi*-immunized monkeys. In a few human trials complete protection was obtained by repeated exposure to biting irradiated mosquitoes infected with either *P. falciparum* or *P. vivax.* In these cases CSP antibodies could be demonstrated, but the number of volunteers was too low to predict protection on the basis of these antibodies. Only the SNA test seems to reflect antisporozoite protection, but this test is unsuitable for use in humans. It is very doubtful that a single test for antibodies can be used to predict the state of protection, since other factors of the immune mechanism, i.e., cell-mediated responses, contribute to it as well (Spitalny *et al.*, 1977; Verhave *et al.*, 1978).

III. THE ANTIBODY RESPONSE AGAINST EXOERYTHROCYTIC FORMS

The fluorescence of EEFs in fluorescent antibody tests seems to be mainly a matter of cross-reactivity with antibodies raised to the erythrocytic stage of the parasite. Antibodies induced by the blood stages of *P. gallinaceum* (Voller and Taffs, 1963; Ingram and Carver, 1963; El-Nahal, 1967), *P. yoelii yoelii* (El-Nahal, 1967), *P. berghei* (Golenser *et al.*, 1977), *P. cynomolgi* (El-Nahal, 1967; Ward and Conran, 1968), *P. knowlesi* (Krotoski *et al.*, 1973a,b), and *P. malariae* (El-Nahal, 1967) fluorescence with the homologous EEF antigen. However, some investigators reported fluorescence with heterologous EEF antigen as well: El-Nahal (1967) found some fluorescence of *P. yoelii* EEFs with sera from rats immune to *P. berghei*, *P. vinckei*, and *P. chabaudi*. Similar serological cross-reactions were seen between strains and subspecies of *P. cynomolgi*. However, *P. cynomolgi* EEF antigen did not react with anti-*P. inui* or anti-*P. shortii* serum. Neither did *P. malariae* EEF antigen cross-react with anti-*P. falciparum* serum or with sera from any other primate, rodent, or bird malaria tested. *Plasmodium gallinaceum* antigen does not cross-react with *P. juxtanucleare* serum (Voller and Taffs, 1963; El-Nahal, 1967). On the other hand, Krotoski *et al.* (1973a) found that *P. knowlesi* EEFs reacted as well as *P. cynomolgi* EEFs with *P. cynomolgi* antiserum. Golenser *et al.* (1977) used the

P. berghei EEF antigen from fixed livers to study the cross-reacting aspects of anti-blood stage antibodies in more detail. It was found that cross-reactivity occurred in the course of a blood-induced infection in rats within a week after inoculation. Rats inoculated with sporozoites and treated with chloroquine to prevent parasitemia did not show antibodies cross-reacting with EEFs unless two or three boosters of sporozoites were given. This might be due to the schizogony of EEFs, which is not prevented by chloroquine. Exposure to sporozoites while animals are under pyrimethamine cover or exposure to ir-radiated sporozoites induces neither the growth of EEFs nor the development of anti-EEF antibodies (Meuwissen *et al.*, 1978). Vanderberg (1973) and Foley and Vanderberg (1977) showed that antisporozoite immune serum did not affect the growth or morphology of established EEFs.

The character of this interstage cross-reactivity has been further studied by using an absorption technique. Absorption of sporozoite immune serum with sporozoites does not affect the fluorescence with EEFs, but absorption with blood schizonts does. It is likely that both sporozoites and blood schizonts have, in addition to their stage-specific determinants, also secondary determinants which are specific for other stages such as the EEFs (Verhave *et al.*, 1980). Further study will be needed before the possibility of the existence of antibody specific for EEF can be categorically denied. It should be noted that the section-ing of EEFs exposes interior antigens which are presumably masked from the host's immune system *in vivo* and therefore probably do not contribute to an immune response to the EEFs.

IV. THE ANTIBODY RESPONSE TO BLOOD STAGES

A. General Background

Within a few days of the invasion of the blood the major serological responses to malaria are initiated. At first antibodies are detectable only by the most sensitive tests, but the levels increase rapidly and become easily measurable. These high antibody levels are maintained well beyond the crisis when the parasite numbers decrease dramatically. In fact the fall in antibody can be so gradual that it can still be detected months or even years after infection. During recrudescences and relapses malaria antibody levels can again rise, this time more rapidly than during the primary attack, and they rise to higher levels which are maintained for a longer time. This is the typical situation for a long-term semiimmune residents in a malaria endemic area. In the serum of such individu-als can be found protective antibody, malaria-specific antibody which does not correlate with protection and serological factors induced by the malaria infection but reactive with nonmalarial material.

B. Protective Antibody

In 1937 Coggeshall and Kumm showed that sera from monkeys which had been repeatedly infected with malaria protected recipient monkeys against challenge with the homologous strain (Coggeshall, 1943). Little attention was paid to this type of work subsequently, until the 1960s when Cohen *et al.* (1961) and Cohen and McGregor (1963) indicated quite convincingly that IgG from West African adults when passively transferred reduced the *P. falciparum* parasitemia in naturally infected recipient young children within a week of treatment. Edozien *et al.* (1962) showed that similar protective antibody was present in the cord blood of Africans in West Africa. Protection between East and West African *P. falciparum* strains was less convincing. Sadun *et al.* (1966) found that West African IgG suppressed infection with the heterologous strain in chimpanzees but had little effect on Southeast Asian *P. falciparum* infections.

Coggeshall (1943) noted that at the time mature schizonts were present the erythrocytic forms of *P. knowlesi* were most affected by the immune sera. Subsequently Cohen *et al.* (1961) reached the same conclusion for *P. falciparum* and further determined the target of protective action of the antisera to be the released merozoite.

It is thus quite clear that the immunoglobulin fraction (particularly IgG) of the sera of immune or semiimmune malaria patients or primates has protective action against homologous malaria parasites. Similar factors have also been shown in the sera of malaria-infected birds and rodents. Protective immunity is dealt with in detail by Kreier and Green this volume, Chapter 3.

C. Nonspecific Serological Factors Induced by Malaria

These represent the serum changes accompanying malaria infections but which are not directly attributable to malarial antibody antigen reactions. The most obvious influence of malaria is seen in the greatly increased serum levels of IgG and IgM, only part of which can be attributed to specific antimalarial antibodies; presumably much of the remainder constitutes the heterophiles, antiglobulins, etc. Adeniyi-Jones (1967) noted the occurrence of antibodies to erythrocytes in human malaria infections, and Kano *et al.* (1968) and Greenwood *et al.* (1970) confirmed that these were heteragglutinins, especially of the IgM type, reactive with foreign species red blood cells and with trypsinized human erythrocytes. They were also found in the sera of rats infected with *P. berghei* (Kreier *et al.*, 1966). It is the presence of these factors that may lead to uninfected erythrocytes being phagocytosed in a malaria infection. Zuckerman (1964) has argued that such autoantibodies can lead to an autoimmune type of hemolytic reaction in malaria, resulting in the excessive anemia often observed, especially in conditions like blackwater fever. This state of autoimmune reactivity may be only transitory (Zuckerman and Spira, 1961) and so might not be detected easily. If this mechanism is correct, then it might be expected that antiglobulin Coomb's tests would be positive, however, this is not always the case. Supportive evidence for antierythrocyte antibodies is given by Rosenberg *et al.* (1973) who found IgM class antierythrocyte antibodies in the sera of *P. falciparum* patients.

Houba and Allison (1966) and Greenwood *et al.* (1971) reported that rheumatoid factor, an IgM antiglobulin, was very common in malarious areas and correlated with the levels of specific antimalarial antibody. Klein *et al.* (1971) also noted the transient occurrence of rheumatoid factor in monkeys with induced malaria infections. The presence of such factors in tropical sera can easily be wrongly interpreted by serologists as indicative of a classic type of autoimmune disease such as rheumatoid arthritis.

In the tropical splenomegaly syndrome (TSS) both the heterophile levels and antiglobulin are reported to be particularly elevated, and Wells (1970) has postulated that these antibodies are induced by the circulating immune complexes of parasitized erythroctye and malarial antibody, respectively.

However, it is also possible that the production of these antibodies is related primarily to work-stimulated hypertrophy of the spleen (Jandl *et al.*, 1965; Pearson *et al.*, 1978). Ziegler (1973) further showed that cryoprecipitates were present in the sera of malarial TSS patients and that they were especially rich in IgM. G. Crane *et al.* (unpublished) stress that the basic abnormality in TSS patients is in the quantitative or qualitative abnormal IgM production.

Yet another autoimmune indicator found in the sera of malaria patients is "speckled antinuclear factor" (ANF). This can be detected by indirect immunofluorescence tests with the nuclei or rat liver as substrate. Greenwood *et al.* (1970) found that speckled ANF correlated with high malarial antibody levels, and Voller *et al.* (1972) noted an association of ANF with total IgM levels and malarial antibody and reported that it was restricted to malarious parts of Tanzania. Crane *et al.* (unpublished) confirmed the association of elevated IgM with elevated IgG malarial antibody levels. Kreier and Dilley (1969) reported the presence of anti-nucleic acid antibodies in rats with *P. berghei* infection, so it may be considered that such antibodies occur in various species during plasmodial infection.

D. The Specific Serological Responses to Malaria

The principle, the practice, and the application of each test will be described. Taken together they will provide a comprehensive guide to the specific immune response to the blood stages and its measurement.

1. Direct Agglutination

Eaton (1938) noted that sera taken from monkeys with chronic *P. knowlesi* infections agglutinated *in vitro* (1) erythrocytes infected with mature schizonts of

P. knowlesi and (2) parasites released from such mature schizonts. These agglutinins, which were species-specific, were present at high levels in monkeys given repeated infections and persisted for more than a year. The agglutinin level reflected the protective capacity of sera used in passive transfer experiments (Coggeshall and Eaton, 1938b).

Several years later Brown and Brown (1965) developed the agglutination method into a highly sensitive, very specific schizont-infected cell agglutination (SICA) test, again with *P. knowlesi* (see below).

It was by using the SICA test that Brown *et al.* (1968) were able to show that the parasites of each relapse or recrudescence in *P. knowlesi* infections was antigenically distinct. Parasites from a particular recrudesence could only be agglutinated by sera taken from the animal after each recrudescence had occurred. Each parasite population type was termed a variant, and the complete process was called antigenic variation. Eventually, after long chronic infections, the sera agglutinated all variants of a given strain but not those of other strains of *P. knowlesi* (Brown *et al.*, 1970a). This corresponded to a lack of cross-immunity to challenge between these strains. In immunized monkeys there was no correlation between the SICA titers and their resistance to challenge (Brown *et al.*, 1970b). Butcher and Cohen (1971) further emphasized that SICA titers were independent of the inhibitory effect of immune sera on *in vitro* growth of *P. knowlesi*.

Technical Details of the Schizont-Infected Cell Agglutination Test. The procedure given below has kindly been provided by K. N. Brown.

1. Collect 2–3 ml of serum from the monkey before infection.
2. When parasitemia is suitable, ideally between 30 and 60%, prepare the agglutination trays. Parasite levels below these values tend to give very low yields. At higher parasitemias parasites may not mature properly or will clump spontaneously in the agglutination tray.
3. From Giemsa-stained smears, determine the time when the majority of parasites are in the schizont (multinucleate) stage.
4. Make up the diluent, consisting of 1% preinfection monkey serum in saline.
5. Add 400 μl to each well of a round-bottomed WHO hemagglutination tray.
6. Add 100 μl of test sera to top wells and make fivefold dilutions. Always include a known parasite control serum and a normal serum.
7. Tranquilize the monkey with Sernylan (phencyclidine hydrochloride) and anesthetize it more fully with intravenous Nembutal (pentobarbitone sodium).
8. Bleed initially by heart puncture with a fairly wide-bore needle (gauge depending on the size of the monkey) into 50-ml syringes containing citrate–saline. When bleeding becomes difficult, open the thoracic cavity, pour in some

citrate saline, and make an incision in the heart. Collect blood from the thoracic cavity with a bulb pipet. It is important to let the heart bleed right out, since the last part of the bleed often contains the highest concentration of schizonts.

9. Dispense the citrated blood in 100-ml centrifuge tubes and spin at 1800 g for 10 minutes.

10. Remove the supernatant and resuspend the cells in Krebs–glucose. Dispense into 10-ml conical centrifuge tubes and centrifuge at 400 g for 15 minutes. The schizont-containing cells will appear as a brown layer under the buffy layer.

11. If there is a sufficient yield of cells, carefully remove the buffy layer and discard it. Then collect the brown layer and dilute it in Krebs buffer (without glucose) to a concentration of 4×10^7/ml.

12. If the yield is poor, take the top cells from each tube, recentrifuge at 400 g for 15 minutes, and collect the brown layer again for dilution in Krebs buffer.

13. Make sufficient cell suspension to add 400 μl to each well, at a concentration of 4×10^7/ml, in Krebs buffer (without glucose). A 3-kg monkey should yield enough parasitized cells for about 500 wells, but this can vary greatly.

Wilson and Phillips (1976) described a method for cryopreserving schizonts in liquid nitrogen for use in schizont agglutination tests. This should prove valuable in avoiding waste of material.

2. In Vitro Growth Inhibition Assay

Cohen *et al.* (1969) showed that sera taken from monkeys immune to *P. knowlesi* inhibited the growth of this parasite *in vitro*. It is of interest to note that there was little effect on the parasite's growth up to the time of schizogony, but at this point immune serum had a dramatic and dose-related effect in stopping the cycle of parasite development after schizogony. Cohen and Butcher (1970) and Cohen *et al.* (1972) interpreted the results of the assay as indicating the host's immune status. They found that both IgG and IgM had significant effects in preventing reinvasion of new red cells by merozoites and that the antibody was mostly, although not always, variant-specific. However, later work by the same group (Butcher *et al.*, 1978) showed that in some situations the level of inhibitory antibody did not reflect the immune status of the monkeys; i.e., vaccinated animals could have antibody and yet were not protected.

Both the SICA test and the growth inhibition assay require a synchronized infection, and this has virtually restricted their application to *P. knowlesi* infections. The exception is the work of Phillips *et al.* 1972 and Wilson and Phillips (1976) who cultured *P. falciparum* with various immune sera from West Africans resident in the same geographic area from which the parasites were obtained. They noted considerable difference in the effects of sera on various parasite isolates, suggesting that several parasite populations were probably present in the same locality.

Technical Details of *In Vitro* Assay of Growth-Inhibiting Antibody. The details of this assay have been provided by G. H. Mitchell.

i. Reagents

Medium 199, supplemented with glucose (2 mg/ml) and penicillin (5 IU/ml) sterilized by filtration
Panel of test sera and known normal control serum. At least 0.2 ml of each serum is necessary; sterile
Tritiated leucine sufficient to give approximately 2 μCi/ml of final culture suspension; sterile
For microscopy sampling: fetal calf serum
For radio-activity harvesting: phosphate-buffered saline (PBS), trichloracetic acid (TCA) (10%), absolute methanol, ether, formic acid (80%), scintillation cocktail.
For drawing blood: heparin, in PBS; sterile; 1 ml/10 ml blood drawn

ii. Procedures (Sterile Technique is Imperative Throughout)

1. On the day before culture dispense 0.1 ml of each serum under test into each of duplicate petri dishes. Store humidified at 4°C.
2. Bleed the parasite donor monkey when the parasitemia is predominantly late trophozoites or early schizonts and at 1% or higher. If the parasitemia is significantly above 1%, bleed a normal red cell donor.
3. Make, fix, and stain a film from the infected blood drawn and accurately count the parasitemia.
4. Discard the plasma (with great care) from the parasitized blood to avoid loss of brown layer parasites.
5. Resuspend the cells in medium to wash, recentrifuge as above, and discard the supernatant.
6. Calculate the volume of medium necessary for cultures: 1 ml/petri dish.
7. Calculate the volume of packed cells needed for culture: 0.1 ml/petri dish.
8. Calculate the ratio of packed infected blood cells to normal cells needed for the resultant parasitemia to be close to 1%, hence actual volumes of packed cells to be added to measured total volume of medium.
9. Calculate and add the required volume of tritiated leucine.
10. Dispense 1 ml of suspension into each petri dish.
11. From the excess suspension make a 0-hour blood film for assessing the actual starting parasitemia.
12. Place the petri dishes in humidified 37°C carbon dioxide incubator on an orbiting table.
13. At 24 hours make films from each dish by spinning 0.1 ml of suspension

down through a small volume of fetal calf serum (300 g for 10 minutes), discarding the supernatant and spreading the pellet in the normal way.

14. Check each culture for sterility at 24 hours.

iii. Preparation for Radioactivity Counting

1. Aspirate the petri dish contents into numbered disposable tubes. Each dish should be washed out twice with PBS, the washings being added to the tube using about 1 ml PBS for each wash.

2. Centrifuge the tubes at 500 g for 10 minutes, discard the (radioactive) supernatant, buzz the pellet, and add 10 ml of 10% TCA per tube. Allow to stand at room temperature overnight.

3. Centrifuge as above, aspirate the supernatant, buzz the pellet, add a further 10 ml of 10% TCA to wash precipitate, and recentrifuge.

4. Repeat washing with absolute alcohol and then absolute ether.

5. After aspirating the ether allow the pellet to dry, add 2 ml formic acid to each tube, and incubate at 50°C overnight.

6. Allow to cool and dispense 0.1 ml of solution into numbered scintillation vials, add scintillant, and count.

7. Calculate inhibitory titre as follows: mean counts in control dishes = 100% growth; express counts with each test serum as a percentage of this. Inhibitory titer of the serum in question equals 100 minus this figure.

3. Agar Gel Methods

Immunodiffusion methods rely on the precipitation in agar gel of complexes formed between diffusing soluble antigen and antibody. The method readily permits the analysis of multiple antigen–antibody systems but is less suitable for quantitative work.

The earliest reported data on agar gel diffusion were those of Zuckerman and Spira (1965) who found that there were both species-specific and shared antigens in different plasmodia. This group of workers extracted the soluble antigens by means of saponin lysis followed by pressure disintegration in a Hughes press. Zuckerman et al. (1969) showed that the precipitins appeared within 1–2 weeks following the inoculation of rats with *P. berghei*. Most sera taken after the crisis of parasitemia contained precipitating antibody. Rats vaccinated with *P. berghei* extracts produced even stronger precipitins. Diggs (1966) drew attention to the fact that immunodiffusion reactions of antisera raised against injected parasitic material must be viewed with caution, as virtually all the precipitin lines given by rabbit antisera against rat-derived *P. berghei* extracts could be attributed to the reaction with rat erythrocytes and rat serum components.

Brown et al. (1970b) also used the gel diffusion method in analyzing the immune response of rhesus monkeys with chronic infections and of those vaccinated with *P. knowlesi* extracts. Monkeys with chronic infections occasionally developed up to three lines of precipitation. Some lines were given by only one strain, and others were shared by the various strains of *P. knowlesi*. The sera of animals vaccinated with schizont extracts and Freund's adjuvant yielded up to four strong precipitin bands. However, the development of precipitins was not correlated with protective immunity.

By far the most extensive immunodiffusion studies are those carried out by McGregor and colleagues in Gambia on sera from individuals exposed to *P. falciparum*. [McGregor et al 1966] Turner and McGregor (1969a) showed that adult Gambians' sera yielded a number of precipitin bands against *P. falciparum* extracts obtained from infected placentas; in addition antigen was detected circulating in the sera following malaria attacks. The same workers (Turner and McGregor, 1969b) reported that the antibodies were predominantly in the IgG fraction of adults' and older children's sera, although some antibody was found in the IgM fraction. Wilson *et al.* (1969) extended the gel diffusion studies on *P. falciparum* in Gambia by classifying the antigens into groups according to their behavior after exposure to heat (see the following tabulation).

Labile (L) antigens	Destroyed by heat at 56°C for 30 minutes	At least 7 identified
Resistant (R) antigens	Survived 56°C for 30 minutes but were destroyed by 100°C for 5 minutes	At least 2 identified
Stable (S) antigens	Survived heating to 100°C for 5 minutes	At least 20 identified

The S antigens were found both in parasitized erythrocyte extracts and in the free soluble form in the sera of patients, especially children, with heavy *P. falciparum* infections (Wilson, 1970). It appears that the antibodies to the subclass La of the labile antigens account for most precipitating antibody (McGregor and Wilson, 1971), and their evolution corresponds most closely to the development of protective immunity. They are present in most newborns and then fall for a year or so, after which they increase until 95% of the population over 5 years have such antibodies in the IgG fraction of their sera (Wilson *et al.*, 1966).

The S antigens are usually present in the sera of young children who can produce a transient antibody response to them, but the main response is seen in adults' IgG and IgM and even so the incidence is much lower than for the La antibody response. Wilson *et al.* (1976) suggested that the use of inadequate panels of S antigens may have led to an underestimation of the incidence of antibodies to S antigens. There was a close epidemiological association between increased serum IgM levels and the presence of antibodies to S antigens (McGregor and Wilson, 1971).

Wilson and Voller (1970, 1972) showed that infected erythrocytes of *Aotus* monkeys with *P. falciparum* infections contained all the classes of precipitin antigens reported in human infections. Moreover, some of the *Aotus*-derived antigens gave reactions of identity with the material derived from human sources.

Soluble antigens have also been described in the plasma of birds infected with avian malaria (Smith *et al.*, 1969).

a. Technical Details of Double Diffusion in Gel for Malaria.   The details provided below have been taken from the World Health Organization (1974).

i. Test Procedure.   Double diffusion by the method of Ouchterlony may be carried out in 1.5% Noble agar in either 0.3 *M* phosphate buffer (pH 8.0) or 0.05 *M* Veronal buffer (pH 8.6) applied to microscope slides. Gels prepared with Veronal buffer tend to give better resolution of complex precipitin reactions. Wells 2 mm in diameter placed 5 mm (center to center) apart have been found satisfactory.

Antigen is extracted from infected blood by a disintegration procedure such as freezing and thawing, sonication, or pressure disintegration with a Hughes press or similar apparatus. Blood infections should be dense (about 50% erythrocytes infected), and most of the parasites should be mature or nearly mature schizonts. Extracts are centrifuged (at 28,000 *g* or more for 20 minutes), and the clear supernatant is taken as antigen. As mature asexual erythrocytic forms of *P. falciparum* are rarely encountered in the peripheral blood of malaria patients, supplies of requisitely infected blood may be obtained (1) from infected human placentas and (2) by *in vitro* cultivation in proprietary media to parasite maturity of trophozoite-infected blood obtained from malaria patients. In each instance the schizont density of the infected blood may be increased by slow centrifugation (at 400 *g*) for 15 minutes and by collecting the schizont-rich, chocolate-colored layer that forms beneath the buffy coat. Erythrocytic lysis prior to antigen extraction is not recommended.

Antigen and antisera are diffused in gels at controlled temperatures—usually 4°C—for 48 hours in a humid chamber, and the slides are then washed in at least two changes of 1% sodium chloride containing about 0.01 *M* sodium azide for up to 48 hours, care being taken to avoid lifting or breaking the gel. When washed, the wet gels may be examined by transillumination for the presence of precipitins. The slides are then rinsed in distilled water for 1 hour, a strip of wet, lint-free filter paper is applied to cover the gel surface, and the slide is allowed to dry slowly at room temperature (usually 16–24 hours). Slides may then be stained with an appropriate dye, e.g., amido black. Stained slides should be examined for precipitin reactions, both macroscopically and with the aid of a hand lens ($\times 8$–$\times 10$) with good illumination against a white background.

As in other antibody tests, appropriate positive and negative control sera should be included in selected test systems.

ii. Mode of Interpretation

1. The simplest is to record the negative and positive results.
2. The number of lines present between individual sera and the antigen well may be counted.
3. The titer of antibody can be established by appropriate dilution of the test sera.

iii. Antigen Storage. Although aqueous extracts of antigen can be stored at −70°C for many weeks with little apparent deterioration in antigen content, it is probably best to store infected blood at −70°C and to disintegrate aliquots of it when the need for antigen extracts arises. Lyophilized infected blood has been stored in this way for 5 years without apparent deleterious effects. At room temperature, lyophilized infected blood appears to keep satisfactorily for a least 1 month. Extracts made from infected blood have been noted to lose potency slowly on storage at −20°C and rapidly at 4°C. Loss of activity of the labile group of antigens usually occurs first.

b. Other Agar Gel and Electrophoresis Methods. One disadvantage of double diffusion is that it is a slow, relatively insensitive technique. The counter current immunoelectrophoresis (CIE) method in which an electric charge is induced across the reaction area is much quicker and is generally more sensitive than double diffusion. Seitz (1975) used this method on cellulose acetate membranes to demonstrate antibodies to *P. berghei* and *P. vinckei* in rodent sera, and Bidwell *et al.* (1973) detected *P. falciparum* antigen and antibody in this way. The main drawback of this method is that it lacks the resolving power of the double diffusion techniques yet still is insensitive in comparison with the labeled reagent tests to be discussed later.

One of the most promising methods for antigenic analysis is crossed immunoelectrophoresis in which the antigenic mixture is first electrophoresed in one direction and then the plate is turned at right angles and a second electrophoresis is carried out into agar-containing antisera. Bjerrum and Bøg Hansen (1976) found this to be an excellent method for characterizing erythrocte membrane proteins. More recently this technique was applied to antigenic analysis of the erythrocyte stages of *P. knowlesi* (Deans *et al.*, 1978; Schmidt-Ullrich and Wallach, 1978). Eleven major antigens were identified; nine were shared by rings, trophozoites, schizonts, and merozoites. However, one specific antigen was formed as the trophozoites developed, and another was restricted to schizonts and merozoites.

4. Complement Fixation

Coggeshall and Eaton (1938a) described a complement fixation (CF) test using as antigen extracts of *P. knowlesi*-infected blood or spleens. These antigens were very anticomplementary and had to be diluted for use in the CF test. This test was not very satisfactory in that it usually gave low titers of 1:2–1:16. Even after repeated challenge, titers only rarely reached 1:64. Application of similar tests to the diagnosis of human malaria was unsatisfactory in that many parasitologically positive individuals were not positive by the CF test (Kligler and Yoeli, 1941; Stratmen-Thomas and Dulaney, 1940). D'Antonio *et al.* (1966) improved the CF test by using an antigen derived by pressure disruption of monkey erythrocytes infected with *P. knowlesi*.

Schindler and Voller (1967) compared the CF test with immunofluorescence for the study of antibody levels in *P. cynomolgi* infections in rhesus monkeys. Both tests became positive about a week after the blood was invaded. After 6–8 months the immunofluorescent antibody levels were still quite high, but the CF test titers had reverted to negative even though the monkeys still had parasitemia. False positive reactions and low sensitivity meant that this test was not acceptable for epidemiological work (Voller and Schindler, 1967). The work of Mahoney *et al.* (1966) suggests that better methods of antigen extraction might improve the values of the CF test. However, the availability of newer, more sensitive techniques has led workers away from the CF test which is troublesome to carry out.

5. Indirect Hemagglutination (Passive Hemagglutination)

The passive hemagglutination test, so successfully applied in various fields of microbiology and immunology for the demonstration of circulating antibodies, was introduced in the field of malaria serology by Desowitz and Stein (1962). The test, called the indirect hemagglutination (IHA) test for malaria, is based on the agglutination of malaria antigen-sensitized carrier erythrocytes in the presence of malarial antibody. Sheep or human red blood cells are treated with tannic acid and exposed to a soluble extract of malaria parasites. The sensitized cells are added to serum dilutions in wells of plastic trays. The different setting patterns of the cells relate to the degree of agglutination. The IHA antibody titer is the last dilution causing agglutination and so provides a semiquantitative indicator of the antibody content of the sample. Because of difficulties with reproducibility, it was several years before this test found application in extensive field studies. Only within a critical range of physicochemical factors can agglutinating antibody molecules link the red cells to form a three-dimensional lattice; therefore the reproducibility of the test involves a wide range of factors, such as properties of the red cells of various species and of individual donors, external conditions related to temperature and pH during preparation of the carrier cells and their sensitization, properties of individual batches of sensitizing antigen, the composition of the suspending medium, and the concentration of the sensitized red cells therein. The sensitizing plasmodial antigen ranks highest in the order of priority of these factors. It is prepared by freezing and thawing or by sonication of parasitized red blood cells. These are obtained from primates inoculated with simian plasmodia or from *Aotus* monkeys infected with human plasmodial species. The water-soluble fraction containing components of parasite as well as host cells is used as sensitizing antigen. Obviously its composition varies, i.e., with the degree of parasitization of erythrocytes, with the degree of parasite development in the erythrocytes, and with the degree of stability of its components.

Successful isolation, purification, and characterization of antigenic components have not yet been achieved. It is clear that this is essential however, for exact standardization of the test procedure. The reproducibility of the test was enhanced by the introduction of a procedure for the production of lyophilized test cells. This was achieved by fixation of the carrier red cell with gluteraldehyde before sensitization (Meuwissen and Leeuwenberg, 1972). Reagents can be prepared in quantities; they are relatively stable, are ready for immediate use, and can be applied even under field conditions since elaborate laboratory equipment is no longer required.

a. The Specificity of the Test. Since the carrier cell is coated with a mixture of host- and parasite-derived antigens, serum samples containing antibodies against the former components can cause false positive agglutination patterns. In a field study in Tanzania it was shown that about 2.5% of the samples contained such nonspecific agglutination factors (Meuwissen and Leeuwenberg, 1972). By absorption of the serum samples with red cells coated with erythrocytic antigens derived from noninfected monkeys this problem can be solved. The absorbed serum samples react specifically with plasmodial antigens on the surface of the carrier erythrocytes. In a study of over 500 healthy blood donors not one seropositive reaction was seen, whereas only one false positive reaction was seen in a series of about 200 samples collected from various patients. H. M. Mathews (personal communication) reported false positive IHA tests in rare cases of patients infected with *Babesia,* but this report was not substantiated (Meuwissen, 1974). With regard to selection of the species of sensitizing plasmodial antigen it was found that the highest IHA titers and therefore the highest degree of sensitivity of the test were obtained with cells coated with homologous antigen (Mahoney *et al.,* 1966; J. H. E. Meuwissen, personal communication; Mathews *et al.,* 1975). If some loss in sensitivity of the test is acceptable, heterologous plasmodial antigens can also be used.

A critical point of the IHA test for malaria is its insensitivity during the first stage of a primary malaria infection. Wilson *et al.* (1971) found that the IFA test detected antibodies slightly more efficiently than the IHA test during the first weeks of primary infections. Also, in a seroepidemiological survey in Tanzania a discrepancy was found between the results of IFA and IHA tests, both carried out with *P. falciparum* antigen (Meuwissen *et al.,* 1974). The mean titers obtained in the IFA test with anti-IgG conjugate were higher than the IHA titers in the younger age groups, but in adults this was reversed. The titer levels in the IFA test started to rise earlier, and the increase occurred more gradually than in the IHA test. Sera collected from parasite carriers showed four times as many negative seroreactors in the IHA test as in the IFA test. Sera of patients with high parasite densities were more often negative in the IHA test than those of individuals with a low parasite density. This aspect was studied further in experimental *P. falciparum* infections in *Aotus* monkeys (Bidwell *et al.,* 1973). Again it was found that IFA titers were higher than IHA titers in the primary phase of the infection, but both tests were consistently positive later in the infection.

In numerous field studies in South America, Africa, and Asia the IHA test has been applied since the first studies of Stein and Desowitz (1964). The test is simple to perform, rapid, specific, and in general rather sensitive. Moreover it has the advantage that it can be applied under field conditions. Therefore the IHA test can be considered a useful epidemiological tool for assessment of the degree of malaria endemicity and for evaluation of malaria control (Kagan, 1972; Meuwissen, 1974).

b. Technical Details of the Passive Hemagglutination Test. The assay described below was taken from the World Health Organization (1974).

i. Antigen. Defibrinated blood or blood taken with an anticoagulant is obtained from infected monkeys or from human placentas. The cells are centrifuged, and the supernatant is discarded. The cells are then washed in PBS (pH 7.2) and resuspended to the original blood volume. To eliminate the white blood cells, an equal volume of 3% high-molecular-weight dextran in PBS is added to the cell suspension and the erythrocytes are allowed to sediment for 1 hour. The supernatant containing white cells is discarded. The aggregated erythrocytes are resuspended to the original volume in PBS. The dextran treatment is then repeated. The sedimented erythrocytes are resuspended in PBS and centrifuged at 1100 *g* for 5 minutes at 4°C. Resuspension and centrifugation are repeated twice more. The packed erythrocytes are then stored in 0.1-ml aliquots in rubber-stoppered vials at −70°C.

Control antigens are prepared in the same way from uninfected erythrocytes preferably obtained, where a monkey is being used, from the same animal before infection.

On the day of the actual test, an ampule is removed from the refrigerator, and 0.9 ml of PBS (pH 5.5) is added to the cells in the ampule. The cells in the suspension are then disrupted either by sonication or, less satisfactorily, by freezing and thawing. The suspension is then centrifuged at 8500 g for 15 minutes at 4°C, and the supernatant is used, undiluted, as the antigen.

ii. Preparation of Sensitized Cells

(1) Fixation of erythrocytes. Blood is collected from a sheep in Alsever's solution and stored at 4°C for up to 8 days. (In the following procedures all solutions are kept sterile and are maintained at a temperature of 4°C.) The erythrocytes are packed by centrifugation and washed three times in sterile PBS. Commercially available 25% stabilized gluteraldehyde solution, kept in a refrigerator at 4°C, is diluted to 1% with a buffer containing 1 volume of 0.15 M PBS (pH 8.2) plus 9 volumes of 0.15 M sodium chloride plus 5 volumes of distilled water. The sheep erythrocytes are mixed to a 1–2% suspension with this diluted gluteraldehyde solution. The suspension is incubated at 4°C for 30 minutes with intermittent stirring. The erythrocytes are sedimented by centrifugation at 400 g for 5 minutes at room temperature. They are then resuspended to give a 20% suspension and washed five times with PBS (pH 7.2) and five times with distilled water. The fixed cells are then made up to a 30% suspension in distilled water and stored in aliquots of 1 ml at 4°C. Human group O cells can also be used.

(2) Tannic acid treatment of fixed cells. When fixed sheep erythrocytes, prepared as above, are to be used for sensitization, the supernatant is decanted and discarded.

One milliliter of PBS (pH 7.2) is added to the erythrocytes in each ampule, and the vial is shaken mechanically; a further 8 ml of the saline solution is then added, and the suspension is centrifuged at 400 g for 5 minutes. This procedure is then repeated.

The 0.3 ml of packed cells is resuspended in 9.7 ml of tannic acid solution (1:40,000 in PBS, pH 7.2) and incubated at 4°C for 15 minutes. The suspension is centrifuged at 400 g for 5 minutes, and the supernatant is discarded. The cells are resuspended in PBS (pH 7.2) and centrifuged. Finally the cells are again resuspended in 9.7 ml of the saline solution.

(3) Antigen titration procedure. The cell suspension is divided into five aliquots and centrifuged. The cells are then washed in PBS (pH 5.5) and centrifuged again, the supernatant being discarded. The contents of the five tubes are resuspended in PBS (pH 5.5) to a total volume of 0.9 ml containing 0, 60, 100, 200, and 300 μl of antigen, respectively. The stoppered tubes are incubated in a water bath at 37°C for 30 minutes.

The tubes are then centrifuged, and the cells resuspended in PBS (pH 7.2) containing 1% inactivated rabbit serum (i.e., diluent). The cells are then packed by centrifuging, resuspended, washed in the same diluent, and recentrifuged. Four mililiters of diluent PBS (pH 7.2) is added to each tube. An aliquot of 0.5

ml from one tube is used to determine the hematocrit value of the suspension. The cells in each tube are then made up to exactly a 1.3% suspension in the same diluent.

Five series of twofold dilutions are made, in a microtiter system, of one negative and three positive reference sera in the range of 1:40–1:5120 with the same diluent. It is imperative to use U-type permanent Lucite (Cooke) plates or U-type disposable 6 (Linbro) plates. Volumes of 0.025 ml from each of the batches of sensitized cells are added to one of the series of diluted sera and to a control well containing only diluent.

The microtiter plates are mechanically shaken immediately for 2 minutes. The hemagglutination patterns are read after incubation at room temperature for 1 hour, and the plates are stored overnight in a refrigerator.

The optimum quantity of sensitizing antigen is the smallest amount that shows the highest hemagglutination titer with the set of positive reference sera, while the sensitized cells tested with the negative reference sera and the unsensitized cells tested with either sera or plain diluent show a negative pattern.

A hemagglutination pattern is considered negative when the well shows a button of sedimented cells. The end point of the test is read as the point where a ring pattern replaces the button pattern.

(4) Sensitization. Cells to be used for the actual test are sensitized with the optimum quantity of antigen as determined in the antigen titration test. This is done for both the test cells, i.e., cells sensitized with malaria antigen, and the cells meant for the preparation of control cells, i.e., cells sensitized with antigen prepared from noninfected erythrocytes (control antigen).

(5) Lyophilization of test and control cells. Sensitized fixed cells suspended in diluent as a 5–20% suspension can be lyophilized when they are not needed for immediate use. For each 3 ml of packed red cells present in the suspension, 0.5 ml of a 12.5% solution of Tween 80 in PBS (pH 7.2) is added. By means of 5-ml Pyrex ampules, 1-ml aliquots of the suspension are prepared and freeze-dried for about 18 hours. The ampules can be vacuum-sealed or sealed after filling with dry nitrogen gas. The lyophilized preparation remains stable for over a year at ambient temperatures, even under tropical conditions. When the lyophilized test and control cells are used, diluent must be added to the lyophilized contents of the ampules. Optimum reconstitution of the cell suspensions from the lyophilized preparations requires that the contents of the ampules be mixed carefully so as to avoid foam formation which would have a deleterious effect on the quality of the cells. Initially, only half the quantity of diluent should be added to the lyophilized control cells, as these cells are the first to be used in the absorption procedure.

(6) Examination of samples by the IHA test. In the actual test, the first step is an absorption procedure for the elimination of nonspecific agglutination activity from the plasma samples to be investigated. In the first well of each row of the

microtiter plate, 2 drops (i.e., 0.05 ml) of the plasma of serum samples diluted 1:10 are mixed with an equal volume of control cell suspension in double strength, i.e., 26%. With only this first row of the microtiter plate filled, the cell suspensions are shaken mechanically for 2 minutes and incubated at room temperature for 1 hour. After this the control cells will have sedimented the bottom of the well. With serum diluters, 0.025 ml of the supernatant (i.e., a 1:20 diluted absorbed sample) is taken from the first well for further twofold serial dilution in diluent. These dilutions of the samples are used for mixing with the 1.3% suspension of test cells. Another volume of 0.025 ml of absorbed sample is serially diluted to 1:40 and 1:80 for the later addition of 0.025 ml of a 1.3% suspension of control cells as a control on the persistence of nonspecific agglutination factors in the sample after absorption. Each plate also includes, as extra control wells, 0.025-ml test and control cell suspensions added to different wells with only 0.025 ml of diluent.

The plates are shaken mechanically for 2 minutes and incubated exactly as described for the antigen titration procedure. For an estimation of the specific antibody titer of the malarious sera in the wells in which the sample dilutions were mixed with the test cells, the sedimentation patterns of all the control wells must be negative.

6. Immunofluorescence

a. The Direct Method. In this method antimalarial immunoglobulin is labeled with a fluorescent dye such as fluorescein. This conjugate will react with malaria parasites or antigen in blood smears or tissue sections. The method was used initially to show the wide antigenic cross-reactivity between the different species of malaria parasites (Ingram et al., 1961; Tobie and Coatney, 1961; Voller, 1962). This method was of little use for the measurement of antibody, since each serum sample had to be individually labeled, which required a large amount of serum and was a time-consuming process.

The major use of direct immunofluorescence has been in immunopathological studies, particularly with respect to identification of the components of immune complexes on the kidney glomerular basement membrane in quartan malaria nephrotic syndrome. Allison et al. (1969), Ward and Kibukamusoke (1969), and Houba et al. (1971) all showed that in the nephrotic syndrome IgM and, less commonly, IgG and βIC were present in the complexes. About one-third of the patients had malarial antigen in their complexes, and this was demonstrable using fluorescein-conjugated antisera to P. malariae. Voller et al. (1973) also found IgM deposits in the glomerular of Aotus with induced quartan malaria infections. Similarly direct immunofluorescence has been invaluable in studying the renal deposition of immunoglobulin, complement, and malarial antigen in P. berghei infections in rodents (Ehrich and Voller, 1972; Suzuki, 1974; Boonpucknavig et al., 1972).

b. The Indirect Method. The IFA method has been the mainstay of malarial serology over the last decade, as it overcomes the disadvantages of the direct method; i.e., very small quantities of serum can be assayed at a very sensitive level and the reagents are commercially available. The IFA test is a two-step method (see Fig. 1) (1) dilutions of the test serum are reacted with slide antigen (thick or thin blood smears of parasitized blood); the unreacted components are then washed away with PBS. (2) A solution of fluorescein-labeled antiglobulin (e.g., anti-human immunoglobulin) is reacted with the slide and attaches to the malarial parasite–antibody complex on the slide. After washing the slide is illuminated by ultraviolet blue light on a fluorescence microscope, and the intensity of fluorescence of the parasites is noted.

Serial dilutions of the test sera are used to establish a visual end point, the titer being the last dilution which yields visible fluorescence. It is readily apparent that this method is subjective; nevertheless experienced workers can produce very reproducible results. There is however, difficulty in comparing results from different laboratories. The IFA is rather labor-intensive, but the easy preparation of antigen slides (blood smears) somewhat compensates for this. Fluorescence microscopes were formerly restricted to sophisticated research centers, but they are now widely available, and so many laboratories have the capability for performing malaria IFA tests. If malarial antigen could be made available together

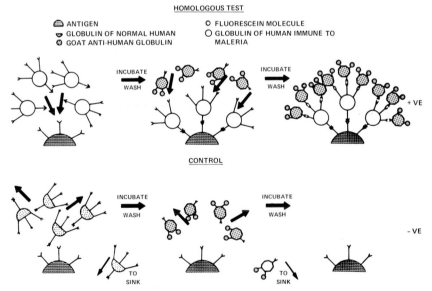

FIG. 1. Diagrammatical representation of the IFA method for malaria. (Reproduced from the Bulletin of the World Health Organization with permission of the authors Voller *et al.* and the publisher.)

with reference antimalarial sera and defined conjugates, it would be easier for new laboratories to establish this test for malaria.

c. Review of Immunofluorescence Applications. At its inception in the early 1960s the IFA test was a novelty, and heroic efforts were required to obtain acceptable results. The following decade and a half have seen a continuous improvement in equipment, reagents, and availability of antigen.

Early investigators were obliged to use optical benches with a normal microscope at one end, carbon arc illumination at the other, and various solutions acting as filters in between. This contraption was very cumbersome and has fortunately been replaced by modern fluorescence microscopes which have a compact built-in high-intensity light source, carefully computed solid filters, and special objectives some of which permit epiillumination. Most diagnostic laboratories now have such microscopes, so immunofluorescence tests can be carried out if malarial antigen is provided to such laboratories.

Fluorescein-labeled antiglobulins have also been much improved over the years. At first each laboratory was obliged to do its own conjugation, but now there are numerous antispecies conjugates (e.g., fluorescein-labeled anti-chicken immunoglobulin, anti-rabbit immunoglobulin, etc.), and well-defined human immunoglobulin class-specific materials (fluorescein-labeled anti-human IgG; anti-human IgM etc.)

Although IFA tests have been performed widely for malarial antibody, it is difficult to make valid comparisons among the results of different laboratories. Generally the results are expressed as titers. These titer values represent the last dilution of the test serum which yields visually detectable fluorescence. It can be readily appreciated that this is a highly subjective value; it will be influenced (1) by the type of antigen used (e.g., whether schizonts are present or absent); (2) by the test conditions (the time and temperature of incubation and washing steps); (3) by the potency and spectrum of reactivity of the antiglobulin conjugate (e.g., whether it is antiimmunoglobulin and anti-IgG); (4) by the microscopical system used (e.g., illumination, filters, condenser type); and (5) by the observer. In theory the use of reference antimalarial sera should permit a large measure of comparability among laboratories, and the use of objective measurements of fluorescence should also assist. However, such reference antisera are not in general use, and the quantitation of the IFA method, because it is time-consuming and requires sophisticated equipment Manawadu and Voller 1971 (Manawadu and Voller, 1978a,b), has not been widely employed. Attempts to use adsorbed soluble antigen with results read objectively on a fluorimeter (Sadun and Gore, 1968) gave promising results but again have not been put into routine practice. The recent improvement of solid-phase immunofluorescence techniques (e.g., FIAX-STIQ, I.D.T. Corporation) may lead to a resurgence of interest in objective immunofluorescence.

The provision of suitable malarial antigen has always been the limiting factor in IFA tests. Initially workers used thin blood smears from infected individuals or primates (Tobie and Coatney, 1961; Voller, 1962). For these to be satisfactory, high parasitemias were required, and only a few tests could be done on each slide. Sulzer *et al.* (1969) made a major practical contribution when they showed that washed infected erythrocytes could be used as thick blood smear antigen. This permitted the use of much lower parasitemias, and multiple thick blood smear spots could be made on each slide, thus allowing many more samples to be tested (Voller and O'Neill, 1971).

It was realized early on that either homologous human plasmodia or closely related simian plasmodia were best used as antigen for detecting antibody in human malaria. This posed problems particularly in relation to the provision of mature schizont forms of *P. falciparum,* which were known to be the most reactive in IFA tests (Targett, 1970) and which do not occur often in the peripheral blood. At first IFA tests were restricted to centers in the tropics where human malaria-infected blood could be obtained or to centers outside the tropics where experimentally induced infections or naturally infected patients were available. This was very unsatisfactory, but the problem was overcome by the adaptation of *P. falciparum, P. vivax,* and *P. malariae* to *Aotus* monkeys. These monkeys support rather high levels of parasitemia, and all stages of the erythrocyte cycle are found in the peripheral blood. Short-term culture of infected blood by the methods of Butcher and Cohen (1971) or by Sulzer and Latorre (1977) will increase the yield of schizonts of *P. falciparum,* thus improving the antigen. The only problem with this source of antigen is the scarcity of *Aotus* monkeys. The supplies of this South American primate are very limited indeed. The recent development of *in vitro* long-term culture of *P. falciparum* (Trager and Jensen, 1976) should finally solve the problems of *P. falciparum* antigen supply. Since the prepared slides can be stored for several years at −70°C, a few centralized facilities could supply all such antigen that might be required.

i. Specificity of the Malaria Indirect Fluorescent Antibody Test.   In the early work on rodent malaria, Voller (1962, 1965) noted that, although there was a fairly strong cross-reaction between *P. berghei* and *P. vinckei,* these species did not cross-react with a group of primate malarias between the members of which there were again cross-reactions. Cox and Turner (1970a) found that there were cross-reactions, albeit at a low level, even between rodent malarias and *Babesia,* although the homologous reactions were always strongest. Kielmann *et al.* (1970) claimed that there was a satisfactory degree of cross-reaction between an avian malaria, *P. gallinaceum,* and sera from individuals with malaria, but this has not been borne out by the experience of other workers.

Voller (1962) reported on IFA cross-reactions between the different primate malarias studied, and Tobie *et al.* (1961) expressed this quantitatively. They found that the titer was always highest in the homologous parasite–antiserum system. This difference between homologous and heterologous IFA systems has been confirmed for many primate and human malarias (Collins *et al.*, 1966a,b, 1967b; Diggs and Sadun, 1965; Wilson *et al.*, 1970). However, although accepting that there are such differences, Garin *et al.* (1966) have suggested *P. cynomolgi*, and Meuwissen (1966, 1968) the simian parasite *P. fieldii*, to be acceptable "all-purpose malarial antigens." Sulzer *et al.* (1969), in detailed comparisons of human malarias by the IFA test, concluded that human malarial parasites should be used wherever possible to yield maximum sensitivity to the test and to give additional information on the probable species of the infecting parasite. The data of Diggs and Sadun (1965) support this viewpoint.

The multispecies malaria slide containing *P. vivax, P. falciparum,* and *P. brasilianum* ($\equiv P. malariae$) of Sulzer *et al.* (1973) provides a suitable antigen for maximum sensitivity in detecting antibody to all these main human malaria infections. Unfortunately difficulties in its production mean that its use will be restricted to a very few centers.

The well-documented study by Ludford *et al.* (1972) confuses even more the story of malaria IFA specificity. They found, with a minority of human parasite sera, extensive and high-level cross-reactions with *Babesia* antigen. Similarly some cattle with *Babesia* reacted strongly with *P falciparum* antigen. This cross-reaction is probably not a serious problem in practice.

ii. Course of Antibody Production as Measured by the Indirect Fluorescent Antibody Test. In one of the earliest publications on malarial IFAs Kuvin *et al.* (1962) outlined the course of antibody production in volunteers infected with *P. vivax* or *P. cynomolgi*. The first appearance of antibody closely followed patent parasitemia; titers rose rapidly over the next 2–3 weeks and then declined, stabilizing at low levels after about 3 months. This was confirmed by Tobie *et al.* (1966) who found that even in sporozoite-induced infections antibody production only began once the blood was invaded. Throughout the prepatent period no antibody could be detected. These authors mentioned that relapses again led to rapid rises in the antibody levels, but Lunn *et al.* (1966) found that only a proportion of the patients reacted this way; in others there was a transient decrease. Schindler and Voller (1967) observed the same antibody patterns in rhesus monkeys with induced infections of *P. cynomolgi*. Collins *et al.* (1967a) studied *P. knowlesi* antibody levels in induced monkey infections and confirmed that higher titers were usually seen in recrudescences. They stressed that individual animals reacted quite differently from a quantitative point of view, so it would be hard to interpret the antibody levels in terms of the status of malaria in their monkeys.

The earliest longitudinal antibody study on *P. falciparum* in nonimmunes was made by Collins *et al.* (1964b). Antibody levels were not high and varied considerably during the course of infection. However, reinoculation of semiimmunes resulted in antibody levels rapidly climbing to stable plateaus (Collins *et al.*, 1964c). Antibody could still be detected almost 2 years later in their patients.

Collins *et al.* (1964a) also titrated antibody to *P. malariae* in induced *P. malariae* infections. In this instance levels were higher and more stable than in the case of *P. falciparum*. Lupascu *et al.* (1966) extended the use of IFA in *P. malariae* infections, showing that the antibody response was related to the length and intensity of the infection. Reinoculations of *P. malariae* resulted in especially high titers.

Meuwissen (1966, 1968) made intensive IFA studies on malaria due to *P. ovale*. Antibody appearance closely followed parasitemia and rose rapidly to reach a plateau within 2–3 weeks.

All these early studies measured the total antibody response without distinguishing the immunoglobulin class components making up the total response. As early as the mid-1960s, Abele *et al.* (1965) and Tobie *et al.* (1966) were drawing attention to the significant changes in IgM and IgG in induced malaria. Collins *et al.* (1971a), with the use of immunoglobulin class-specific conjugates, were able to measure the antibody content of the IgG, IgM, and IgA separately. The IgM and IgA antibody responses were transient, but the IgG antibody was much more persistent.

Targett (1970) also used class-specific conjugates in his study on *P. falciparum* in Gambia. The sera of residents there had significant amounts of antibody in the IgG and IgM fractions and lesser amounts in IgA. None was detected in IgE. Ambroise-Thomas *et al.* (1971) studied a monkey with an induced *P. cynomolgi* infection, and they too found early antibody in the IgM but later virtually all the antibody was in the IgG fraction.

Fewer studies have been carried out on the serological response to rodent malarias using the IFA test. Voller (1965) reported on a transient antibody response in rats infected with *P. berghei*. Waki and Suzuki (1974) found a similar response in *P. berghei*-infected mice, the IgM antibody levels in particular declining very rapidly. However, Cox *et al.* (1969) and Cox and Turner (1970b) noted that, with *P. berghei yoelii* and *P. vinckei* in mice, the initial development of antibody was similar to that reported by earlier workers, but thereafter both IgG and IgM antibodies remained at a plateau level.

For the proper interpretation of malarial IFA tests it would be nice to know how long the antibody persists. It is generally agreed that antibody is detectable throughout the patent parasitemia, but there is disagreement on its persistence after spontaneous cure or following therapy. It seems that the persistence of antibody is dependent on the length and intensity of the infection and on the frequency of exposure. Some studies have indicated that antibody can be detectable 7–15 years after infection (Collins *et al.*, 1968a; Kuvin and Voller, 1963; Luby *et al.*, 1967; Bruce-Chwatt *et al.*, 1972; Fasan *et al.*, 1976), but following radical cure of relative short infections it usually drops from the highest levels within a month or two (Wilson *et al.*, 1970), and even following *P. malariae* infections most cured patients will be serologically negative within a couple of years (Lupascu *et al.*, 1969).

iii. Applications in Nonendemic Areas. There is little value in the use of the IFA test for diagnosis of acute attacks of malaria—conventional parasitological techniques will always result in the detection of parasites in these cases. However, chronic malaria may be suspected in patients who have been in the tropics recently and who have suggestive symptoms such as hepatosplenomegaly, and here the serology can be most useful in confirming or more often in ruling out a diagnosis of malaria. The detection of malaria in blood donors is another obvious use. It is neither necessary nor practical to screen all donors for malaria in nonendemic areas, but high-risk donors can be tested. Dranga *et al.* (1969), using the IFA test, detected potential transfusion threats in *P. malariae* carriers in an area that had been subjected to malaria eradication many years earlier. It has also been possible by the IFA method to identify the responsible donor following posttransfusion-induced malaria (Fisher and Schultz, 1969; Bruce-Chwatt, 1974; Najem and Sulzer, 1976). Similarly the IFA test can be used to identify drug addicts with low malaria infections who have been responsible for "needle-transmitted" malaria.

In all these instances cited, parasites would have been circulating in the blood but may well not have been detected by routine parasitological methods because their densities were at such a low level.

iv. Applications in Areas Where Malaria Is or Has Been Endemic. The situations where serology, especially the IFA test, can be useful in this context have been given by the World Health Organization (1974) as follows (1) to establish malarial endemicity—especially age-specific indexes; (2) to assess changes in transmission during or after antimalaria programs; (3) to delineate malarious areas; and (4) to identify areas or people requiring treatment for malaria, especially during control programs.

It is in the area of malaria seroepidemiology that the IFA test has been most intensively applied and has proved to be useful in addition to parasitological examination. Parasitological screening indicates the point prevalence of malaria, and previously this was supplemented by spleen rates to give period prevalence data of exposure to malaria. However, spleen rates are nonspecific in that they are affected by other concurrent diseases and are very variable following chemotherapy. More precise period prevalence data relating to malaria can be given by serological methods such as the IFA test.

Voller and Bray (1962) first demonstrated that antibody could be detected in virtually all inhabitants of a malaria hyperendemic area of Liberia, and they also showed that antibody levels increased with age. McGregor and colleagues (1965) made a much more detailed study of the malaria IFA response in Gambia, West

Africa. Children were born with high levels of antibody which then declined over the first few weeks of life. Thereafter the levels increased throughout childhood into adult life. If pregnant women are given antimalarial protection and if their newborn children are maintained on malaria prophylaxis, they do not develop antibody detectable by the IFA test (Voller and Wilson, 1964). The work in Gambia and other early studies in North Africa (Coudert *et al.*, 1966), in Nigeria (Voller and Bruce-Chwatt, 1968), and in Malaysia (Collins *et al.*, 1968b) led to the realization that the population's antibody profile could be used as a measure of their malarial experience. This information could be of value in indicating actual malarial endemicity as well as changes following control measures (Collins *et al.*, 1968b; Lelijveld, 1971). Some of the clearest results emerge from the East African work on the altitude delination of malaria transmission. Both in Ethiopia (Collins *et al.*, 1971b) and in Tanzania (Voller *et al.*, 1971) there was a clear difference in IFA response in people living above and below the critical altitude for transmission.

Draper and Voller (1972) published a mathematical model for interpreting age-related antibody prevalence rates, and it was evaluated reasonably successfully in East Africa and Brazil. A much improved statistical method was later prepared by Van der Kaay (1975) and was validated in Surinam.

The precision of the IFA test in identifying malarial foci has been attested to by numerous publications of which those by Edrissian and Afshar (1974) in Iran, by Warren *et al.* (1975) in Central America, and by Sulzer *et al.* (1978) on work in Peru can be taken as good examples. The serology made possible the localization of endemic foci in remote areas. Logistic difficulties meant that blood slide examination would not have been feasible on the same scale.

The IFA test has been shown to reflect changes in malaria transmission. Bruce-Chwatt and Draper (1973) and Bruce-Chwatt *et al.* (1975) were able to show by IFA methods that malaria was no longer being transmitted in Mauritius and Greece, respectively. Similarly Ambroise-Thomas *et al.* (1972) showed the absence of malaria in most of Corsica following eradication activities, and the remaining transmission areas were readily identified.

Ambroise-Thomas and colleagues (1976) also followed the progress of a large antimalarial campaign in Tunisia. They found the IFA test most useful when parasite rates were under 1%.

In virtually all these studies it is stressed that the IFA test should supplement and not replace slide examination. This is important, since occasionally negative results can be obtained even with IFA methods (although to a lesser extent than with the other serological test) in people, especially children, with patent parasitemia.

d. Technical Details of the Indirect Fluorescent Antibody Method for Malaria.   The antigen consists of thick or thin blood films containing mature malaria parasites. At present these are best prepared from *Aotus* monkeys infected with *P. falciparum, P. vivax,* or *P. brasilianum* ($\equiv$ *P. malariae*).

Infect monkeys with an appropriate species of parasite. Monitor the parasitemia daily and, when it is over 1%, determine the precise cycle of development by frequent blood smears so that the blood can be harvested when the parasites are mature. Take the blood into heparin–saline or citrate–saline anticoagulant, wash it three times in PBS (pH 7.2–7.4), and discard the washings. Make up the sediment of erythrocytes to about 3% in PBS. Distribute drops of this suspension onto microscope slides (12–16 drops per slide) and air-dry. Complete the drying of the slides over calcium chloride in a desiccator and then wrap the slides in packets of 5 or 10 in absorbent paper. The packets of antigen slides can be stored at $-70°C$. The test can be performed according to the method outlined by the World Health Organization (1974).

1. Packets of antigen slides are removed from the freezer and allowed to warm to room temperature in a desiccator or in their plastic covering before being unwrapped. This avoids damage to the antigen by hemolysis.

2. Serial dilutions of the test plasma or serum samples are made in PBS (pH 7.2). A dilution of 1:20 is a commonly used starting point. Measured quantities of the serum dilutions are then transferred to each antigen spot. The subsequent processing of the slides is carried out as follows at 20°–37°C. (a) Incubate with serum dilutions in a humid chamber for 30 minutes. (b) Wash with PBS with agitation and three changes of 5 minutes each. (c) Pour off the excess saline and dry the slides, except for the antigen spots. (d) Apply the diluted fluorescein-labeled antiglobulin conjugate. Incubate in a humid chamber for 30 minutes. (e) Wash as in (b). (f) Mount slides with coverslips in 10% glycerol in PBS (or with a commercial mountant, particularly if permanent preparations are required.) (g) Examine with a fluorescence microscope permitting ultraviolet blue excitation and with barrier filters allowing observation of yellow-green fluorescence.

The end point of the IFA titration is the last serum dilution that results in more intense fluorescence of the schizonts than that observed with schizonts reacting with negative control serum.

The day-to-day sensitivity and specificity of the test must be monitored by the inclusion of positive and negative control sera.

7. Enzyme-Linked Immunosorbent Assay

There is an indirect method of ELISA for the detection of malarial antibody, and it is analogous to the IFA test except that an enzyme is used to label the antiglobulin instead of fluorescein; a colorimetric estimation of the enzyme by means of a chromogenic substrate replaces the visual, microscopical estimation of fluorescence in the IFA test.

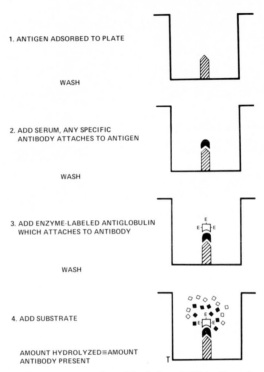

1. ANTIGEN ADSORBED TO PLATE

WASH

2. ADD SERUM, ANY SPECIFIC
ANTIBODY ATTACHES TO ANTIGEN

WASH

3. ADD ENZYME-LABELED ANTIGLOBULIN
WHICH ATTACHES TO ANTIBODY

WASH

4. ADD SUBSTRATE

AMOUNT HYDROLYZED≡AMOUNT
ANTIBODY PRESENT

FIG. 2. Diagrammatical representation of the indirect ELISA. (Reproduced from the Bulletin of the World Health Organization with permission of the authors Voller *et al.* and the publisher.)

In the indirect ELISA for malaria (Fig. 2) soluble malarial antigen is passively adsorbed to plastic test tubes or to the wells in microplates. The test serum is then reacted with the sensitized solid phase and, after washing, an enzyme-labeled antiglobulin is incubated. After a further washing step the enzyme substrate is added. Its color change can be estimated visually or photometrically and is proportional to the amount of antibody in the test serum.

Voller *et al.* (1975) used ELISA with *P. knowlesi* antigen, and they were able to measure malarial antibody levels in human populations in Iran and Tanzania. However, the microplate method with *P. falciparum* antigen was more convenient and sensitive (Voller *et al.*, 1974). This latter method allowed the identification of malarious areas in New Guinea, and malaria control activities were reflected by lower ELISA values (Voller *et al.*, 1976). Recently this same method was used to follow antibody levels in *Aotus* monkeys infected with *P. falciparum*, and it was found that such animals became ELISA-positive within a week of patent parasitemia. Studies using the ELISA to measure antibody levels to *P. knowlesi* following vaccination show that ELISA values do not accurately reflect protective immunity.

Technical Details of the Enzyme-Linked Immunosorbent Assay for
Malaria Antibody

i. Antigen Preparation. Take *P. falciparum*-infected blood in heparin from
an *Aotus* monkey when the parasitemia is over 20%. If necessary, culture 18–24
hours until the parasites reach the schizont stage. Wash the infected erythroctyes
in PBS. Centrifuge at 3000 rpm for 10 minutes and discard the supernatant.
Repeat the washing and centrifuging. Store the pellet at −70°C.

Make up the pellet in a minimal quantity of PBS. Sonicate 20 seconds at 4°C.
Centrifuge at 10,000 rpm for 30 minutes and discard the residue. The supernatant
is the stock antigen. Store at −70°C in small aliquots. Test dilutions of antigen
against positive–negative reference sera to determine the optimum coating dilution.

ii. The Test

1. 200 µl of soluble malarial antigen in coating buffer is added to each well of
a polystyrene microplate. The plate is covered and left overnight at 4°C. The
plates are then washed in PBS–Tween three times, each washing being of 3
minutes duration; the plates are then shaken dry.

2. 200 µl of test plasma or serum diluted 1/200 in PBS–Tween is added and
incubated for 2 hours at room temperature. The plates are washed again.

3. 200 µl of diluted enzyme (usually alkaline phosphatase or peroxidase)-
labeled anti-human immunoglobulin is added to each well, and the plates incubated 3 hours at room temperature. The plates are then washed.

4. 200 µl of the enzyme substrate [*p*-nitrophenyl phosphate (PNP) for alkaline phosphatase or *o*-phenylenediamine (OPD) for peroxidase] is added to
each well of the plate, and 30 minutes later the enzyme reaction is stopped by the
addition of 50 µl strong alkali or acid, depending on the substrate used.

The results are read visually, colored wells being positive. Samples can be
removed from the wells, and the absorbance can be read spectrophotometrically
at the wavelength giving maximum absorbance for the particular substrate used
(405 nm for PNP and 492 nm for OPD). Positive readings are those significantly
higher than those given by sera from uninfected individuals.

iii. Materials

Carrier surface: disposable polystyrene microhemagglutination plates (Dynatech
    M29 AR MicroELISA plates)
Coating buffer: carbonate–bicarbonate (pH 9.6): 1.59 g of Na_2CO_3, 2.93 g of
    NaHCO, and 0.2 g of NaN_3 made up to 1 liter with distilled water. Store at
    4°C for not more than 2 weeks.

PBS–Tween: consisting of 8.0 g of NaCl, 0.2 g of KH_2PO_4, 2.9 g of $Na_2HOP_4 \cdot 12H_2O$, 0.2 g of KCl, 0.5 ml of Tween 20, and 0.2 g of NaN_3 in 1 liter of distilled water, pH 7.4. Store at 4°C.

Conjugates (a) Alkaline phosphatase-labeled sheep anti-human IgG. Store in concentrated form at 4°C with NaN_3 as preservative. Dilute stock solution in PBS–Tween immediately before use. (b) Horse radish peroxidase-labeled sheep anti-human IgG. Store in a lyophilized state or in solution at −20°C. Make up the amount needed and dilute in PBS–Tween immediately before use.

Substrates (a) For alkaline phosphatase conjugates: Diethanolamine buffer (10%) consisting of 97 ml of diethanolamine, 800 ml of water, 0.2 g of NaN_3, 100 mg of $MgCl_2 \cdot 6H_2O$; 1 M HCl is added until the pH is 9.8. The total volume is made up to 1 liter with water. Store at 4°C in the dark. Remove a sufficient amount 1–2 hours before the substrate solution is to be used and allow to warm to room temperature. The substrate solution is PNP (1 mg/ml). Tablets (5 mg) are stored at −20°C in the dark until used. Immediately before use, one (5 mg) tablet is dissolved in each 5 ml of 10% diethanolamine buffer which has been warmed to room temperature. It must be used the same day. The reaction-stopping solution is 3 M NaOH. (b) For peroxidase conjugates: Phosphate citrate buffer (pH 5.0) consisting of 24.3 ml of 0.1 M citric acid (19.2 g/1000 ml), 25.7 ml of 0.2 M phosphate (28.4 g Na_2HPO_4/1000 ml), and 50 ml of H_2O. The Substrate solution is OPD made up freshly *immediately* before use. Dissolve 40 mg OPD in 100 ml of the above buffer and add 0.15 ml of 30% H_2O_2. This substrate is light-sensitive and must be used at once. The reaction-stopping solution is 2 M H_2SO_4.

8. Radioimmunoassay

Rather surprisingly, radioimmunoassay has not been used extensively even in malaria research. The little work which has been done is based on indirect methods analogous to the ELISA or the IFA test but with ^{125}I as the label on the antiglobulin indicator.

Stutz *et al.* (1974) fixed soluble *P. falciparum* antigen on sheep erythrocytes. These were reacted with test sera thought to contain malarial antibody, and after washing a ^{125}I-labeled anti-human globulin solution was added. This reacted with the malarial antibody fixed to the antigen-coated erythrocytes which could be centrifuged down, and their radioactivity could be measured in a gamma counter.

Voller *et al.* (1977) described a more convenient isotopic assay carried out in microplates in the same way as the ELISA, except that an ^{125}I-conjugated antiglobulin was used as the indicator reagent.

These isotopic assays were very sensitive and yielded results comparable with the ELISA. However, the short shelf life of ^{125}I and the necessity for complex equipment may restrict their wider application.

Houba *et al.* (1976) also used an isotopic assay to measure the amount of malarial antibody in immune complexes. They labeled specific antimalarial antibody with ^{125}I and then injected it into subjects with the nephrotic syndrome. The uptake of the labeled material into immune complexes gave an indication of the important role of malarial antibody and antigen, especially that due to *P. malariae*. This, however, is not a technique for the general assessment of malarial antibody.

9. Summary

There is a wide range of tests available for measurement of the immune response in malaria. Some of these are suitable for experimental laboratory work, whereas others are more applicable to fieldwork. These tools have enabled us to obtain a better understanding of the complexity of the humoral response to malarial infection, and they have also been of practical use in supplementing parasitological examinations in the field. It can be anticipated that, should a successful vaccine be developed, there will be a new role for serology in assessing the immune response to such vaccines and there will be an urgent need for a rapid and simple method for measuring the protective immune response in malaria.

REFERENCES

Abele, D. C., Tobie, J. E., Hill, G. J., Contacos, P. G., and Evans, C. B. (1965). Alterations in serum proteins and 17S antibody production during induced malarial infections in man. *Am. J. Trop. Med. Hyg.* **14**, 191–197.

Adeniyi-Jones, C. (1967). Agglutination of tanned sheep erythrocytes by serum from Nigerian adults and children. *Lancet* **1**, 188–190.

Allison, A. C., Houba, V., Hendrickse, R. G., de Petris, S., Edington, G. M., and Adeniyi, A. (1969). Immune complexes in the nephrotic syndrome of African children. *Lancet* **1**, 1232–1237.

Ambroise-Thomas, P., Kien Truong, T., and Saliou, P. (1971). Evolution des anticorps fluorescents au cours du paludisme expérimental des singes. *Bull. W.H.O.* **44**, 719–728.

Ambroise-Thomas, P., Quilici, M., and Ranque, P. (1972). Réapparition du paludisme en corse. *Bull. Soc. Pathol. Exot.* **65**, 533–542.

Ambroise-Thomas, P., Wernsdorfer, W., Grab, B., Bertagna, P., and Cullen, J. (1976). Longitudinal sero-epidemiological studies on malaria in Tunisia. *Bull. W.H.O.* **54**, 355–367.

Bawden, M. P., Palmer, T. J., Beaudoin, R. L., and Leef, M. G. (1978). Development of a serologic test specific for malaria sporozoites. *Bull. Wld. Hlth. Org.* **57**, Suppl. 1, 205–209.

Beaudoin, R. L., Strome, C. P. A., Mitchell, F., and Tubergen, T. A. (1977). *Plasmodium berghei* immunization of mice against the ANKA strain using the unaltered sporozoite as an antigen. *Exp. Parasitol.* **42**, 1–5.

Bidwell, D. E., Voller, A., Meuwissen, J. H. E., and Leeuwenberg, A. (1973). Comparison of IHA and IFA for malarial antibody in *Aotus monkeys infected with P. falciparum*. *Bull. W.H.O.* **49**, 313–316.

Bjerrum, O. J., and Bøg Hansen, T. (1976). The immunochemical approach to the characterization of membrane proteins. *Biochim. Biophys. Acta* **455**, 66–69.

Boonpucknavig, S., Boonpucknavig, V., and Bhamapravati, N. (1972). Immunological studies on *P. berghei* infected mice: Immune complex nephritis. *Arch. Pathol.* **94**, 322–330.

Brown, I. N., Brown, K. N., and Hills, L. A. (1968). Immunity to malaria: The antibody response to antigenic variation by *Plasmodium knowlesi* malaria. *Immunology* **14**, 127–138.

Brown, K. N., and Brown, I. N. (1965). Antigenic variation in chronic infections of *Plasmodium knowlesi. Nature (London)* **208**, 1286–1288.

Brown, K. N., Brown, I. N., and Hills, L. A. (1970a). Protection against *P. knowlesi* shown by monkeys sensitized with drug suppressed infections or by dead parasites in Freund's adjuvant. *Exp. Parasitol.* **28**, 304–317.

Brown, K. N., Brown, I. N., Trigg, P., Phillips, R. S.,and Hills, L. A. (1970b). Serological response of monkeys sensitized by drug suppressed infections or by dead parasitized cells in Freund's complete adjuvant. *Exp. Parasitol.* **28**, 318–338.

Bruce-Chwatt, L. J. (1974). Transfusion malaria. *Bull. W.H.O.* **50**, 337–346.

Bruce-Chwatt, L. J., and Draper, C. C. (1973). Sero-epidemiological evidence of eradication of malaria from Mauritius. *Lancet* **2**, 547–551.

Bruce-Chwatt, L. J., Draper, C. C., Dodge, J. S., Topley, E., and Voller, A. (1972). Sero-epidemiological studies on populations previously exposed to malaria. *Lancet* **1**, 512–515.

Bruce-Chwatt, L. J., Draper, C. C., Avramidis, D., and Kazandzoglou, C. (1975). Sero-epidemiological surveillance of disappearing malaria in Greece. *J. Trop. Med. Hyg.* **78**, 194–200.

Butcher, G. A., and Cohen, S. (1971). Short term culture of *Plasmodium knowlesi. Parasitology* **62**, 309–320.

Butcher, G. A., Mitchell, G. H., and Cohen, S. (1978). Antibody mediated mechanisms of immunity to malaria induced by vaccination with *P. knowlesi* merozoites. *Immunology* **34**, 77–86.

Clyde, D. F., McCarthy, V. C., Miller, R. M., and Woodward, W. E. (1975). Immunization of man against falciparum and vivax malria by use of attenuati sporozoites. *Am. J. Trop. Med. Hyg.* **24**, 397–401.

Cochrane, A. H., Aikawa, M., and Nussenzweig, R. S. (1976). Antibody induced ultrastructural changes of malaria sporozoites. *J. Immunol.* **116**, 859–867.

Coggeshall, L. T. (1943). Immunity in malaria. *Medicine (Baltimore)* **22**, 87–98.

Coggeshall, L. T., and Eaton, M. D. (1938a). The complement fixation reaction in monkey malaria. *J. Exp. Med.* **67**, 871–883.

Coggeshall, L. T., and Eaton, M. D. (1938b). The quantitative relationship between immune serum and infective dose of parasites as demonstrated by a protection test in monkey malaria. *J. Exp. Med.* **68**, 29–41.

Coggeshall, L. T., and Kumm, H. W. (1937). Demonstration of passive immunity in experimental monkey malaria. *J. Exp. Med.* **66**, 177–190.

Cohen, S., and Butcher, G. A. (1970). Properties of protective malarial antibody. *Immunology* **19**, 369–383.

Cohen, S., and McGregor, I. A. (1963). Gamma globulin and acquired immunity to malaria. *In* "Immunity to Protozoa" (P. C. C. Garnham, *et al.,* eds.), p. 123–159. Blackwell, Oxford.

Cohen, S., McGregor, I. A., and Carrington, S. P. (1961). Gamma globulin and acquired immunity to human malaria. *Nature (London)* **192**, 733–737.

Cohen, S., Butcher, G. A., and Crandall, R. B. (1969). Action of malarial antibody *in vitro. Nature (London)* **223**, 368–371.

Cohen, S., Butcher, G. A., and Mitchell, G. H. (1972). *In vitro* studies of malarial antibody. *Helminth. Soc. Washington* **39**, 231–237.

Collins, W. E., Jeffery, G. M., and Skinner, J. C. (1964a). Development of antibodies to *P. malariae*. *Am. J. Trop. Med. Hyg.* **13**, 1–5.

Collins, W. E., Jeffery, G. M., and Skinner, J. C. (1964b). Development and persistence of antibodies to *P. falciparum*. *Am. J. Trop. Med. Hyg.* **13**, 256–260.

Collins, W. E., Jeffery, G. M., and Skinner, J. C. (1964c). Development of antibodies to *P. falciparum* in semi-immune patients. *Am. J. Trop. Med. Hyg.* **13**, 777–782.

Collins, W. E., Jeffery, G. M., Guinn, E., and Skinner, J. C. (1966a). Fluorescent antibody studies. IV. Cross reactions between human and simian malaria. *Am. J. Trop. Med. Hyg.* **15**, 11–15.

Collins, W. E., Skinner, J. C., and Guinn, E. G. (1966b). Antigenic variations in the plasmodia of lower primates as detected by immunofluorescence. *Am. J. Trop. Med. Hyg.* **15**, 483–485.

Collins, W. E., Contacos, P. G., Skinner, J. C., Chin, W., and Guinn, E. (1967a). Development of antibodies to *P. knowlesi*. *Am. J. Trop. Med. Hyg.* **16**, 1–6.

Collins, W. E., Skinner, J. C., and Coiffman, R. E. (1967b). Fluorescent antibody studies on human malaria. V. Response of Nigerians to five *Plasmodium* antigens. *Am. J. Trop. Med. Hyg.* **16**, 568–571.

Collins, W. E., Skinner, J. C., and Jeffery, G. M. (1968a). Studies on the persistence of malarial antibody response. *Am. J. Epidemiol.* **87**, 592–598.

Collins, W. E., Warren, McW., Skinner, J. C., and Fredericks, H. J. (1968b). Studies on the relationship between fluorescent antibody response and ecology of malaria in Malaysia. *Bull. W.H.O.* **39**, 451–463.

Collins, W. E., Contacos, P. G., Skinner, J. C., Harrison, A. J., and Gell, L. S. (1971a). Patterns of antibody and serum components in experimentally induced human malaria. *Trans. R. Soc. Trop. Med. Hyg.* **65**, 43–58.

Collins, W. E., Warren, McW., and Skinner, J. C. (1971b). Serological survey of Ethiopian highlands. *Am. J. Trop. Med. Hyg.* **20**, 199–205.

Coudert, J., Garin, J. P., and Ambroise-Thomas, P. (1966). Perspective nouvelles sur l'immunologie paludréenne. *Bull. Soc. Pathol. Exot.* **59**, 558–565.

Cox, F. E. G., and Turner, S. A. (1970a). Antigenic relationships between malaria parasites and piroplasms of mice. *Bull. W. H. O.* **43**, 337–340.

Cox, F. E. G., and Turner, S. A. (1970b). Antibody levels in mice infected with *P. berghei yoelii*. *Ann. Trop. Med. Parasitol.* **64**, 175–180.

Cox, F. E. G., Crandall, C. A., and Turner, S. A. (1969). Antibody levels detected by the fluorescent antibody technique in mice infected with *P. vinckei* and *P. chabaudi*. *Bull. W. H. O.* **41**, 251–260.

D'Antonio, L. E., von Doenhoff, A. E., and Fife, E. H. (1966). Serological evaluation of the specificity and sensitivity of purified malaria antigens made by a new method. *Mil. Med.* **131**, Suppl., 1152–1166.

Deans, J. A., Dennis, E. D., and Cohen, S. (1978). Antigenic analysis of sequential erythrocytic states of *Plasmodium knowlesi*. *Parasitol.* **77**, 333–344.

Desowitz, R. S., and Stein, B. (1962). A tanned red cell haemagglutination test using *P. berghei* and homologous antisera. *Trans. R. Soc. Trop. Med. Hyg.* **56**, 257–262.

Diggs, C. L. (1966). Immunodiffusion studies of *P. berghei*. Interactions of an extract of the erythrocytic flow with rabbit antisera. *Exp. Parasitol.* **19**, 237–243.

Diggs, C. L., and Sadun, E. H. (1965). Serological cross-reactivity between *Plasmodium vivax* and *P. falciparum* as determined by a modified fluorescent antibody tests. *Exp. Parasitol.* **16**, 217–233.

Dranga, A., Marinov, R., and Miha, M. (1969). Contribution á l'etude de l'immunité residuelle au paludisme en Roumanie. *Bull. W. H. O.* **40**, 753–761.

Draper, C. C., and Voller, A. (1972). The epidemiological interpretation of serologic data in malaria. *Am. J. Trop. Med. Hyg.* **21**, 696–703.

Eaton, M. D. (1938). The agglutination of *Plasmodium knowlesi* by immune serum. *J. Exp. Med.* **67**, 857–861.

Edozien, J. C., Gilles, H. M., and Udeozo, I. O. K. (1962). Adult and cord blood gamma globulin and immunity to malaria in Nigerians. *Lancet* **2**, 951–952.

Edrissian, G. H., and Afshar, A. (1974). Serological and parasitological observations on malaria in southern Iran. *Iran. J. Public Health* **3**, 27–39.

Ehrich, J. H., and Voller, A. (1972). Studies on kidneys of mice with rodent malaria. I. Deposition of gamma globulins in early disease. *Z. Trop. Med. Parasitol.* **23**, 147–152.

El-Nahal, H. M. S. (1967). Fluorescent antibody technique applied to the study of serological cross-reactions of exo-erythrocytic schizonts of avian rodent and simian malaria. *Bull. W.H.O.* **37**, 154–160.

Fasan, P. O., Sulzer, A. J., Lobel, H., and Kagan, I. G. (1976). IFA and HA antibodies to malaria in Nigerian students resident in Washington D.C., U.S.A. *Afr. J. Med. Sci.* **5**, 149–153.

Fisher, G. U., and Schultz, M. G. (1969). Unusual host parasite relationships in blood donors responsible for transfusion induced falciparum malaria. *Lancet* **2**, 716–718.

Foley, D. A., and Vanderberg, J. P. (1977). *Plasmodium berghei:* Transmission by intraperitoneal inoculation of immature exo-erythrocytic schizonts from rats into rats, mice and hamsters. *Exp. Parasitol.* **43**, 69–81.

Garin, J. P., Rey, M., and Ambroise-Thomas, P. (1966). Cross serological reactions between *P. falciparum* and *P. c. bastianellii*. *Bull. Soc. Pathol. Exot.* **59**, 316–325.

Golenser, J., Heeren, J., Verhave, J. P., Van der Kaay, H. J., and Meuwissen, J. H. E. (1977). Cross-reactivity with sporozoites, exo-erythrocytic forms and blood schizonts of *Plasmodium berghei* in indirect fluorescent antibody tests with sera of rats immunized with sporozoites or infected blood. *Clin. Exp. Immunol.* **29**, 43–51.

Golenser, J., Verhave, J. P., de Valk, J., Heeren, J., and Meeuwissen, J. H. E. (1978). Studies on the role of antibodies against sporozoites in *Plasmodium berghei* malaria. *Science* **14**, 606–610.

Greenwood, B. M., Herrick, E. M., and Holborrow, E. J. (1970). Speckled ANF in African sera. *Clin. Exp. Immunol.* **7**, 75–83.

Greenwood, B. M., Muller, A. S., and Valkenburg, F. (1971). Rheumatoid factor in Nigerian sera. *Clin. Exp. Immunol.* **9**, 161–173.

Hansen, T. (1980). In preparation.

Houba, V., and Allison, A. C. (1966). M-Antiglobulin factors (RF) and other gamma globulins in tropical parasitic infections. *Lancet* **1**, 848–849.

Houba, V., Allison, A. C., Adeniyi, A., and Houba, J. E. (1971). Immunoglobulin classes and complement in biopsies of Nigerian children with nephrotic syndrome. *Clin. Exp. Immunol.* **8**, 761–774.

Houba, V., Lambert, P. H., Voller, A., and Soyanno, M. A. O. (1976). Clinical and experimental investigations of immune complexes in Malaria. *Clin. Immunol. Immunopathol.* **6**, 1–12.

Ingram, R. L., and Carver, R. K. (1963). Malaria parasites: Fluorescent antibody technique for tissue study. *Science* **139**, 405–406.

Ingram, R. L., Otken, L. B., and Jumper, J. R. (1961). Staining of malaria parasites by FA technique. *Proc. Soc. Exp. Biol. Med.* **106**, 52.

Jandl, J. H., Files, N. M., Barnett, S. B., and MacDonald, R. (1965). Proliferative response of the spleen and liver to haemolysis. *J. Exp. Med.* **122**, 299–303.

Kagan, I. G. (1972). Evaluation of indirect haemagglutination test as an epidemiologic technique for malaria. *Am. J. Trop. Med. Hyg.* **21**, 683–689.

Kano, K., McGregor, I. A., and Milgram, F. (1968). Haemagglutinins in sera of Africans in Gambia. *Proc. Soc. Exp. Biol. Med.* **129**, 849–853.

Kielmann, A., Weiss, N., and Savasin, G. (1970). *P. gallinaceum* as antigen in human malaria. *Bull. W.H.O.* **43**, 617–622.

Klein, F., Mattern, P., and Meuwissen, J. H. E. (1971). Experimental anti-γ globulin in infectious disease. *In* "Human Anti-γ Globulins" (J. B. Grubb, ed.), p. 63. Pergamon, Oxford.

Kligler, I. J., and Yoeliz, M. (1941). The diagnostic and epidemiological significance of the complement fixation test in human malaria. *Am. J. Trop. Med.* **21**, 531–540.

Kreier, J. P., and Dilley, D. A. (1969). *Plasmodium berghei:* Nucleic acid agglutinating antibodies in rats. *Exp. Parasitol.* **26**, 175–180.

Kreier, J. P., Shapiro, H., Dilley, D., Szilvassy, I. P., and Ristic, M. (1966). Autoimmune reactions in rats with *P. berghei* infections. *Exp. Parasitol.* **19**, 155–162.

Krotoski, W. A., Jumper, J. R., and Collins, W. E. (1973a). Immunofluorescent staining of E.E. schizonts of simian plasmodia in fixed tissue. *Am. J. Trop. Med. Hyg.* **22**, 159–162.

Krotoski, W. A., Collins, W. E., and Jumper, J. R. (1973b). Detection of early E.E. schizonts of *P. cynomolgi* by immunofluorescence. *Am. J. Trop. Med. Hyg.* **22**, 443–451.

Kuvin, S. F., and Voller, A. (1963). Malarial antibody titres of West Africans in Britain. *Br. Med. J.* **2**, 477–479.

Kuvin, S. F., Tobie, J. E., Evans, C. B., Coatney, G. R., and Contacos, P. G. (1962). Fluorescent antibody studies on course of antibody production in volunteers infected with human and simian malaria. *Am. J. Trop. Med. Hyg.* **11**, 429–435.

Lelijveld, J. L. M. (1971). Sero-epidemiological studies on malaria in Tanzania. Doctoral Thesis, p. 1. University of Nijmegen.

Luby, J. P., Collins, W. E., and Kaiser, R. (1967). Persistence of malarial antibody! Findings in patients infected during an outbreak of malaria in California. *Am. J. Trop. Med. Hyg.* **16**, 255–257.

Ludford, C. G., Hall, W. T. K., Sulzer, A. J., and Wilson, M. (1972). *Babesia argentina, P. vivax* and *P. falciparum* antigenic cross-reactions. *Exp. Parasitol.* **32**, 317–326.

Lunn, J. S., Chin, W., Contacos, P. F., and Coatney, G. R. (1966). Changes in antibody tests during prolonged infections with vivax or falciparum malaria. *Am. J. Trop. Med. Hyg.* **15**, 3–12.

Lupascu, G., Bossie, A., Bona, C., Ionid, L., Smolinski, M., Negulici, E., and Florescu, C. (1969). Fluorescent antibody technique in estimation of immunity in patients with *P. malariae* infections. *Trans. R. Soc. Trop. Med. Hyg.* **60**, 201–207.

Lupascu, G., Bossie, A., Bona, C., Ionid, L., Smolinski, M., Ngulici, E., and Florescu, C. (1969). The development of the serological response to *P. malariae* infections. *Bull. W.H.O.* **40**, 312–319.

McCarthy, V. C., and Clyde, D. F. (1977). *Plasmodium vivax:* Correlation of circumsporozoite precipitation (CSP) reaction with sporozoite-induced protective immunity in man. *Exp. Parasitol.* **41**, 167–172.

McConnell, E. (1978). The effect of single bites of *Anopheles stephensi* mosquitoes infected with *Plasmodium berghei* on the level of sporozoite-specific IFAT antibody in white mice previously immunized with irradiated sporozoites. *Proc. Int. Congr. Parasitol., 4th, 1978* Sect. E, p. 111.

McGregor, I. A., and Wilson, R. J. M. (1971). Precipitating antibodies and immunoglobulins in *P. falciparum* infections in the Gambia. *Trans. R. Soc. Trop. Med. Hyg.* **65**, 136–145.

McGregor, I. A., Williams, K. Voller, A., and Billewicz, W. Z. (1965). Immunofluorescence and the measurement of immune response to hyperendemic malaria. *Trans. R. Soc. Trop. Med. Hyg.* **59**, 395–414.

McGregor, I. A., Hall, P. J., Williams, K., Hardy, C. L. S., and Truner, M. W. (1966). Demonstration of circulating antibodies to *Plasmodium falciparum* by gel-diffusion techniques. *Nature (London)* **210**, 1384–1386.

Mack, S. R., Vanderberg, J. P., and Nawrot, R. (1978). Colum separation of *Plasmodium berghei* sporozoites. *J. Parasitol.* **64**, 166–168.

Mahoney, D. E., Redington, B. C., and Schoenbechler, M. J. (1966). The preparation and serologic activity of plasmodial fractions. *Mil. Med.* **131**, 1141–1151.

Manawadu, B. R., and Voller, A. (1971). The use of a fibre optic system in malarial IFA tests. *Trans. R. Soc. Trop. Med. Hyg.* **65,** 693.

Manawadu, B. R., and Voller, A. (1978a). Standardization of IFA for malaria. *Trans. R. Soc. Trop. Med. Hyg.* **72,** 456-462.

Manwadu B. R., and Voller, A. (1978b). Detection and measurement of species-specific malarial antibodies. *Trans. R. Soc. Trop. Med. Hyg.* **72,** 463-466.

Mathews, H. M., Fried, J. A., and Kagan, I. G. (1975). The indirect haemagglutination test for malaria. *Am. J. Trop. Med. Hyg.* **24,** 417-422.

Meuwissen, J. H. E. (1966). Antibodies in human malaria especially in *P. ovale. Trop. Geogr. Med.* **18,** 250-259.

Meuwissen, J. H. E. (1968). Antibody response in patients with natural malaria to human and simian plasmodium antigens measured by fluorescent antibody test. *Trop. Geogr. Med.* **20,** 137-140.

Meuwissen, J. H. E. (1974). The indirect haemagglutination test for malaria and its application to epidemiological surveillance. *Bull. W.H.O.* **50,** 277-286.

Meuwissen, J. H. E., and Leeuwenberg, A. D. E. M. (1972). Indirect haemagglutination test for malaria with lyophilized cells. *Trans. R. Soc. Trop. Med. Hyg.* **66,** 666-667.

Meuwissen, J. H. E., Leeuwenberg, A. D. E. M., Voller, A., and Matola, Y. (1974). Specificity of the indirect haemagglutination test with *Plasmodium falciparum* test cells. Comparison of indirect haemagglutination and fluorescent antibody tests on African sera. *Bull. W.H.O.* **50,** 513-519.

Meuwissen, J. H. E., Golenser, J., and Verhave, J. P. (1978). Development of effective anti-sporozoite immunity by natural bites of *Plasmodium berghei* infected mosquitoes in rats under prophylactic treatment with various drug regimens. *Isr. J. Med. Sci.* **14,** 601-605.

Moser, G., Brohn, F. H., Danforth, H. D., and Nussenzweig, R. S. (1978). Sporozoites of rodent and simian malaria purified by anion exchange retain their immunogenicity and infectivity. *J. Protozool.* **25,** 119-124.

Mulligan, H. W., Russell, P. F., and Mohan, B. N. (1940). Specific agglutination of sporozoites. *J. Malar. Inst. India* **3,** 513-521.

Najem, G. R., and Sulzer, A. J. (1976). Transfusion induced malaria from an asymptomatic carrier. *Transfusion* **16,** 473-476.

Nardin, E. H., and Nussenzweig, R. S. (1978). Stage-specific antigens on the surface membrane of sporozoites of malaria parasites. *Nature (London)* **274,** 55-57.

Nussenzweig, R. S. (1977). Immunoprophylaxis of malaria: Sporozoite-induced immunity. *In* "Immunity to Blood Parasites of Animals and Man" (L. H. Miller, J. A. Pino, and J. J. McKelvey, Jr., eds.), p. 75-87. Plenum, New York.

Nussenzweig, R. S., and Chen, D. (1974). The antibody response to sporozoites of simian and human malaria parasites: Its stage and species specificity and strain cross-reactivity. *Bull. W.H.O.* **50,** 293-297.

Nussenzweig, R. S., Vanderberg, J. P., and Most, H. (1969). Protective immunity produced by the injection of X-irradiated sporozoites of *Plasmodium berghei.* IV. Dose response, specificity and humoral immunity. *Mil. Med.* **134,** 1176-1182.

Nussenzweig, R. S., Vanderberg, J., Sanabria, Y., and Most, H. (1972a). *Plasmodium berghei:* Accelerated clearance of sporozoites from blood as part of immune-mechanism in mice. *Exp. Parasitol.* **31,** 88-97.

Nussenzweig, R., Vanderberg, J., Spitalny, G. L., Rivera, C. I. O., Orton, C., and Most, B. (1972b). Sporozoite-induced immunity in mammalian malaria: A review. *Am. J. Trop. Med. Hyg.* **21,** 722-728.

Nussenzweig, R. S., Montuori, W., Spitalny, G. L., and Chen, D. (1973). Antibodies against sporozoites of human and simian malaria produced in rats. *J. Immunol.* **110,** 600-601.

Pearson, H. A., Johnson, D., Smith, K. A., and Touloukian, R. J. (1978). The born-again spleen: Return of splenic function after splenectomy for trauma. *N. Engl. J. Med.* **298,** 1389-1392.

Phillips, R. S., Trigg, P. I., Scott-Finnigan, T. J., and Bartholomew, R. K. (1972). Culture of *P. falciparum in vitro:* Subculture technique for demonstrating anti-plasmodial activity in serum from some Gambians resident in a malarious area. *Parasitology* **65**, 525–535.

Richard, W. H. G. (1966). Active immunization of chicks against *Plasmodium gallinaceum* by inactivated homologous sporozoites and erythrocytic parasites. *Nature (London)* **212**, 1492–1494.

Rosenberg, E. B., Strickland, G. T., Yang, S. L., and Whalen, G. E. (1973). IgM antibodies to red cells and autoimmune anaemia in patients with malaria. *Am. J. Trop. Med. Hyg.* **22**, 146–152.

Sadun, E. H., and Gore, R. W. (1968). Mass diagnostic test using *P. falciparum* and chimpanzee erythrocyte lysate. *Exp. Parasitol.* **23**, 277–285.

Sadun, E. H., Hickman, R. L., Wellde, B. T., Moon, A. T., and Udcozo, I. O. K. (1966). Active and passive immunization of chimpanzees infected with West African and S.E. Asian strains of *P. falciparum. Mil. Med.* **131**, Suppl., 1250–1262.

Schindler, R., and Voller, A. (1967). A comparison of CFT and IFA methods in a longitudinal study of simian malaria infections. *Bull. Wld. Hlth. Org.* **37**, 669–674.

Schmidt-Ullrich, R., and Wallach, D. F. H. (1978). *P. knowlesi* induced antigens in plasma membranes of parasitized rhesus monkey erythrocytes. *Proc. Natl. Acad. Sci.* **75**, 4949–4943.

Seitz, H. M. (1975). Counter-current immunoelectrophoresis for demonstration of malarial antibodies and antigens in the sera of rats and mice. *Trans. R. Soc. Trop. Med. Hyg.* **69**, 88–90.

Smith, A. R., Lykins, J. D., Voss, E. W., and Ristic, M. (1969). Identification of an antigen and specific antibody in the sera of chickens infected with *P. gallinaceum. J. Immunol.* **103**, 6–14.

Sodeman, W. A., and Jeffery, G. M. (1964). Immunofluorescent staining of sporozoites of *Plasmodium gallinaceum. J. Parasitol.* **50**, 477–478.

Spitalny, G. L., and Nussenzweig, R. S. (1972). Effect of various routes of immunization and methods of parasite attenuation on the development of protection against sporozoite-induced rodent malaria. *Proc. Helminthol. Soc. Wash.* **39**, 506–514.

Spitalny, G. L., and Nussenzweig, R. S. (1973). *Plasmodium berghei:* Relationship between protective immunity and anti-sporozoite (CSP) antibody in mice. *Exp. Parasitol.* **33**, 168–178.

Spitalny, G. L., and Nussenzweig, R. S. (1976). *Plasmodium berghei:* The spleen in sporozoite induced immunity to mouse malaria. *Exp. Parasitol.* **40**, 179–184.

Spitalny, G. L., Verhave, J. P., Meuwissen, J. H. E., and Nussenzweig, R. S. (1977). *Plasmodium berghei:* T cell dependence of sporozoite-induced immunity in rodents. *Exp. Parasitol.* **42**, 73–81.

Stein, B., and Desowitz, R. S. (1964). The measurement of antibody in human malaria by a formalized tanned sheep cell haemagglutination test. *Bull. W.H.O.* **30**, 45–49.

Stratman-Thomas, W. K., and Dulaney, A. D. (1940). Complement fixation in human malaria. *J. Immunol.* **39**, 257–265.

Stutz, D. R., McAlister, R. O., and Diggs, C. L. (1974). Estimation of anti-malaria antibody by radioimmunoassay. *J. Parasitol.* **60**, 539–542.

Sulzer, A. J., and Latorre, C. R. (1977). A simplified method for *in vitro* production of schizonts of primate malarias as antigen for serological tests. *Trans. R. Soc. Trop. Med. Hyg.* **71**, 553.

Sulzer, A. J., Wilson, M., and Hall, C. (1969). An evaluation of a thick smear antigen in the IFA test for malarial antibodies. *Am. J. Trop. Med. Hyg.* **18**, 199–205.

Sulzer, A. J., Wilson, M., Turner, A., and Kagan, I. G. (1973). A multi-species malaria antigen for use in IFA. *Trans. R. Soc. Trop. Med. Hyg.* **67**, 55–58.

Sulzer, A. J., Sulzer, K. R., Cantella, R. A., Colichon, H., Latorre, C. R., and Welch, M. (1978). Study of coinciding foci of malaria and leptospirosis in the Peruvian Amazon area. *Trans. R. Soc. Trop. Med. Hyg.* **72**, 76–83.

Suzuki, M. (1974). *P. berghei:* Experimental model for malarial renal immunopathology. *Exp. Parsitol.* **35**, 187–195.

Targett, G. A. T. (1970). Antibody response to *P. falciparum* malaria: Comparison of immunoglobulin concentration, antibody titres and antigenicity of different asexual stages of the parasite. *Clin. Exp. Immunol.* **7**, 501–517.

Tobie, J. E., and Coatney, G. R. (1961). Fluorescent antibody staining of human malaria parasites. *Exp. Parasitol.* **11**, 128–132.

Tobie, J. E., Abele, D. C., Hill, G. J., Contacos, P. G., and Evans, C. B. (1966). Fluorescent antibody studies on immune response in sporozoite and blood induced vivax malaria. *Am. J. Trop. Med. Hyg.* **15**, 676–683.

Trager, W., and Jensen, J. R. (1976). Human malaria parasites in continuous culture. *Science* **193**, 673–675.

Turner, M. W., and McGregor, I. A. (1969a). Studies on the immunology of malaria. I. Preliminary characterization of antigens of *P. falciparum. Clin. Exp. Immunol.* **5**, 1–16.

Turner, M. W., and McGregor, I. A. (1969b). Studies on the immunology of malaria. II. Characterization of antibodies to *P. falciparum. Clin. Exp. Immunol.* **5**, 17–27.

Vanderberg, J. P. (1973). Inactivity of rodent malaria anti-sporozoite antibodies against exoerythrocytic forms. *Am. J. Trop. Med. Hyg.* **22**, 573–577.

Vanderberg, J., Nussenzweig, R. S., and Most, H. (1969). Protective immunity produced by the injection of X-irradiated sporozoites of *Plasmodium berghei*. V. *In vitro* effects of immune serum on sporozoites. *Mil. Med.* **134**, 1183–1190.

Van der Kaay, J. H. (1975). Malaria in Surinam. A sero-epidemiological study. Doctoral Thesis, University of Leiden.

Verhave, J. P. (1975). Immunization of sporozoites. An experimental study of *Plasmodium berghei* malaria. Ph.D. Thesis, Catholic University Nijmegen, The Netherlands.

Verhave, J. P., Meuwissen, J. H. E., and Golenser, J. (1978). Cell-mediated reaction and protection after immunization with sporozoites. *Isr. J. Med. Sci.* **14**, 611–616.

Verhave, J. P. *et al.* (1980). In preparation.

Voller, A. (1962). Fluorescent antibody studies on malaria parasites. *Bull. W.H.O.* **27**, 283–287.

Voller, A. (1965). Immunofluorescence and humoral immunity to *P. berghei. Ann. Soc. Belge Med. Trop.* **45**, 385–396.

Voller, A., and Bray, R. S. (1962). Fluorescent antibody staining as a measure of malaria antibody. *Proc. Soc. Exp. Biol. Med.* **110**, 907–910.

Voller, A., and Bruce-Chwatt, L. J. (1968). Serological malaria surveys in Nigeria. *Bull. W.H.O.* **39**, 883–897.

Voller, A., and O'Neill, P. (1971). Immunofluorescence method suitable for large-scale application to malaria. *Bull. W.H.O.* **45**, 524–529.

Voller, A., and Schindler, R. (1967). An evaluation of CFT and IFA with a simian malarial antigen in a study of malarial antibody levels in a malaria endemic area. *Bull. W.H.O.* **37**, 675–678.

Voller, A., and Taffs, L. F. (1963). Fluorescent antibody staining of exoerythrocytic stages of *Plasmodium gallinaceum. Trans. R. Soc. Trop. Med. Hyg.* **57**, 32–33.

Voller, A., and Wilson, H. (1964). Immunological aspects of a population under prophylaxis against malaria. *Br. Med. J.* **2**, 551–552.

Voller, A., Lelijveld, J. L. M., and Matola, Y. G. (1971). Immunoglobulin and malarial indices at different altitudes in Tanzania. *J. Trop. Med. Hyg.* **74**, 45–52.

Voller, A., O'Neill, P., and Humphrey, D. (1972). ANF and malaria indices in Tanzania. *J. Trop. Med. Hyg.* **75**, 136–139.

Voller, A., Davies, D. R., and Hutt, M. S. R. (1973). Quartan malarial infection in *Aotus* with special reference to renal pathology. *Br. J. Exp. Pathol.* **54**, 457–468.

Voller, A., Bidwell, D. E., Huldt, G., and Engvall, E. (1974). A microplate method of enzyme linked immunosorbent assay and its application to malaria. *Bull. W.H.O.* **51**, 209–210.

Voller, A., Huldt, G., Thors, C., and Engvall, E. (1975). A new serological test for malaria. *Br. Med. J.* **1**, 659–661.

Voller, A., Bartlett, A., and Bidwell, D. E. (1976). Enzyme immunoassays for parasitic diseases. *Trans. R. Soc. Trop. Med. Hyg.* **70**, 98–106.

Voller, A., Bidwell, D. E., Bartlett, A., and Edwards, R. (1977). A comparison of isotopic and enzyme immunoassays for tropical parasitic diseases. *Trans. R. Soc. Trop. Med. Hyg.* **71**, 431–437.

Waki, S., and Suzuki, M. (1974). Development and decline of anti-plasmodial IFA in mice infected with *P. berghei. Bull. W.H.O.* **50**, 521–526.

Ward, P. A., and Conran, P. B. (1968). Application of fluorescent antibody to exo-erythrocytic stages of simian malaria. *J. Parasitol.* **54**, 171–172.

Ward, P. A., and Kibukamusoke, J. W. (1969). Evidence for soluble immune complexes in the pathogenesis of the glomerulonephritis of quartan malaria. *Lancet* **1**, 283–285.

Warren, McW., Collins, W. E., Jeffery, G. M., and Skinner, J. C. (1975). The seroepidemiology of malaria in middle America. *Am. J. Trop. Med. Hyg.* **24**, 749–754.

Wells, J. (1970). Immunological studies in tropical splenomegaly syndrome. *Trans. R. Soc. Trop. Med. Hyg.* **64**, 531–546.

Wilson, M., Sulzer, A. J., and Runcik, K. (1970). Malarial antibody patterns as determined by the IFA test in U.S. servicemen after chemotherapy. *Am. J. Trop. Med. Hyg.* **19**, 401–404.

Wilson, M., Sulzer, A. J., Rogers, W. A., Jr., Fried, J., and Mathews, H. M. (1971). Comparison of the indirect fluorescent antibody and indirect haemagglutination tests for malaria antibody. *Am. J. Trop. Med. Hyg.* **20**, 6–13.

Wilson, R. J. M. (1970). Antigens and antibodies associated with *P. falciparum* infections in West Africa. *Trans. R. Soc. Trop. Med. Hyg.* **64**, 547–554.

Wilson, R. J. M., and Phillips, R. S. (1976). Methods to test inhibitory antibody in human sera to wild populations of *P. falciparum. Nature (London)* **263**, 132–134.

Wilson, R. J. M., and Voller, A. (1970). Malarial "S" antigens from man and owl monkeys infected with *P. falciparum. Parasitology* **61**, 461–464.

Wilson, R. J. M., and Voller, A. (1972). A comparison of malarial antigens from human and *Aotus* monkey blood infected with *P. falciparum. Parasitology* **64**, 191–195.

Wilson, R. J. M., McGregor, I. A., Hall, P. J., Williams, K., and Bartholomew, R. (1969). Antigens associated with *P. falciparum* infections in man. *Lancet* **2**, 201.

Wilson, R. J. M., McGregor, I. A., Williams, K., Hall, P. J., and Bartholomew, R. K. (1976). Precipitating antibody response to malarial "S" antigens. *Trans. R. Soc. Trop. Med. Hyg.* **70**, 308–312.

World Health Organization (1974). Serological testing in malaria. *Bull. W.H.O.* **50**, 527.

Ziegler, J. L. (1973). Cryoglobulinaeria in tropical splenomegaly syndrome. *Clin. Exp. Immunol.* **15**, 65–78.

Zuckerman, A. (1964). Autoimmunization and other types of indirect damage to host cells as factors in some protozoan diseases. *Exp. Parsitol.* **15**, 138–183.

Zuckerman, A., and Spira, D. (1961). Blood loss and replacement in plasmodial infections. *J. Infect. Dis.* **108**, 339–348.

Zuckerman, A., and Spira, D. (1965). Immunoelectrophoretic comparison of plasmodial antigens. *W.H.O. Malar. Doc.* **449**, 65–70.

Zuckerman, A., Goberman, V., Ron, N., Spira, D., Hamburger, J., and Burg, R. (1969). Antiplasmodial precipitins demonstrated by double diffusion in agar gel in the serum of rats infected with *P. berghei. Exp. Parasitol.* **24**, 299–312.

The Vertebrate Host's Immune Response to Plasmodia

Julius P. Kreier and Theodore J. Green

I. INTRODUCTION

The vertebrate immune response may be considered to be a triggered cellular cascade, analogous to the molecular cascades which result in blood clotting and complement activation (Hobart and McConnell, 1978). The function of such cascades in multicellular animals is usually the amplification, direction, and modulation of some primitive function of the organism. From an evolutionary standpoint the most primitive component of the immune system, i.e., that which was developed earliest, is phagocytosis. Phagocytic cells which may be considered analogous to macrophages are present in sponges (Stuart, 1970) and are present in all more advanced animals. In vertebrates, macrophages still perform the functions they perform in sponges. In all animals macrophages monitor the organism, ingesting dead and dying cells and denatured protein molecules, and with varying success they destroy foreign cells. The recognition of senescent erythrocytes at least requires the mediation of serum globulin (Kay, 1975) and is thus under control external to the macrophage. It is possible that in higher animals no recognition of material to be removed is made directly by macrophage membrane receptors without the mediation of appropriate serum proteins (Pearsall and Weiser, 1970). It is certainly true that a few defined receptors such as fc and C' receptors (Mantovani *et al.*, 1972) and receptors for noninducible serum opsonins (Pearsall and Weiser, 1970) serve to mediate macrophage recognition of a wide range of structures. One may assume, however, that at least in modified form the primitive phagocytic function of the phagocytic cells has survived in the vertebrate. Direct receptors for some configurations of denatured protein molecules could, for example, be present in the macrophage membrane.

Modified versions of the phagocytic function of the macrophage are involved in both the initial induction phase of the immune response and in the final effector phase as well. The antigen presentation function of the macrophage (Mosier, 1976) triggers the cascade, and the activities of the activated macrophage represent the amplified effects resulting from the cascade. These effects are not only amplified by the lymphokines responsible for macrophage activation but are also directed, modulated, and amplified by cytophilic and opsonic antibodies. It is probable that natural or noninducible opsonins and complement activated through the alternate pathway contribute to the initial macrophage recognition of the antigen or foreign cell via the fc receptors, while complement activation through the classical pathway is tied into the effector phase of the system through the same receptor.

The consequences of the immunological activation are, on balance, usually helpful to the organism but may often cause harm by, for example, deposition of immune complexes and complement activation in the kidneys, or by other allergic and hypersensitivity reactions which may result in too severe inflammation with consequent vascular and tissue damage (see Volume 2, Chapter 2). To minimize the undesirable consequences of the immunological response the system has built-in homeostatic mechanism that limit the progress of the triggered changes and return the entire system to its resting equilibrium. Recent work on the immune response during malarial infection indicates that even the macrophage, the cell that triggers the cascade, is involved in its modulation (Wyler, 1978), while some of the lymphocytes in the intermediate stages of the cascade are modulators or suppressors as well as amplifiers of the response (Gravely *et al.*, 1976). Macrophage activation, a consequence of the immune response, may in itself, by causing macrophages to ingest and destroy antigen efficiently, reduce the stimulus for further response.

From a slightly different point of view the immunological response may be considered one of the homeostatic mechanisms of vertebrates. A successful consequence of the immunological response would thus be the return of the animal to the state which existed before the antigenic stimulus, except of course for those changes which permit the animal to respond more rapidly to the next exposure to the same antigen.

Like all physiological responses the immune response increases with increasing stimulation only within limits. There is usually a threshold below which the system will not be triggered and, if the stimulus is too great or of too long duration, the system may shut off or even collapse. Even if the stimulus is moderate and the system is working well, there are limits to how far the amplification of the response is permitted to proceed before inhibitory factors are brought into play. The much reported suppression of the immune response to heterologous antigens which occurs in animals with malaria (Terry, 1977) may be a glimpse we have obtained of one phase of the homeostatic control to which the immunological cascade, triggered by the parasite, is subjected. We may even be seeing the failure of the already maximally stimulated or already overloaded or exhausted system to respond to further or different stimulation.

One of the early events in the development of the cells which produce antibody is cellular proliferation. In all multicellular animals cellular proliferation is under rigid control. Appropriate stimuli, such as antigenic stimulation in the case of the immune response, release the inhibition of proliferation but soon inhibition is reestablished. As we know that proliferation of cells of any type cannot continue indefinitely without destroying the organism, the inhibition of further proliferation following continuing antigenic stimulation must become progressively stronger. We observed for example, that the more normal lymphocytes normal rats received, the more susceptible to malaria they became; the reverse was true with immune lymphocytes (Gravely and Kreier, 1976). This observation is best explained by postulating an inhibition of the requisite proliferation step in the immunological cascade by cell population control mechanisms brought into play as a result of overcrowding produced by the transferred cells.

It will be the purpose of this chapter to analyze literature on the vertebrate host's immune response to plasmodial infection from the point of view that the immune response is a homeostatic physiological response that changes constantly as the disease progresses. This point of view implies that the system is not only a dynamic cellular cascade which changes as the disease progresses, but that when the result is death it may change in ways different than when the result is recovery. It also implies that the bits of evidence we have can only be interpreted properly if they are fitted into the proper place in the system.

The volume of literature on the immune response is huge and rapidly growing; that on the immune response to plasmodia is smaller but still large and rapidly growing. Our selection of literature to be cited is therefore arbitrary, resulting partly from chance encounter and partly from deliberate selection to fit the theme presented here.

II. THE IMMUNE RESPONSE AGAINST PLASMODIA

A. Role of Macrophages in the Induction and Regulation of the Immune Response

One of the most important functions performed by macrophages during the induction of an immune response may be the presentation of antigen to antibody-forming cell precursors in a molecular form appropriate for lymphocyte activation (Mosier, 1976). Much of our knowledge of the role of the macrophage in antigen presentation has been derived from *in vitro* studies (Pierce and Knapp, 1976). From these studies it appears that macrophage presentation is required for the initiation of response to most antigens but is more prominent with T cell-dependent antigens than with T cell-independent antigens. In addition to their role in antigen presentation macrophages play a role in immunoregulation (Nelson, 1976). Macrophages are not the seat of specificity of the immune response. This role resides in the lymphocyte population. Antigens of any specificity are processed by the same macrophages and must compete for them. On presentation to lymphocytes each antigen reacts with a distinct subset of the lymphocyte population, and competition for the same lymphocytes does not occur.

While it is certainly true that antigen presentation to lymphocytes by macrophages serves to initiate the cellular cascade which is the immune response (Rosenstreich and Oppenheim, 1976), the macrophage does not serve as a simple trigger for the cascade but plays a regulatory role as well. More or less antigen may be degraded, which affects the extent and duration of the stimulus. Soluble products from macrophages may stimulate lymphocyte transformation or suppress it. Such soluble products have been demonstrated in rats with plasmodial infections (Wyler, 1978).

When activated, macrophages appear to be the source of substances which suppress lymphocyte reproduction (Nelson, 1976). If a multicellular organism is to survive, it must not only activate cell systems such as those involved in the immune response but also stop their reproduction at an appropriate time. The macrophage activates the lymphocyte system and is in turn activated by it. The suppressor substances from the activated macrophage may thus be part of the homeostatic control of the immune response.

Various mechanisms have been described by which phagocytic cells bind and ingest antigens before the immune response is initiated. Such antigen recognition may be mediated by noninducible serum proteins (DiLuzio *et al.*, 1972). One well-characterized constitutive opsonic protein is an α-2-globulin (Allen *et al.*, 1973; Blumenstock *et al.*, 1976). Complement may also serve as a constitutive opsonin in the early stages of some infections (Winkelstein *et al.*, 1975; Guckian *et al.*, 1978). Complement activation in the early stages of infection may take place by the alternate pathway and may involve properdin, another constituve serum protein (Götze and Müller-Eberhard, 1976). It has been suggested that antigen handling by macrophages occurs in a "nonspecific" fashion (Unanue, 1972) presumably by macrophage membrane receptors of very broad specificity, possibly receptors for denatured protein configurations.

Our knowledge of how the macrophage ingests malarial antigens before immunity develops is limited. Macrophages do bind and ingest plasmodial parasites in the absence of antibody specific for the parasites (Chow and Kreier, 1972; Green and Kreier, 1978). The encapsulated merozoite, however, is rarely phagocytized in the absence of specific antibody, and extracellular trophozoites are phagocytized to some degree even in the absence of normal serum (Brooks and Kreier, 1978). There is evidence that erythrocyte membrane fragments or parasite materials may activate the alternate C' pathway (Krettli et al., 1976). Only a minor enhancement of plasmodial parasitemia, however, was observed in cobra venom factor-treated rats (Diggs et al., 1972b). This suggests that, if complement activation by the alternate pathway contributes to antigen binding by macrophages in malarious animals during the initial stages of infection, there must be additional recognition systems which may perform the same function in the absence of complement.

The demonstration of a macrophage cytophilic antibody capable of binding plasmodia to macrophages but only weakly stimulating phagocytosis (Green and Kreier, 1978) suggests a mechanism for amplification of antigen presentation once the immune response is initiated, but does not help to explain the initial presentation. An amplification role for cytophilic antibody has been proposed previously on the basis of studies using dinitrophenyl–guinea pig albumin as antigen (Cohen et al., 1973). Data supporting a role for antiplasmodial antibody in the presentation of plasmodial antigens by macrophages is available (Green, 1978). The experiments providing this evidence were based on the observation that weaning CDF rats were quite susceptible to Plasmodium berghei while adults were quite resistant (Gravely et al., 1976). The differences in susceptibility of young and mature rats permit studies on the role of cells in enhancing the young rats' immune response by cell transfer from mature to young rats (Gravely and Kreier, 1976). Two of four weanling rats given buffer alone died following challenge with P. berghei, and all developed a severe infection. While the infections were as severe in weanling rats given adult macrophages as in those given buffer, no deaths occurred following challenge in weanling rats receiving adult macrophages. Infections following challenge in weanling rats given adult macrophages incubated with free parasites were considerably milder than infections in rats receiving buffer or adult macrophages alone, while infections following challenge in weanling rats given adult macrophages preincubated with free parasites and immune serum were very mild. That the effect was not just from the immune serum in the preparation of macrophages and free parasites is apparent from the fact that immune serum alone had less effect than immune serum with adult macrophages and parasites and because immune serum alone delayed development of the parasitemia while the immune serum–macrophage–antigen treatment did not delay initial development of the parasitemia. This suggests that in the latter rats the transferred antibody was not free to act on the developing parasites directly but rather played a role in increasing the efficiency of the development in the weanling rats of their own active immunity.

It is probably fair to say that we have little information about the mechanisms by which the macrophages of the nonimmune animal recognize plasmodial antigens, process them, and present them to the lymphocytes. Macrophages apparently can recognize and ingest normally intracellular forms of the parasite, and host and parasite debris produced when the parasite ruptures the host cell before immunity develops. Antigens which resist phagocytosis, such as capsular material, may be carried into macrophages with more easily phagocytized membrane fragments. It is probably this scavenged antigen that is presented by macrophages to the lymphocytes to initiate the immune response. Cytophilic and opsonic antibody, when produced, may increase the ability of the macrophage to interact with plasmodial antigens, and this may result in amplification of the presentation function of macrophages. Further work will have to be done to determine the role of noninducible serum factors and macrophage receptors in the initial recognition of malarial antigens by macrophages.

A number of individuals have approached the problem of the role of the macrophage in induction and regulation of the immune response by study of the ability of the host during plasmodial infection to respond to heterologous antigens (Wedderburn, 1974; Terry, 1977; Wyler, 1978). Early in plasmodial infection and during recovery the ability to mount an immune response to heterologous erythrocytes is normal or enhanced, while during the acute phases of infection this ability, is depressed (Loose and DiLuzio, 1976). The cell controlling these responses is the macrophage (Loose et al., 1972; Warren and Weidanz, 1976). Macrophages in the spleen appear to be more severely affected in their ability to respond to heterologous erythrocytes during acute plasmodial infection than those in the lymph nodes (Weidanz and Rank, 1975), suggesting that direct exposure of macrophages to the massive amounts of blood-borne antigens during the acute stages of infection is a cause of the effect (Loose and DiLuzio, 1976). Organ distribution of phagocytized heterologous erythrocytes was not significantly different in infected and noninfected animals (Loose et al., 1972; Loose and DiLuzio, 1976). Thus in infected animals sufficient antigen to stimulate a response was probably ingested by splenic macrophages, which are in close proximity to lymphocytes, and the depressed response to foreign erythrocytes during acute infection cannot be considered to result from the diversion of antigen to liver macrophages where it may be degraded without presentation to lymphocytes.

That macrophages and macrophage products may either stimulate or repress the immune response to plasmodial antigens depending on the stage of infection is apparent from the paper by Wyler (1978). It would help interpretation of Wyler's observations if it were known whether clones of lymphocytes secreting antiplasmodial antibody had already been produced when the macrophages producing repressor substances were obtained.

Herman (1977) has shown that lymphocytes from animals immune to *P. berghei* cluster around macrophages which have ingested *P. berghei* antigens. Significant clustering has not been seen with normal lymphocytes and macrophages digesting *P. berghei* antigen. This may indicate simply that lymphocytes with appropriate receptors on their surfaces are not present in sufficient numbers before immune stimulation and clonal expansion to be detected by the clustering technique.

Terry (1977) observes that a number of protozoan infections in rodents, such as those caused by *Plasmodium yoelii, Babesia microti,* and *Trypanosoma musculi* are acute and rapidly controlled by an effective immune response. In these infections he notes that, while immune responses to heterologous antigens are depressed at the height of parasitemia, they are rapidly restored once the blood has been cleared of parasites. This pattern is compatible with antigenic competition for macrophages by antigens, as the immunological response to the antigens of the parasites is obviously working satisfactorily. The inability of liver macrophages from rodents acutely infected with plasmodia to detoxify endotoxin (Loose *et al.,* 1971) has been explained in terms of exhaustion of lysosomal enzymes and suggests a mechanism by which macrophage processing of antigen may fail. The situation in animals such as mice infected with uniformaly lethal *P. berghei* parasites may be different. Seitz (1976) has observed that mice dying of *P. berghei* develop much antibody to *P. berghei* antigens. The antibody just is not protective. He reports further that mice protected from death by various treatments develop antibody to soluble antigens present in the serum of dying mice. This suggests antigenic competition between parasite antigens stimulating protection and those irrelevant to protection, or possibly a high dose tolerance reaction, or even a simple swamping of the protective immune response by antigen.

Terry (1977) points out the difficulty in interpreting the significance of immunodepression to heterologous antigens during parasitoses which are long-lasting and ultimately fatal. In these cases the parasites possess various mechanisms for escaping the host immune defenses, such as antigenic variation, antigenic disguise, and rapid reproduction, and one cannot determine if the ultimate fatal outcome of the infection is due to immunodepression or simply failure of the immunoregulatory system.

Resolution of the questions concerning the role of the macrophage in initiating the immune response and in its regulation require information on the very early events in the immune response to the parasite, as well as events during the later phases of the response. To determine if depression of the immune response to heterologous antigens during acute plasmodial infection is a form of immunoregulation designed to concentrate a limited physiological capacity upon the major problem of responding to the parasites and its products, we will need to measure the response of the host to the parasite antigens at the same time we measure its response to the heterologous antigens. Only the development and use of a test for the immune response to plasmodial antigen providing information of a type comparable to that provided by the Jerne plaque test for response to sheep red blood cells will provide the information needed to evaluate the regulatory role of the macrophage in the animal's response to plasmodial parasites. To be of greatest value such a test should be based on antigens shown to stimulate the protective response, not just the response to any plasmodial antigen.

B. Role of Lymphocytes in the Induction and Regulation of the Immune Response

The production of specific antibody against plasmodia begins when macrophages process antigen and present it to T lymphocytes. Phagocytosis of antigen by macrophages may be unaided or may be enhanced by nonspecific opsonins such as microglobulins or properdin, or even by cross-reacting "natural" antibodies. However, when macrophage presentation of antigen to lymphocytes occurs, the process becomes antigen-specific, as only antigen-specific clones of lymphocytes are capable of being activated by the process. Soluble macrophage products are released which nurture and enhance the proliferation of clones of T cells, which in turn stimulate specific B cells to proliferate and subsequently transform into antibody-producing plasma cells.

The cellular interactions which occur during the induction of immunity have been the subject of intensive research, and the elements of these cellular interactions are now known. Katz and Benacerraf (1972) have shown that the humoral immune response to many antigens requires the participation of both T and B lymphocytes and that the T cells act as "helpers" to the B cells. Jayawardena *et al.* (1977) reported that, in T cell-deprived mice, the antibody response to *P. yoelii* was severely reduced and the development of germinal centers in the spleen was severely impaired. The immunological defect in T cell-deprived mice could be partially corrected by T-cell reconstitution. These results indicate a helper role for T cells in the induction of immunity to plasmodia.

Recovery from malarial infection is dependent upon a proliferation of splenic T cells (Gravely *et al.*, 1976), a phenomenon not observed in animals with fatal infections (Clark and Allison, 1974; Krettli and Nussenzweig, 1974). In young rats infected with *P. berghei,* for example, a collapse of the T-cell population associated with thymic involution results in a lack of immune responsiveness.

The poor immune response and T-cell failure are probably responsible for the severe malarial infections seen in these animals (Gravely *et al.*, 1976; Krettli and Nussenzweig, 1974). Gravely *et al.* (1976) have shown that, after the proliferation of T cells, the immune response to *P. berghei* in adult rats is characterized by hypertrophy of the B-cell system. This sequence of events also suggests a helper cell role for the T cells.

Miller (1977) has suggested that a very vigorous T-cell response may be necessary to ensure production of antiplasmodial antibody in quantities sufficient to control the parasite. Roberts *et al.* (1977) have demonstrated a relationship between thymic function and the prevention of recrudescent *P. yoelii* malaria in mice. Their data suggest that the prevention of recrudesence requires T cells in a helper function for the production of protective antibody, since the role of the T cell could be fulfilled by the injection of polyvalent hyperimmune serum. The physical interaction of syngeneic mouse macrophages, which had digested *P. chabaudi,* with splenic lymphocytes was investigated by Herman (1977). He demonstrated specific antigen-mediated binding of immune lymphocytes to the macrophage membranes, which he considered to indicate a mechanism of interaction of macrophages and T cells in rodents with malaria.

Protection results from the transfer of immune lymphoid cells to nonimmune recipients (Stechschulte, 1969; Phillips, 1970; Gravely and Kreier, 1976). Mixed splenic lymphoid cells have been more commonly used in cell transfer experiments in malaria than have lymphoid cells from other sources. Stechschulte (1969) found that immune lymphoid cells obtained from lymph nodes were as effective in transferring immunity to *P. berghei,* as were mixed lymphoid cells from immune spleens. However, thoracic duct lymphocytes were not protective. Thoracic duct lymphocytes are primarily memory T cells.

In a series of adoptive transfer experiments in rats in which the splenic lymphoid cells were separated into T and B types, Gravely and Kreier (1976) demonstrated that differentiated B lymphocytes were primarily responsible for the transfer of immunity to *P. berghei* from immune to susceptible young rats, presumably by virtue of their ability to produce specific antibody. Similarly, Brown *et al.* (1976a,b) found that adoptive transfer of immune rat T cells alone was less effective than transfer of immune T and B cells in conferring immunity on mice infected with *P. berghei,* but that T cells did provide some protection, probably as a result of their ability to stimulate B cells to produce antibody to new variants of the parasite. The observation that immune lymphocyte suspensions depleted of B cells could still confer some protection to *P. berghei* was made by transfer of immune T cells to rats with B cells. Results of experiments on the transfer of T cells to rats without B cells similar to the work on mice by McDonald and Phillips (1978b) would be required to obtain definitive answer to the question of the role of T cells in immunity to malaria.

In their series of adoptive transfer experiments using mice immune to *P.*

chabaudi, McDonald and Phillips (1978b) found some immunity to reside in glass wool-filtered immune spleen cells, as well as immune T and B cells. Transferred T cells gave the least protection, and no synergism could be demonstrated in irradiated mice between the transferred immune T and B cells. If the role of T cells were restricted to a helper function and if the B cells were already differentiated, the effect of the T cells would not be apparent in this type of transfer experiment.

T cells mediate the activation of macrophages (Mackaness, 1969; Krahenbuhl *et al.*, 1973) to a hyperphagocytic state (Brown, 1971). North (1973) has shown that a rapidly replicating population of short-lived θ-positive T cells in the spleen mediates an increase in the population of activated splenic macrophages. These T cells initiate the events which cause the development of splenomegaly (Roberts and Weldanz, 1978), which is always associated with recovery from malarial infection. No long-lived memory cells result from this T-cell–macrophage interaction.

Macrophages may serve to present antigen continuously in a nontolerogenic form and thus stimulate continuous clonal proliferation of lymphocytes. The macrophages may do this in part by producing factors which ensure the viability and differentiation of the developing lymphocyte clone (Rosenstreich and Oppenheim, 1976). Helper T cells will proliferate under the influence of macrophages, which may serve both to process and present malarial antigens to the lymphocytes and to produce macrophage factors essential for successful proliferation of the sensitized lymphocyte clones. The observations of Green and Kreier (1978) and Brooks and Kreier (1978) suggest that specific cytophilic antibodies which serve to arm macrophages for antigen binding may well play a role in the presentation of an antigen by macrophages to lymphocytes.

Antimalarial protective antibody has been found in both the IgM and IgG classes, with IgG antibodies being predominant in established infections (Cohen and Butcher, 1971; Cohen, *et al.*, 1977). B lymphocytes producing antimalarial IgM will become IgG producers under continuing antigenic stimulation and with the help of helper T cells. The time interval required for the conversion of IgM-producing lymphocytes to IgG-producing cells is approximately 6 days (Sterzl and Nordin, 1971).

Solid immunity to malaria seldom appears even after repeated infections. Two possible methods by which parasites may evade the immune response are antigenic variation and immunosuppression of the protective immune response (Voller and Rossan, 1969; Wilson and Phillips, 1976). A suppressive activity by spleen cells may prevent the complete cure of *P. inui* in intact rhesus monkeys, since splenectomized monkeys cure their chronic infections while intact ones do not (Wyler *et al.*, 1977). Yet the protective effect of passive transfer of antiserum is reduced by T-cell depletion or splenectomy of rats (Brown and Phillips, 1974; Golenser *et al.*, 1975). Because of their lack of sensitivity to antilymphocyte serum (ALS) suppressor cells have been identified as T1 lymphocytes, whereas the ALS-sensitive helper cell is a T2 lymphocyte (Raff and Cantor, 1971). Poels and Van Niekerk (1977) suggested that malarial immunosuppression and related immune disturbances may be due to a combination of severe T-cell depletion, polyclonal mitogenic recruitment of B cells, and consequent macrophage dysfunction.

It has been suggested that malarial antigens may possess mitogenic properties as well as the ability to elicit specific antibody responses (Greenwood and Vick, 1975). Rosenberg (1978) has shown that specific antibody responses can occur concurrently with large nonspecific polyclonal B-cell responses; both responses are T cell-dependent. Rosenberg (1978) does not interpret his results to indicate a direct mitogenic stimulation of B lymphocytes, but rather a mitogen-induced T-cell proliferation resulting in release of lymphokines which in turn stimulate B-cell proliferation nonspecifically.

Williamson and Greenwood (1978) found that often malarious children could not be successfully vaccinated against *Salmonella typhi* and meningococcus and that the duration of the refractory state varied. However, circulating T cells from patients with malaria have been shown to proliferate when exposed to malarial antigens (Wyler and Brown, 1977). Freeman (1978) found that delayed-type hypersensitivity reactions in mice infected with *P. berghei* and *P. yoelii* were weak and that the weakness was in expression rather than in T-cell sensitization and did not therefore reflect impaired T-cell function. T-cell proliferation may be reduced during malaria, however, causing a depression of the inflammatory response. These results suggest that the poor heterologous responses in individuals with malaria may not indicate general immunosuppression.

If antigenic variation is a feature of malaria, as suggested by Cox, (1959), Brown (1965), and Briggs et al. (1968), then successive rapid rises in variant-specific antibodies would be required to control the infection. Transferred immune cells would be able to respond to new variants and thus to control the infection, while passively transferred serum would not be able to control new variants that would arise.

The immune system produces both humoral and cell-associated responses to malaria as a result of immunization with malarial antigen in Freund's complete adjuvant; both these types of response may be required for a fully expressed immune response (Brown et al., 1970a). Playfair et al. (1977) demonstrated that protection against malarial infection was dependent in part upon T cells, but that helper T cells were not necessary for the resistance to reinfection found in recovered animals. Rank and Weidanz (1976) found that bursectomized agammaglobulinemic chickens were immune to reinfection with *P. gallinaceum* following drug cure. Similarly drug-rescued B cell-deficient mice were found to be resistant to subsequent challenge with *P. yoelii* despite the lack of detectable antiplasmodial antibody (Roberts and Weidanz, 1979). These latter observations indicate that a non-antibody-mediated immunity may be present in animals immune to plasmodia. It has been proposed that T cells are somehow capable of mediating a type of malarial immunity that is distinct from antibody production. No mechanisms for such an effect have yet been demonstrated. It has been proposed, however, that activated macrophages are induced by activated T cells to secrete substances that cause the destruction of both malaria and babesia parasites in the intraerythrocytic location (Clark *et al.*, 1976; Allison and Clark, 1977).

There are difficulties in assessing the role of killer lymphocytes in malarial immunity. Immune lymphocytes have been shown not to be directly antiparasitic when tested *in vitro* (Phillips *et al.*, 1970; Cohen and Butcher, 1971). An increase in the proportion of null cells in blood lymphocyte populations from acutely infected children has been reported by Greenwood *et al.* (1977). These null cells (K cells) destroyed chicken red cells *in vitro*, however, purified T cells were not cytolytic for chicken erythrocytes in these tests. Allison and his associates (Allison and Clark, 1977) feel that K cells may contribute to malarial immunity. Coleman *et al.* (1975) described cytotoxic effects attributable to immune T cells and null cells. In the experiments by Coleman and his associates specific antibody enhanced the destruction of infected red cells by immune lymphocytes and also induced normal lymphocytes to destroy erythrocytes.

C. Course of Appearance of Antibody during Plasmodial Infection

Studies on the course of plasmodial infection in susceptible nonimmune humans (Powell *et al.*, 1972), primates (Schmidt, 1978a,b), birds (Seed and Manwell, 1977), and rodents (Carter and Diggs, 1977) have made it clear that after infection the number of plasmodia in the blood of immunologically competent hosts increases rapidly for a limited time. After reaching a peak level there is generally a crash in the population, referred to as the crisis, and then, if the host does not die, a period of variable duration occurs when the parasites persist in the blood but their number is obviously controlled quite effectively by some system newly acquired by the host.

Many attempts have been made to determine if there is a positive correlation between development of this clinical immunity and the presence of specific antiplasmodial antibody in the plasma. Almost any serological test can be used to demonstrate the antibody response of a host to infection with plasmodia (Fife, 1971, 1972; this volume, Chapter 2). The problem of obtaining a suitable antigen in sufficient quantity for the procedure chosen (Kreier, 1977) is usually the major factor considered in deciding which test is to be used. The direct agglutination procedure (Kreier *et al.*, 1965; Kortmann *et al.*, 1971), because it requires large amounts of a purified parasite preparation as antigen, has not been much used.

The earliest workers used complement fixation (CF) tests in their attempts to demonstrate antibody to plasmodia in infected animals. This test was probably selected because it does not require highly purified antigens. Complement-fixing antibodies have been shown to occur in the serum of mice (Schindler and Dennig, 1962), birds (Davis, 1948), monkeys (Coggeshall and Eaton, 1938), and humans (Dulaney and Stratman-Thomas, 1940) with malaria.

The pattern of infection and complement-fixing antibody response in rhesus monkeys is typical of that seen in most species. In rhesus monkeys infected with *P. knowlesi* specific complement-fixing antibodies appear early in the course of the infection and persist during the course of the chronic infection which may be induced by quinine treatment. The first appearance of complement-fixing antibodies occurs during acute infection when parasites are present in the blood. The titer rises to fairly high levels at first and then slowly drops. During the first months of infection there is no apparent relationship between the number of circulating parasites and changes in complement-fixing titer. During the later stages of chronic infection there is a fall in titer preceding each parasitic relapse, and after the relapse terminates there is an elevation in the complement-fixing titer (Coggeshall and Eaton, 1938). Coggeshall and Eaton (1938) note that there is a wide variation in the degree of production of complement-fixing antibodies among monkeys and that in general there does not seem to be a good correlation between levels of complement-fixing antibodies in the serum and immunity. A wide variety of parasite antigen–host antibody pairs may fix complement. The antibody measured during the chronic phase of infection may be protective, that during the acute phase almost certainly is not.

Hemagglutination (HA) tests have been extensively used for the demonstration of antiplasmodial antibody (Desowitz and Saave, 1965; Matthews *et al.*, 1975; Meuwissen *et al.*, 1972). The HA test has been used more for the demonstration of antibody as a diagnostic aid than for studies on the relationship between antibody and immunity.

Precipitins specific for plasmodial antigens have been reported to occur in the plasma of rats and mice (Goberman and Zuckerman, 1966; Zuckerman *et al.*, 1969a) and humans (McGregor *et al.*, 1966) during the course of infection with plasmodia. The precipitation is usually carried out in gels. Precipitins developed in all but one of a group of 46 rats infected with *P. berghei* (Zuckerman *et al.*, 1969a). Precipitins appeared between days 3 and 17 after infection with erythrocytic parasites and in general were present thereafter with occasional negative periods for as long as the rats were tested. Tests were conducted for up to 51 days. The one rat which did not develop precipitins died of a fulminating infection. Precipitins develop not only as a result of infection but also as a result of artificial immunization (Weiss and A. Zuckerman, 1968; 1971). Partial protection and precipitins can be transferred with serum either by serum injection or naturally from mother to offspring (McGregor *et al.*, 1966; Zuckerman *et al.*,

1969a; Zuckerman, 1970). It has been suggested that the precipitation reaction measures protective antibody (Zuckerman, 1970). This suggestion is supported by the observation that precipitins for soluble antigens present in the serum of mice acutely infected with *P. berghei* develop in mice which become immune to *P. berghei* following drug treatment but do not develop in mice which die from *P. berghei* infection (Seitz, 1976). Seitz (1976) also has observed that antibodies to intraerythrocytic parasites, demonstrable by the indirect fluorescent antibody (IFA) technique, are present in mice which die of the infection as well as those which become immune. There is of course no reason to assume that precipitins may only develop to antigens important in protection.

The IFA technique for the detection of antibodies to plasmodial parasites (Ingram *et al.*, 1961; Collins and Skinner, 1972) has been used extensively to measure antibody response to plasmodial infection. This test has been used to measure antibody response in mice (Finerty *et al.*, 1972), in monkeys (Collins *et al.*, 1967) and in humans (Collins *et al.*, 1964; Tobie and Coatney, 1964; Tobie *et al.*, 1966a,b). The test is particularly convenient because the antigen is simply a thin blood film (Collins and Skinner, 1972). Lunn *et al.* (1966) and Tobie *et al.* (1966b) reported particularly complete studies on the relation of antibody titers determined by the IFA technique to parasitemia in humans infected for the first time with *P. vivax* or *P. falciparum* parasites. In humans whose infections were induced by injections of *P. vivax* sporozoites, antibodies were not detected until 3–6 days after parasites were detected in the blood, and maximum titers occurred 8–16 days after parasites were detected. Titers fell slightly during remission but went up again following parasitic relapse. Maximum titers, which occurred during the early acute phases of the infection, ranged from 1:640 to 1:2560. During the chronic phases of the infection titers between 1:10 and 1:160 occurred. These titers persisted throughout the period of observation which in one case was for 252 days after the onset of parasitemia. Antibody was detected before parasites in humans infected by injection of frozen infected blood (Tobie *et al.*, 1966b). Antigen from the parasites killed by the freezing procedure may have stimulated this early response. IgG concentrations increased in parallel with antibody. Increases were 30–40% over control levels. Albumin concentration in the plasma decreased during parasitic relapse. α-1-Globulin concentrations increased when parasites were increasing in number, and α-2-globulins decreased (Lunn *et al.*, 1966; Sadun *et al.*, 1966).

In general the antibody response patterns of individuals infected with *P. falciparum* sporozoites were similar to those of patients with *P. vivax* infection. Lunn *et al.* (1966) observed that there appeared to be little correlation between globulin levels and antibody levels. Abele *et al.* (1965) observed a correlation between B_2M macroglobulins and early antibody response to *P. vivax* infection and commented that this observation was consistent with the observation of an early IgM response to many antigens. Later antibody responses are generally IgG

(Tobie *et al.*, 1966a). The same authors observed little change in IgA levels during *P. vivax* infections. Poels and Van Niekerk (1977) emphasize the presence of elevated levels of antibodies which are not specific for plasmodia in mice with *P. berghei* infection. Some of these antibodies are autoantibodies to erythrocyte membrane components (Kreier *et al.*, 1966; Seed and Kreier, 1969; Rosenberg *et al.*, 1973) or to nucleic acids (Kreier and Dilley, 1969), or are heterophilic antibodies (Houba *et al.*, 1974). Individuals living in malarious areas generally have elevated globulin levels. Some of this globulin may be a result of malaria infection, and some may be a result of other infections common in such areas (Curtain *et al.*, 1965). A factor present in the serum of animals with acute malaria has been demonstrated by electroabsorption techniques. It may be acute phase globulin and be one of the materials which contribute to the elevated globulin levels of malarious individuals (D'Antonio *et al.*, 1969). The recently developed enzyme-linked immunoabsorbent assay for malarial antibody (Voller *et al.*, 1975), like all other serological tests, detects antibodies to whatever antigens are used in the test.

Serological tests could be used to determine the immune status of the individual tested if pure preparations of the antigen stimulating the protective response were available and if it were the case that immunity to plasmodia is antibody-dependent, as has been recently suggested (Heuman *et al.*, 1979). At present we of course do not know for sure which of the multitude of antigens of the blood stages of the parasite stimulate the development of protective antibodies, but there is evidence that merozoite surface proteins are of major importance in induction of immunity (Saul and Kreier, 1977; Grothaus and Kreier, 1980).

D. Demonstration of Protective Activity in Immune Serum

The demonstration by means of various serological tests of antibodies to plasmodial antigens in the serum of infected animals was soon followed by the realization that the presence of these antibodies did not ensure immunity. Coggeshall and Kumm (1937) demonstrated by transfer that at least some of the antibodies to *P. knowlesi* present in the serum of monkeys with chronic infections were protective, but they also observed (Coggeshall and Kumm, 1938) that only incomplete immunity was transferred with serum and that superinfection, if too traumatic, could reduce the potency of the serum in a monkey. They found that monkeys given single superinfections followed by a month's rest yielded the most potent immune serum.

The reasons for the poor correlation between the protective capacity of immune serum on transfer to nonimmune animals and antibody titer in serological tests are to this day a matter of dispute. Plasmodia are a complex mosaic of potentially antigenic substances (Kreier, 1977). The host's immune system may produce antibodies to many of them, but many of these antibodies may only contact their antigens after the parasite is dead and has disintegrated, possibly because the antigens are located inside the living plasmodium. Antibodies to such internal antigens could react in serological tests using disrupted parasites as antigen but would not be important in protective immunity. That merozoite surface antigens are important in immunity was suggested by Miller *et al.* (1975b) by Brooks and Kreier (1978), and by Grothaus and Kreier 1980), although Miller *et al.* (1975b) suggested that the antibodies to the surface coat acted by inhibition of penetration of the host cell, and Brooks and Kreier (1978) suggested that they improved the efficiency of phagocytic ingestion of the merozoites. The two suggested modes of action may of course both occur and complement each other.

Coggeshall (1940) suggested that antibody may not be effective against plasmodia because of the intracellular location of the parasite during most of its residence in the host. He considered that the erythrocyte membrane prevented the antibody from acting on the parasite effectively. He observed that the parasite rapidly invaded a new host cell and that release and reinvasion may occur in protected sites in the body. In his experiments, Coggeshall (1940) demonstrated that serum from humans infected with *P. knowlesi* protected rhesus monkeys from infection by *P. knowlesi*. He concluded that the relatively ineffective and temporary immunity he was able to demonstrate by serum transfer in his experiments should not be interpreted to indicate that immune substances were present in low concentration in the serum but that the immune substances present were unable to exert their influence against the parasite because of the parasites ability to evade their action.

Some authors (Allison and Clark, 1977; Roberts and Weidanz, 1979) have provided evidence for an immune control of plasmodia not mediated by antibody. This evidence will be discussed in Section II, K.

Since the original demonstration that protection against plasmodia could be transferred by transfer of immune serum, many additional passive protection studies have been done (Briggs *et al.*, 1966; Diggs and Osler, 1969a,b, 1975; Stechschulte *et al.*, 1969; Phillips and Jones, 1972; Diggs *et al.*, 1972a; Lourie and Dunn, 1972; Wells and Diggs, 1976; Hamburger and Kreier, 1975, 1976). Causse-Vaills *et al.* (1960) reported that the protective capacity in rat serum was associated with β- and γ-globulins but absent from fractions containing α-globulins and albumin. Diggs and Osler (1969a) found most of the protective activity of hyperimmune rat serum to reside in 7 S immunoglobulins. Stechschulte *et al.* (1969) confirmed this observation and reported in addition that protection resided in the IgG and IgA components of 7 S immunoglobulin. Stechschulte *et al.* also detected protective activity in the 19 S component of serum collected early in the course of an infection. Phillips and Jones (1972) observed that the maximum levels of protective activity occurred in the serum of rats at the time *P. berghei* parasites were eliminated from the host. They interpreted this to indicate that a high level of protective antibody was one essential factor for complete elimination of the parasite. Diggs and co-workers (1972a,b) demonstrated that serum from West Africans infected with *P. falciparum*-protected *Aotus* monkeys infected with an Asian strain of *P. falciparum*. Hamburger and Kreier (1975) demonstrated that immune serum from rats hyperimmune to *P. berghei* contained antibodies which acted against free parasites but not parasitized erythrocytes and that antiserum effectiveness was partially controlled by the test host. They found that some strains of rats had a greater ability to destroy parasites in the presence of antibody than other strains. Wells and Diggs (1976) demonstrated protective antibody in the serum of mice immunized with five doses of irradiated parasitized erythrocytes, although Saul and Kreier (1977) observed by an indirect method that rats immunized with disrupted free parasites only activated the effector arm of their immune system after the challenge infection has already developed. Many individuals (e.g., Desowitz, 1973; Palmer, 1978) have demonstrated the natural transfer of protective antibody from mother to offspring. It has also been observed that injection of immune serum will in part compensate for damage to the host's defense systems. Thus, for example, immune serum injection will partially compensate for the effects of bursectomy (Stutz *et al.*, 1972a,b) or the injection of antithymocyte serum (Lourie and Dunn, 1972).

E. Mechanisms of Antibody Action against Plasmodia

1. Introduction

There are a number of times during the parasite's development in the blood at which antiplasmodial antibody may act against the parasite. The antibody may, for example, act against the parasite while it is inside the erythrocyte either directly after passing through the erythrocyte membrane or indirectly by reaction with plasmodial antigens in the erythrocyte membrane. Alternately, antibody could act against the parasite during the brief period when it passes from one host erythrocyte to another.

There are also a number of ways in which antiplasmodial antibody may affect the parasite after it combines with it or its products in the host cell membrane. A mode of action could be physical coating of the parasite's surface. Such a coat could physically interfere with membrane function. The antibody coating could change the adhesive characteristics of the parasite, or it could block receptor sites, or it could interfere with the parasite's movement. All these actions would affect the parasite's ability to find and penetrate a new host cell or could interfere with membrane transport and nutrition. Interference with membrane transport and thus the parasite's nutrition could also result from antibody coating of the host cell. Antibody bound to host or parasite membrane could initiate the complement cascade and cause membrane damage. The binding of antibody could facilitate phagocytosis of the antibody-coated organisms or host cell and possibly affect the organism's fate once in a phagosome. Phagocytosis of the erythrocyte–host cell complex would as effectively remove the parasite as would phagocytosis of the free parasite. In this section evidence available concerning these various modes of action of antibody in hosts infected with plasmodia will be discussed.

2. Site of Antibody Action

Diggs and Osler (1975) have observed that serum which protects rats against *P. berghei* infection does not sensitize parasitized erythrocytes for *in vivo* destruction. Chow and Kreier (1972), Hamburger and Kreier (1976), Green and Kreier (1978), and Brooks and Kreier (1978) observed that serum which protected rodents from *P. berghei* and which facilitated phagocytosis of free parasites *in vitro* did not facilitate phagocytosis of parasitized erythrocytes *in vitro*. Diggs and Osler (1975) were unable to demonstrate any difference in efflux of a radioactively labeled hemoglobin from parasitized erythrocytes incubated in normal serum or in serum which protected rats. The addition of complement to the cultures did not change this result. These workers were unable to reduce the protective activity of immune serum by absorption with parasitized erythrocytes but did observe consumption of protective antibody *in vivo* during infection. These results were interpreted to indicate that antibody did not bind to the parasitized erythrocyte but to parasites and their products at the time of rupture of schizonts. This interpretation is supported by the observations of Jerusalem *et al.* (1971) and Hamburger and Kreier (1976) who used fluorescent antibody to globulin to demonstrate that antiplasmodial antibody did not bind to the membranes of fresh, unfixed *P. berghei*-parasitized erythrocytes or penetrate the erythrocyte membrane, but did bind to free parasites released by erythrocyte rupture. The cyclic decreases in complement levels which occur at the time of schizont rupture in monkeys with *P. knowlesi* infection (Fogel *et al.*, 1966) and humans with *P. falciparum* infection (Greenwood and Brueton, 1974) also support the assumption that the bulk of antibody binding during most plasmodial infections takes place at the time of schizont rupture. Cohen *et al.* (1961) and McGregor *et al.* (1963) treated *P. falciparum*-infected West African children with IgG from West African adults immune to falciparum malaria. They observed that the globulin injections ameliorated the infections in the children and that the parasites were not much affected by the globulin until the time of schizont rupture. This observation was interpreted to indicate that either mature schizonts or released merozoites were the target of antibody action.

3. Antibody-Mediated Inhibition of Erythrocyte Invasion

Brown *et al.* (1968) and later Cohen *et al.* (1972) demonstrated that *in vitro*
P. knowlesi parasites grew and differentiated inside red blood cells in the presence of immune serum but that reinvasion was prevented. Phillips *et al.* (1972)
similarly found that immune serum did not affect intracellular growth and differentiation of *P. falciparum* in culture but did interrupt reinvasion by the parasites. Cohen and his associates (1974; Cohen, 1977) suggested that the
merozoite-blocking antibody (an antibody inhibitory to invasion) detectable in *in
vitro* blocking tests is a protective antibody *in vivo*. Miller *et al.* (1977b),
however, reported no correlation between functional immunity and *in vitro* inhibition of invasion of erythrocytes by serum of monkeys immune to *P. knowlesi*.
Further tests correlating the capacity of serum to inhibit the ability of merozoites
to invade erythrocytes with the immune status of the serum donor and the ability
of the serum passively to confer immunity on susceptible animals will be needed
to resolve the question of the relationship between the *in vitro* inhibition of red
cell invasion by merozoites and clinical immunity.

The various observations on patients given immune serum (Cohen *et al.*,
1961; McGregor *et al.*, 1963) and on the effects of immune serum on plasmodial
growth *in vitro* (Brown *et al.*, 1968; Cohen *et al.*, 1972; Phillips *et al.*, 1972)
make it quite clear that one mode of action of antiplasmodial antibodies in
inhibition of merozoite penetration of erythrocytes. The mechanisms of this
inhibition have been the subject of various studies. To understand how antibody
inhibits penetration of erythrocytes one must understand the penetration process.
Ladda (1969) has shown by electron microscopy that a merozoite can only enter a
red cell if its anterior, apical complex-bearing end makes contact with the erythrocyte membrane. Entry is then by a phagocytic process. Ladda (1969) observed that material on the surface of the merozoite is squeezed off as the parasite
passes into the vacuole it produces. The process was subsequently observed in
culture and recorded by cinematography (Dvorak *et al.*, 1975). Aikawa *et al.*
(1978) described a moving junction between the merozoite and the erythrocyte
membrane during penetration and observed that the surface coat material covering the merozoite was absent from that portion of the merozoite inside the
vacuole.

Red blood cells including those of animals suffering from malaria (Miller *et
al.*, 1972) have a negative charge. The charge on red cells is largely determined
by sialic acid groups. Miller *et al.* (1973b) observed that erythrocytes bound
positively charged acetic acid–ferric oxide hydrosols at pH 1.8, an indication of
the presence of exposed sialic acid on the red cell, but that free parasites did not.
These results were interpreted to indicate that there was a difference in surface
charge between erythrocytes and red cells, and the suggestion was made that the

low surface change on the parasites permitted close apposition to the host cell and might facilitate invasion. Seed *et al.* (1974) confirmed that plasmodia had less exposed sialic acid than erythrocytes and also demonstrated that parasites stained more intensely with lipophilic iron colloids than erythrocytes. Seed and Kreier (1976) measured the charge on parasites and parasitized erythrocytes at physiological pH values and observed no significant differences in charge between the two types of cells. They further demonstrated by a lipid extraction procedure that the charge on the parasite could be extracted with the membrane lipid but that the charge on the red cell could not. These results do not support a role for charge differences in bringing about apposition of parasites and red cells.

Ladda (1969) described a layer of material, granular in appearance, in their electron micrographs, which covered the surface of the merozoite. In later studies this layer of material, outside the plasmalemma of the merozoite, was called the surface coat (Miller *et al.*, 1975b; Bannister, 1977). It was reported that this surface coat appeared on the plasma membrane of freed merozoites when they were exposed to culture medium (Miller *et al.*, 1975b), but that it was of parasite origin (Mason *et al.*, 1977). Bannister (1977) has described the surface coat of merozoites not exposed to immune serum as consisting of bristlelike filaments about 20 nm in height which in thin-section electron micrographs appear to be T- or Y-shaped. The material of the surface coat binds antiplasmodial antibody present in immune serum, and merozoites exposed to immune serum agglutinate. Miller *et al.* (1975b) observed that agglutinated merozoites could still attach to erythrocytes by their anterior ends, but that the agglutinated mass could not enter the red cells. Miller *et al.* (1973a, 1975a, 1977a) demonstrated specific receptors for malaria merozoites on erythrocytes. Miller *et al.* (1975b) have considered that, if their *in vitro* observations of penetration inhibition by immune serum are indicative of events in the immune host, then antibody blocks erythrocyte penetration by agglutination, not by neutralization of merozoite receptors for the erythrocyte.

Kilejian (1978) has isolated a material from *P. lophurae* which will induce immunity. This material may have a function in merozoite penetration (Kilejian, 1976). There is no evidence of the role, if any, of antibody to this material in the control of plasmodia under natural conditions.

The evidence available at present thus indicates that antibodies do interfere with the plasmodial merozoite's ability to penetrate the red cell. This appears to take place by physical interference with penetration by the mass of material accumulated on the outside of the merozoite, not by highly specific blocking of the parasite's erythrocyte receptors (Miller *et al.*, 1975a). The observation of Hamburger and Kreier (1975) that transfer of antibody-mediated protection to rats required that antibody be injected into the rats to supplement antibody bound to the parasites if protection is to occur also supports the suggestion that antibody does not protect simply by specific blocking of parasite receptors for erythrocytes.

4. Role of Complement in Malaria

Complement may aid in destroying parasites in concert with antibody. The complement is then activated by the classical pathway, and the activation may result in lysis of the parasite or in facilitated phagocytosis. Complement may act independently of induced antibody, either being directly activated by some component of the parasite or being activated by a noninducible serum factor such as properdin. Again the result may be lysis of the parasite or facilitated phagocytosis. The extent to which these mechanisms of complement action contribute to host defense against plasmodia has been the subject of several studies. Complement activity of sera from monkeys with *P. knowlesi,* hamsters with *P. berghei,* and chickens with *P. gallinacium* infections was greatly reduced in comparison to the complement activity of normal sera from the same animals. The degree of reduction in C′ levels generally correlated well with the severity of the infections. In animals with synchronized *P. knowlesi* infections complement concentrations decreased greatly at the time of merozoite release (Fogel *et al.,* 1966). The decreases in complement levels at the time of merozoite release were interpreted as indicating complement fixation by the complexes formed when antibody reacted with antigen released at the time of schizogony (Cooper and Fogel, 1966; Glew *et al.,* 1975). Complement is also activated in children with acute *P. falciparum* infections, probably through the classical pathway (Greenwood and Brueton, 1974). Complement levels in these children return to normal rapidly after parasitological cure (Ree, 1976).

While complement is thus clearly consumed during plasmodial infection, there is no evidence that the binding of complement by antiparasitic antibody–antigen complexes facilitates antibody-mediated parasite clearance. Diggs *et al.* (1972b) and Atkinson *et al.* (1975) found that depression of C3 levels in the serum of infected hosts by cobra venom factor did not diminish antibody-mediated protection. Williams *et al.* (1975) found no difference in the course of infection between mice of strains deficient in complement because of a genetic defect and mice of types syngeneic except that their genes were functional at the locus for complement synthesis.

While there is thus no evidence that complement is a factor in antibody-mediated parasite destruction in malaria, it has been suggested that it may be involved in the hemolysis which occurs during malaria (Ree, 1976) and that complement depletion during infection may contribute to some of the immune complex diseases occurring concomitantly with or as sequellae to malaria (Krettli *et al.,* 1976).

F. Reticuloendothelial Function in Malaria

Gingrich (1941) studied the effect of injection of large numbers of foreign avian erythrocytes upon the course of *P. cathemerium* infection in canaries. On each of three consecutive days he injected 1 ml of a 50% suspension of washed foreign erythrocytes of one species into canaries; he then repeated the procedure for the next 3 days with erythrocytes of a different species, and so on. The reason for changing the type of erythrocyte every 3 days was to avoid the effects of the immune response to the foreign erythrocytes, which became apparent after 3 days. Gingrich (1941) monitored parasitemia as a measure of the effect of the injections. He considered that his experiments determined the effect of "reticuloendothelial blockade" upon the ability of the host to control the plasmodia. His experiments were thus in a sense the reverse of those done later in which the ability of the host to clear colloidal carbon or some other particle during infection was studied. Gingrich (1941) found that the injection of foreign erythrocytes had no effect on the rate of increase in parasitemia during the period of acute rise in parasitemia and concluded from this observation that phagocytosis was not a primary factor in determining the rate of parasite increase during this period. He found, however, that birds which received foreign erythrocytes either had a delayed or aborted crisis and a delayed or aborted recovery. He also was able to produce relapses by the injection of foreign erythrocytes into canaries which were controlling their infections. His conclusion was that "phagocytosis (whatever its relation to humoral factors may be) is an active process and a major factor in acquired immunity to malarial infection in birds." This conclusion was based on the assumption that the reticuloendothelial system was "blockaded" by the injected erythrocytes and that, when phagocytosis was invoked to control the infection during and after crisis, it was inadequate in the "blockaded" canaries. A more modern explanation would be that the foreign red cells caused immunosuppression which prevented the host from developing an immune response to the parasites.

Goble and Singer (1960) similarly found that intravenous injection of india ink did not affect the rate of parasite increase in mice infected with *P. berghei* during the first 6 days of infection but did interfere with their ability to control parasitemia thereafter. In the injected mice the parasitemias were higher after 6 days of infection, and death occurred sooner than in the uninjected mice that served as controls.

In the broadest sense, thus the mice injected with india ink and the canaries injected with foreign red cells were "immunosuppressed," and their ability to control the parasites was reduced by the injection of foreign materials. Whether this immunosuppression was a result of blocked phagocytosis, as was believed at the time, or delayed and poor development of a specific antiparasitic response is not clear. The absence of an effect from the blockage during the early stages of infection and the deleterious effect of blockage just at the time the immune response would have been expected to occur in "unblocked" mice and canaries suggests that immunosuppression may have occurred as a result of the injection of foreign materials.

While the earlier studies on reticuloendothelial activity in animals with malaria such as those by Gingrich (1941) and Goble and Singer (1960) just discussed were concerned with the effect of reticuloendothelial blockage on the course of the disease, most of the more recent work was designed to determine the effect of the disease on the phagocytic capacity of the reticuloendothelial system. Cox *et al.* (1963a,b) observed initial stimulation of reticuloendothelial activity in chicks infected with *P. gallinaceum* and mice infected with *P. vinckei* malaria; late in the infection they observed a rapid decrease in reticuloendothelial activity. The rate of clearance of intravenously injected colloidal carbon was the measure of the reticuloendothelial activity. The infections in the hosts and with the parasites chosen were uniformly fatal.

Lucia and Nussenzweig (1969) compared carbon clearance in uninfected mice and in *P. chabaudi*- and *P. vinckei*-infected mice. Their results were different from those of Cox *et al.* (1963a,b). The rates of carbon clearance were high during the early stages of infection, as were those observed by Cox *et al.*, at least after the parasitemias passed 10%; however, Lucia and Nussenzweig did not observe a subsequent depression of the rate of carbon clearance even in mice which died. Some of the *P. chabaudi*-infected mice recovered from the infection. In these mice during acute infection the carbon clearance rate was elevated during periods of chronic infection and recovery; however, carbon clearance rates often returned to normal.

The studies of Cantrell *et al.* (1970) and Elko and Cantrell (1970) were designed to determine the relationships between reticuloendothelial function and drug treatment. They concluded that the two factors were independent. Their carbon clearance data lend some support to the observation of an infection-related depression of carbon clearance which occurs following the initial stimulation (Cox *et al.*, 1963a,b). Cantrell and Elko (1970) observed that early in infection carbon clearance was abnormally rapid. As infections progressed; however, many rats lost their ability to clear carbon from their circulation rapidly, despite the fact that parasitemia remained high. They observed, however, that loss of the ability to clear carbon from the circulation rapidly did not bear any relationship to the ability of the rats to recover from the infection.

In humans (Sheagrin *et al.*, 1970) clearance of an injected particle, in this instance microaggregated human serum albumin, was also abnormally high during acute malaria. The clearance rates returned to normal following treatment and recovery.

Loose *et al.* (1973a,b) studied the effects of depression and stimulation of the reticuloendothelial system on the course of *P. lophurae* infections in the chicken.

In general, treatments which depressed the system increased the parasitemias over those seen in untreated controls (Loose *et al.,* 1973a). In their studies on chickens they found that zymosan, a stimulant to the reticuloendothelial systems of mammals, was a depressant of the system in chickens (Loose *et al.,* 1973a). They also observed that treatment with the estrogen diethylstilbestrol, a substance that does not affect the mammalian reticuloendothelial system, profoundly depressed the reticuloendothelial system of chickens. In general the observations of Loose *et al.* (1973a,b) that depression of the reticuloendothelial system depressed host defense against malaria are in agreement with those of earlier workers but emphasize the importance of understanding the characteristics of this system before interpreting and generalizing the results.

Kitchen and DiLuzio (1971) have also carried out a study that emphasizes the pitfalls of data interpretation with particular relevance to interpretation of carbon clearance studies. They confirmed the observation of enhanced carbon clearance by plasmodium-infected rats but found no change with infection in the rate of clearance of another material, a gelatinized lipid emulsion. On the basis of very ambiguous and contradictory data they concluded that alteration of humoral recognition factors, not changes in phagocytic capacity during infection, were responsible for the results obtained in carbon clearance studies.

Greenwood *et al.* (1971) and Loose and DiLuzio (1976) attempted to relate reticuloendothelial function alterations to immune capacity in rodents with malaria. Greenwood *et al.* (1971) did not find a significant difference in splenic uptake of labeled sheep erythrocytes between mice with malaria and uninfected mice, while Loose and DiLuzio (1976) found a profound increase in the rate of vascular clearance in the infected mice, with a shift toward hepatic sequestration and away from the splenic sequestration. Both groups of workers found that the spleens of malarious mice injected with sheep red cells contained fewer lymphocytes secreting anti-sheep red cell antibody than the spleens of normal mice injected with equal numbers of sheep red cells. Loose and DiLuzio (1976) suggest that hepatic localization of antigen may reduce the antigen available to stimulate splenic lymphocytes, and Greenwood *et al.* (1971) propose the existence of a defect in the cells transporting antigen to the general centers. This latter suggestion was based on the observation that aggregated human IgG did not accumulate in germinal centers of spleens of mice with malaria. One wonders if germinal centers specific for plasmodial antigens are not deficient in lymphocytes capable of binding other antigens. If germinal centers are clones expanded by stimulation with a given antigen, this should be expected.

G. Role of Macrophages in Parasite Destruction

Macrophages may remove parasites from the circulation either when they are free of the host erythrocyte or by ingesting the parasitized erythrocyte. It is probable that the mechanisms by which these two means of destruction are mediated are distinct. Zuckerman (1945) was not able to demonstrate opsonins for chicken erythrocytes in the serum of chickens infected with or recovering from plasmodial infection. She did, however, demonstrate that erythrocytes of chickens with very high parasitemias and chickens undergoing post-peak anemia (ie crisis) were more readily phagocytized *in vitro* by macrophages than erythrocytes from chickens with early rising parasitemia or chickens with low-grade chronic infections. Phagocytosis-stimulating substances were also present in reduced amounts in the serum of chickens undergoing the crisis. The opsonin for homologous erythrocytes present in the serum of the hyperimmunized chickens described in the same report was almost certainly antibody to blood group antigens, not an autoantibody and quite irrelevant to the plasmodial infection.

Kretschmar and Jerusalem (1963) and Jerusalem (1965) observed significant erythrophagocytosis in smear preparations and in sections of spleens of mice infected with *P. berghei*. The erythrophagocytosis was most prominent on days 10–14 after infection, a time at which parasitemia was very high and the mice were in a crisis. In other studies reporting significant erythrophagocytosis *in vivo* (Aikawa and Sprinz, 1971) and *in vitro* (Seitz *et al.*, 1977) during plasmodial infection, insufficient data were provided to determine the relationship between the stage of the infection and the degree of erythrophagocytosis observed.

Kreier and Ristic (1964) and later Lustig *et al.* (1977) observed globulin coating on erythrocytes of mice after day 10 of infection with *P. berghei*, just when erythrophagocytosis is prominent. These results suggest opsonization of the erythrocytes during the crises. The presence of globulins specific for enzyme-modified and fixed erythrocytes in the serum and on the erythrocytes of rats (Kreier *et al.*, 1966; Kreier and Leste, 1967, 1968), chickens (Kreier, 1969; Gautam *et al.*, 1970), and humans (Rosenberg *et al.*, 1973) with severe plasmodial infections has been demonstrated. At least some of these globulins are specific for lipids exposed by the action of proteolytic enzymes on the erythrocyte membrane (Seed and Kreier, 1969).

Normal noninfected animals can clear trypsin-modified erythrocytes from their circulation (Kreier, 1969), probably with the aid of an opsonin normally present (Kay, 1975). Zuckerman's (1945) observations and those of Kreier *et al.* (1966) strongly suggest that much of the erythrophagocytosis occurring in animals and humans with plasmodial infections is probably the result of erythrocyte membrane damage caused either by parasite proteolytic enzymes or host proteolytic enzymes activated as a result of antigen–antibody and complement reactions. The rapidity with which erythrocyte destruction returns to normal rates after specific antiparasite therapy is good evidence against a true autoimmune or hypersplenic mechanism for erythrocyte destruction in malaria (Swann and Kreier, 1973).

Some of the erythrophagocytosis may result from the action of opsonic antibody directed against parasite antigens in and on the erythrocyte membrane. This mechanism is most completely described in *P. knowlesi* malaria in which the membrane-associated antigens are variant-specific (Brown *et al.*, 1970c; Butcher and Cohen, 1972; Butcher *et al.*, 1978). That phagocytosis of parasitized erythrocytes is an effective mechanism for killing parasites, even those of an avian plasmodium, was demonstrated by Alvarez (1952). A more complete discussion of the mechanisms of erythrocyte destruction in malaria can be found in Volume 2, Chapter 1.

Trubowitz and Masek (1968) were probably the first to describe phagocytosis of a living plasmodial merozoite. The phagocytosis by a polymorphonuclear leukocyte was recorded by time-lapse cinematography. The specimen studied was a drop of blood from a patient who had undergone a relapse of a latent *P. falciparum* infection. Trubowitz and Masek (1968) observed that leukocytes did not move toward parasitized erythrocytes, even those containing mature schizonts, but moved rapidly toward and ingested the merozoites released when a schizont-containing erythrocyte ruptured. This study was made on whole blood from an immune individual, so opsonins may have been present, although they were not considered by the authors.

Chow and Kreier (1972) and later Hamburger and Kreier (1975, 1976) also observed that *in vitro* phagocytes were more likely to ingest free parasites than parasitized or nonparasitized erythrocytes. Chow and Kreier (1972) reported the preferential uptake of free parasites from a crude mixture of free parasites and parasitized and uninfected erythrocytes prepared by forcing blood cells from *P. berghei*-infected rats through a fine-gauge needle, while Hamburger and Kreier (1975, 1976) used free *P. berghei* prepared by continuous-flow sonication (CFS) (Kreier *et al.*, 1976). In these studies by Kreier and his associates it was observed that immune serum increased the amount of phagocytosis of free parasites but had little or no effect on erythrophagocytosis. In all cases free parasites were ingested even in normal serum. Chow and Kreier (1972) also reported that macrophages from immune rats were more efficient in picking up free parasites than macrophages from normal rats, that complement did not appear to be necessary for phagocytosis, and that trypsinization prevented adhesion and phagocytosis by immune macrophages. Chow and Kreier (1972) observed that incubation in immune serum restored the capacity of macrophages to ingest parasites lost as a result of trypsinization. These results were rather a surprise, for the studies were undertaken to evaluate erythrophagocytosis, and phagocytosis of free parasites was not even being considered.

The studies by Green and Kreier (1978) and Brooks and Kreier (1978), unlike those of Chow and Kreier (1972), were undertaken to determine the interactions of macrophages, antibody, and free *P. berghei* parasites. In these studies parasites freed by CFS treatment were used (Kreier *et al.*, 1976). Green and Kreier (1978) demonstrated that a macrophage cytophilic antibody and an opsonic antibody were both present in immune rat serum. The cytophilic antibody was characterized as an IgG1 type which bound to the macrophage before it could bind to its antigen. The cytophilic antibody mediated parasite adhesion to the macrophage but only weakly stimulated internalization. The opsonic antibody was an IgG2 type and facilitated phagocytosis. If, as Strossel (1976) suggests, phagocytosis proceeds by movement of pseudopods around the particle from one recognition site to the next and if the antibody molecules are the main recognition sites in this system, then it is reasonable to expect that the opsonic antibody which coats the parasite would facilitate ingestion while the cytophilic antibody, localized on a few points on the macrophage membrane would not be efficient in promoting ingestion.

By passive protection tests Green and Kreier (1978) demonstrated that the cytophilic and opsonic antibodies acted synergistically in conferring protection on susceptible rats.

The high degree of phagocytosis of free parasites even in the absence of immune serum was puzzling in the studies by Kreier and his associates, because in nonimmune rats and mice parasitemias increase at first almost in proportion to the reproduction rate of the plasmodia. This observation suggests that in the absence of antibodies parasites are not destroyed *in vivo*. The solution to this problem was obtained by electron micrographic studies of the ingestion process (Brooks and Kreier, 1978). These studies demonstrated that in the absence of specific antibody almost all the phagocytic ingestion which occurred involved unencapsulated trophozoites, while substantial numbers of merozoites were only ingested in the presence of immune serum. As the merozoite is the only form of the parasite that can infect new erythrocytes, their ingestion would affect the course of the disease. Ingestion of trophozoites, on the other hand, is a scavenging process and not a host defense mechanism. Brooks and Kreier (1978) have proposed that the merozoite capsule (i.e., surface coat of Ladda, 1969) is an antiphagocytic defense.

H. Spleen Function

Our understanding of the role of the spleen in host defense against malaria is complicated by the fact that it has multiple functions and by the fact that all of its functions may be carried out by other systems in its absence. Splenectomy is thus not invariably or necessarily fatal even in the presence of an infection such as malaria. Many studies (Zuckerman and Yoeli, 1954; Box and Gringrich, 1958; Kretschmar and Jerusalem, 1963; El-Nahal, 1966; Todorovic *et al.*, 1967; Wyler *et al.*, 1977) on blood stage parasite-initiated plasmodial infection in intact and splenectomized animals show clearly that animals without spleens are less able to control their infections than intact animals. The presence of a spleen also enhances the animal's ability to develop immunity following immunization with irradiated parasitized erythrocytes (Wellde *et al.*, 1972) or irradiated sporozoites (Spitalny *et al.*, 1976).

The spleen increases greatly in size during plasmodial infection in all species (Volume 3, Chapter 3). In the mouse and rat in particular some of this hypertrophy can be accounted for by the development of erythropoietic cells. With continuing infection and anemia the proportion of the cells of the spleen engaged in erythropoiesis progressively increases (Singer, 1954b). The apparently anomalous observation that splenectomized mice and rats infected with *P. berghei* may develop parasitemias more slowly than intact ones, but are ultimately less able to control the infection, is a result of the requirement of *P. berghei* for the immature erythrocytes supplied by the hypertrophic spleen (Singer, 1954a; Zuckerman and Yoeli, 1954). The great degree to which the spleens of rats and mice may become devoted to erythropoiesis has been shown by studies on polyribosome profiles of spleens of immunized, infected, or anemic mice (Poels, 1977) and by studies on radioiron uptake by spleen cells (Frankenberg *et al.*, 1977). Frankenberg *et al.* (1977) suggested that the ability of the infected animal to mount an immune response to the parasite would be reduced by a shift of stem cells to the formation of erythropoietic rather than immune-oriented cells in the spleen. Gravely *et al.* (1976), however, suggested that the shift to erythropoiesis, while certainly shaping the course of the disease, was more likely a consequence of the poor immune response of the highly susceptible rodents rather than its cause.

The spleen is a major site of phagocytic cells appropriately positioned to ingest foreign and damaged autologous cells present in the blood (Singer, 1954b). Splenic phagocytes, unlike liver phagocytes, are appropriately positioned to interact with lymphocytes. Weidanz and Rank (1975) have shown that during acute plasmodial infection the ability of these macrophages to present a heterologous antigen to lymphocytes is reduced, while this activity by lymph node macrophages is normal. Weidanz and Rank suggested that the phagocytic load on the splenic macrophages was responsible for the effect. It is of course not to be assumed that the ability of the splenic macrophages to present malaria antigen is necessarily reduced just because their ability to process red cells is reduced.

During the crisis stage of infection, but probably not during the early period of rapid rise of the parasitemia (Gingrich, 1941) or during convalescence, substantial phagocytosis of erythrocytes occurs in the spleen (Kretschmar and Jerusalem, 1963; Jerusalem, 1965). Both parasitized and nonparasitized erythrocytes may be ingested (Kretschmar and Jerusalem, 1963; Jerusalem, 1965; Mungyerova and Jerusalem, 1966; Spira and Zuckerman, 1965). It has been shown that the membranes of the erythrocytes at the crisis are damaged and may be sensitized by an IgM (Kreier *et al.*, 1966; Rosenberg *et al.*, 1973) or an IgG antibody (Lustig *et al.*, 1977). It is probably an error therefore to speak of phogocytosis of normal red cells at the crisis, as the evidence available indicates that the phagocytosis at the crisis is of erythrocytes that have substantial membrane damage (Kreier *et al.*, 1966) and are opsonized. A means by which erythrocytes could incur such damage is suggested by the observation that the erythrocytes of some children with falciparum malaria and anemia gave positive tests with antisera to C3b and C3d (Greenwood *et al.*, 1978).

Antibody-mediated immunity to plasmodia involves a splenic component. Various workers (Brown and Phillips, 1974; Golenser *et al.*, 1975) have shown that antibody-mediated protection against plasmodia is less in splenectomized than in intact rodents. One probable contribution of the spleen to antibody-mediated immunity to malaria is phagocytic. Jerusalem *et al.* (1971), Miller *et al.* (1975b), and Hamburger and Kreier (1976) have shown that *in vitro* exposure of parasites to antibody does not kill them. Jerusalem *et al.* (1971), and Hamburger and Kreier (1976) have further demonstrated that antibody-coated parasites are destroyed after injection into an appropriate host. Green and Kreier (1978) demonstrated opsonic and cytophilic antibody in immune rat sera, while Brooks and Kreier (1978) demonstrated that phagocytosis of free merozoites required these antibodies. At least part of the splenic contribution to antibody-mediated antiplasmodial immunity (Brown and Phillips, 1974; Golenser *et al.*, 1975) is almost certainly the phagocytosis by cytophilic antibody-armed macrophages of opsonized merozoites.

Increased red cell rigidity at the crisis may also be responsible for phagocytosis of red cells in the spleen (Areekul, 1973). Red cells must be readily deformable in order to traverse the narrow, circuitous macrophage-lined cords and squeeze through the small fenestrations of the basement membrane between cords and sinuses. Not only may rigid erythrocytes be retained and phagocytized while attempting passage through the spleen, but the removal of parasites from the erythrocytes has also been reported to occur (Schnitzer *et al.*, 1972).

Zuckerman *et al.* (1969b) suggested that erythrophagocytosis in excess of normal might be a direct result of the hypersplenism associated with malaria. It is doubtful that this is a major factor, however, because erythrocyte destruction rates return to normal after parasitemia is arrested by treatment more rapidly than splenomegaly is resolved (Swann and Kreier, 1973).

Whatever the consequences of splenomegaly may be for erythrocyte and parasite destruction, splenomegaly and phagocyte accumulation in the spleen are immunologically mediated phenomena. Coleman *et al.* (1976) demonstrated the secretion of macrophage migration inhibition factor by splenic lymphocytes exposed to plasmodial antigens, and Wyler and Gallin (1977) demonstrated a mononuclear cell chemotactic factor in spleens of animals with malaria. Wyler and Gallin (1977) observed that the chemotactic factor and the migration inhibition factor acting jointly could provide a mechanism for macrophage accumulation in the spleen. The immunological mechanisms controlling splenomegaly and enhanced phagocytosis and associated anemia were shown by Roberts and Weidanz (1978) to be thymus-dependent responses.

A major function of the spleen in animals with plasmodial infection is to provide a site for the interaction of antigen and the various cells responsible for the immune response. This function has been studied most thoroughly by means of spleen cell transfer between immune and susceptible rodents of inbred strains. The subject of the interaction of the various types of lymphocytes in the induction of immunity to malaria is discussed in Section II,B. Here a brief treatment of the subject will be made to emphasize the role of the spleen in induction of the immune response. It should be remembered that the cellular interactions which result in the induction of an immune response occur at other sites in the body as well as in the spleen, although the greater susceptibility of splenectomized animals to malaria suggests that the spleen is an important site for their occurrence.

Immune serum transfer confers on susceptible individuals only a moderate degree of resistance to plasmodia. It was almost certainly the hope of individuals undertaking spleen cell transfer studies to identify an immune effector cell that would confer more effective immunity than immune serum.

Stechschulte (1969) and Phillips (1970) found that in fact that transfer of immune spleen cells to susceptible inbred rats was a more effective means of transfer of immunity than transfer of immune serum. A consensus now seems to be emerging, however, that splenic T cells do not act directly on the parasites or parasitized erythrocytes but indirectly on splenic B cells to yield an effective and flexible antibody-mediated method of parasite control (Brown *et al.*, 1976a,b; Gravely and Kreier, 1976; McDonald and Phillips, 1978b). How the nonantibody-mediated immunity reported to occur in B cell-deficient mice (Roberts and Weidanz, 1979) and chickens (Rank and Weidanz, 1976) will be related to the antibody-mediated immunity which has been more thoroughly defined is at present uncertain.

Wyler *et al.* (1977) observed that splenectomized monkeys developed much more severe parasitemia than intact monkeys. This observation is in agreement with other observations on the effect on splenectomy on malaria. In this study on *P. inui* infection in rhesus monkeys, however, Wyler *et al.* (1977) observed that splenectomized monkeys cleared their infections in less than 1 year, while in intact monkeys the infections persisted for 1–13 years. These observations were interpreted to suggest that the spleen exerts a protective role during the acute stage and a suppressive role during the chronic stage of *P. inui* infections in rhesus monkeys. A similar dual role for the spleen in the control of malaria does not exist in rats. Zuckerman and Yoeli (1954) observed that no splenectomized rat which survived *P. berghei* infection was capable of suppressing the infection to latency at a time when parasites were no longer demonstrable in intact control rats. In several splenectomized rats parasites persisted for more than a year after infection. Phillips (1970) similarly observed that 75% of intact rats surviving *P.*

berghei infection cleared their infections within 4–6 months, while all splenectomized rats maintained chronic infections for at least 6 months.

I. Infection Immunity or Premunity

The concept of infection immunity, i.e., premunity, is familiar to individuals working with blood parasites. The concept of an immunity associated with a continuing infection was formulated and developed by Sergent *et al.* (1924, 1934, 1945) and dominated thought on immunity to blood parasites for many years. Callow (1977) believes that the immune mechanisms by which infection immunity is mediated are not basically different from those operative in other types of immunity.

It need not in fact be assumed that the premune state is implemented by immune mechanisms different from those induced by nonliving antigens. If the antigens important in the immune response are weak antigens, it is possible that a constant stimulation by antigens released by the living parasite would be needed to maintain adequate immunity. If the important antigens were labile or only present in small amounts or at certain times during the life cycle of the parasite, it could again be necessary to have a growing parasite population constantly releasing antigen to induce and sustain the immunity (Schindler, 1966).

Experimental support for the maintenance of immunity in premune animals by constant antigenic stimulation is provided by studies on the fading of immunity in premune mice following drug cure (Eling, 1978a,b,c). Eling did not observe a sudden loss of immunity in cured mice but rather a slow decay— exactly what would be expected if continuous stimulation by a weak antigen were needed to maintain the immune state of the premune animals.

Hamsters recovered from clinical *B. microti* infection continue to maintain a low-level parasitemia for several months. Parasitemia in such blood does not increase when the blood is placed in culture. If, however, the plasma is removed and replaced with plasma from a normal hamster before culture, then parasitemia increases rapidly (Bautista and Kreier, 1979). These results indicate that antibody in the serum is a significant factor in the control of parasitemia in preimmune hamsters. It is probable that serum functions similarly in humans premune to malaria.

In a paper on immunity to malaria, Brown *et al.* (1970a) reported that rhesus monkeys saved from death by treatment of their *P. knowlesi* infections with drugs developed long-lasting chronic infections, while monkeys immunized with killed schizonts of *P. knowlesi* in Freund's complete adjuvant (FCA) developed a sterile immunity if they survived the initial parasitemia after challenge.

Cohen and his colleagues (Mitchell *et al.*, 1975) confirmed and extended these findings by demonstrating that *P. knowlesi* merozoites in FCA produced the same type of immunity to challenge as the schizont preparations. The injection of schizonts or merozoites in other adjuvants, even Freund's incomplete adjuvant (FIA), did not induce an immunity capable of eradicating the challenge infections (Brown et al., 1970b; Mitchell et al., 1975). Even the observation that schizonts or merozoites in FCA induce an effective sterilizing immunity against P. knowlesi malaria in rhesus monkeys (Brown et al., 1970a; Mitchell et al., 1975) while natural infection only induces a clinical immunity associated with a long-lasting chronic infection is compatible with the hypothesis that the sterilizing immunity is induced by an immune response to a poor antigen acting in conventional ways. In this case the adjuvant causes the animal to do quickly what it would otherwise do very slowly.

In Section II,H evidence was cited (Zuckerman and Yoeli, 1954; Phillips, 1970) which indicated that rats without spleens were not only more likely to die of P. berghei infection but were also more likely to develop a persistent low-level infection than were rats with spleens. Intact rhesus monkeys, on the other hand, are reported to be better able to control acute P. inui infection than splenectomized ones, but the intact monkeys which survive the initial infections develop a persistent infection while the splenectomized ones do not (Wyler et al., 1977). Malaria in intact humans, like malaria in splenectomized rats or intact rhesus monkeys, is frequently chronic. The infection is characterized by relapse and recrudescence—relapse if the parasite reenters the blood from an extrahemic site and recrudescence if the surge of parasitemia orginates from a persistent low-level parasitemia (Coatney, 1976).

Manipulation of the immune system of rhesus monkeys (Brown et al., 1970a) so that they rapidly develop a sterile immunity on challenge with P. knowlesi instead of a chronic infection has raised the hope that similar manipulation of the immune system of humans will be possible (Cox, 1974b). Attempts to determine in what way the adjuvant changed the immune system to prevent the parasites from surviving have not been fruitful (Brown et al., 1970a,b; Phillips et al., 1970). Both monkeys which were immunized with FCA and erradicated their infections after challenge and those which did not, developed agglutinins and opsonins for schizont-infected cells and precipitins for soluble parasite antigens. Neither group of monkeys developed serum lysins for erythrocytes (Brown et al., 1970a,b). Some degree of delayed hypersensitivity to plasmodial antigens was present only in the FCA-sensitized monkeys, but no specific cytoxic activity of immune spleen cells on infected erythrocytes could be demonstrated in any of the experimental monkeys (Phillips et al., 1970). Wyler et al. (1977) has suggested that the rhesus spleen contains a population of cells which suppresses the immunological response after it is induced, but no experimental support for this hypothesis is yet available.

Premune animals limit expression of the clinical features of the disease caused by the parasites they harbor (McGregor, 1972). McGregor (1972) observed that one of the early signs of acquisition of immunity to malaria was the ability to curtail the clinical signs of the disease while a relatively dense parasitemia persisted. In this context premunity may represent a situation in which the host develops the ability to clear the products of the parasite's growth efficiently while not developing an effective mechanism for destroying the parasite itself. Parasites such as plasmodia have complex antigenic natures (Kreier, 1977). A poorly antigenic capsule and an intracellular location could protect the parasite even when the host has developed an effective immune-mediated system for eliminating the products of the parasite's metabolism. Experimental support for such a hypothesis can be drawn from the observation that an immune response to a variety of plasmodial antigens not associated with an effective antiparasitemic immunity occurs in mice dying of malaria, while an immune response to other antigens only occurs in mice which have developed an effective antiparasitic immunity (Seitz, 1975, 1976).

J. Mechanisms of Evasion of the Host Defense by the Parasites

That plasmodia may survive and reproduce for substantial periods of time in their hosts despite the best efforts of the host to eliminate them (McGregor, 1972) is one of the few hard facts available in any discussion of evasion by plasmodia of the host defenses. Cohen (1976) listed possible mechanisms of immune evasion by parasites in a recent review of literature on the survival of parasites in the immunized host. The following list of mechanisms was freely adapted from his paper. The mechanisms are antigenic variation; release of soluble blocking antigens; interference by the parasite with the host's immune response, including stimulation of the production of blocking antibody, blocking of K cells, activation of suppressor cells, induction of immune tolerence, and polyclonal activation of lymphocytes; antigenic disguise; and growth in a protected location, for example, intracellularly.

Antigenic variation in erythrocytic plasmodia has been described for *P. berghei* (Cox, 1959), for *P. knowlesi* (Brown and Brown, 1965), and for *P. lophurae* (Corwin et al., 1970). Chronic infections with *P. knowlesi* in rhesus monkeys occur as successive waves of parasitemia, the parasites of which are antigenically distinct from those present previously (Brown et al., 1968). It has been reported that antibody which inhibits plasmodial penetration of erythrocytes *in vitro* is predominantly specific for the variant antigens (Butcher and Cohen, 1972), but Cox (1974a) states that antibody specific for variant antigens has nothing to do with protection. The occurrence in monkeys of successive waves of parasitemia, each milder than the preceding one and each of a distinct antigenic type (Butcher and Cohen, 1972; Brown and Brown, 1965), and the final resolution of the infection by the development of a protective immunity transcending variation, lead one to consider that the immune response to the variants has some role in protection even if it does not have an overriding one. Whether antigenic variation occurs in plasmodia of humans and, if it occurs, whether it has a role in immunity is at present unknown.

Soluble antigens of parasite origin are present in the plasma of animals (Eaton, 1939; Dooris and McGhee, 1975; Seitz, 1976) and humans (McGregor *et al.*, 1968) with acute plasmodial infections. In Gambian children the antigen usually ceased to be demonstrable within 7 days of drug cure (Wilson *et al.*, 1975). Antigens appeared to be released from human red cells infected with *P. falciparum* at the time of schizont rupture. Immune complexes formed if antibody was present, and immune serum opsonized parasite debris from ruptured erythrocytes (Wilson and Bartholomew, 1975). Incomplete protection was produced by the immunization of rhesus monkeys with soluble *P. knowlesi* antigens obtained from plasma (Collins *et al.*, 1977). While it is appealing to suggest that soluble plasmodial antigens in the plasma may block immune effector mechanisms (Wilson, 1974), at present there are no data to support this claim.

The interference by the parasite with the host's immune response is a subject to which much speculation has been devoted (Wedderburn, 1974; Greenwood, 1974; Terry, 1977; Playfair, 1978). Host responses to heterologous antigens injected during the course of acute or chronic infection are commonly depressed but, as noted by Terry (1977), the significance of this depression in the control of the parasite is quite unclear. It can be expected that animals dying of malaria probably are not producing a satisfactory response to parasite antigens, although as Seitz (1976) notes they may be producing an immune response which is not of any use to them. Jerusalem *et al.* (1971) and Hamburger and Kreier (1976) demonstrated an antibody in immunized rodents which under certain conditions appeared to enhance the severity of infection. Most passive transfer tests, however, as noted earlier in this chapter, have demonstrated antibody which mediates at least partial protection in the host.

As far as blocking of K-cell action (Cohen, 1976) is concerned, the action of K cells in malaria has yet to be demonstrated. There has been one report of what is probably antibody-mediated erythrocyte cytotoxicity in malaria (Coleman *et al.*, 1975), but other workers have not been able to obtain consistent evidence of cyotoxic activity in malaria (Playfair, 1978). Thus demonstration of a mechanism of evasion of cell-mediated parasite killing by cells other than macrophages in malaria will have to await the demonstration of parasite destruction by such cells.

The experimental evidence for suppressor cell activity in malaria and for the development of immune tolerance to plasmodial antigens ranges from indirect to nonexistent. Dorris and McGhee (1975) induced tolerance to serum antigen in newly hatched chickens, but what relationship this may have to natural infection in adult animals is unclear. Mice (Krettli and Nussenzweig, 1974) and young rats (Gravely *et al.*, 1976) dying of malaria do not undergo clonal expansion of their

T cells, while mature rats do (Gravely *et al.*, 1976). While it has been suggested that suppressor T cells may be the cause of the failure of the mice and young rats to expand the T-cell populations, no proof has been forthcoming. Playfair (1978) states that, in mice infected with *P. berghei* where nonspecific immunosuppression is particularly intense, he has not been able to find convincing evidence for suppressor cells.

There is evidence for polyclonal B-cell activation during plasmodial infection (Freeman and Parrish, 1978), and it may be that plasmodia produce a mitogenic factor (Greenwood and Vick, 1975; Strickland, 1978). General polyclonal lymphocyte activation could possibly interfere with the specific antiplasmodial response, but again data supporting such an effect are lacking.

There is at present no evidence that plasmodia, like some trypanosomes, can assume an antigenic disguise by coating themselves with host materials (Desowitz, 1970).

The final mechanism on the list, growth in a protected location, i.e., intracellularly, is probably the mechanism of evasion for which there is the best experimental evidence. Plasmodia, unlike toxoplasma and certain other parasites, do not reside in phagocytes. Erythrocytes have no intracellular defenses, and liver parenchymal cells and vascular endothelial cells may not either. It is thus not even necessary to demonstrate a mechanism by which the parasite protects itself from the host cell's defense mechanisms to propose that intracellular growth of plasmodia is growth in a protected location.

Coggeshall (1940) quite early suggested that the intracellular location of the parasite protected it from the action of antibody. Cohen *et al.* (1961) and McGregor *et al.* (1963) showed that immune globulin had its main effect *in vivo* at the time of schizont rupture. Later Cohen *et al.* (1972) and Phillips *et al.* (1972) showed quite clearly that immune serum did not affect intracellular growth of the parasites but inhibited reinvasion. Additional studies on antibody action by Jerusalem *et al.* (1971), Diggs and Osler (1975), and Hamburger and Kreier (1976), among many others, all confirm Coggeshall's (1940) suggestion that the intracellular location of the parasite during most of its life cycle shields it from antibody action fairly effectively. The killing of the parasite in the erythrocyte, which occurs at the crisis, will be discussed in the next section.

K. The Crisis

In most individuals with malaria there is a period after parasitemia develops during which clinical signs of the infection are not severe. During this period parasite numbers may increase quite rapidly. This period is usually ended by development of the crisis (Taliaferro and Taliaferro, 1944; 1947; Thompson, 1944; Zuckerman and Yoeli, 1954). A rapid fall in the packed erythrocyte volume, a rapid fall in the parasitemia, and the appearance of pycnotic and degenerating parasites in erythrocytes are characteristic of the crisis. It has been assumed that an immune response is responsible for the crisis, but little is known of the actual mechanisms inducing it (Barnwell and Desowitz, 1977).

Barnwell and Desowitz (1977) have suggested that the immunity inducing postcrisis refractivity may be very different from the processes inducing the crisis. The studies by the Taliaferros (1944, 1947) certainly suggest that such is the case, for they note that intraerythrocytic death of parasites occurs during crisis but is not an obvious feature of the low-grade parasitemias which may persist after the crisis in clinically recovered individuals.

Taliaferro and Taliaferro (1944) suggest that antibody may be responsible for crisis forms. This suggestion should not be rejected out of hand, for crisis forms occur most frequently in advanced trophozoites and schizonts, and host cells of these forms at the crisis may be quite permeable (Homewood and Neame, 1974; Neame and Homewood, 1975). The Taliaferros further suggest that many of the clinical signs of the crisis are the result of intense antigen–antibody reactions.

The hematological aspects of the crisis are dealt with in Volume 2, Chapter 1. In the remainder of this section only the mechanisms of intraerythrocytic killing of parasites during the crisis will be considered further.

There is considerable evidence that some intraerythrocytic killing of parasites during the crisis may be mediated by a soluble factor which is not a specific antiparasitic antibody. Intravenous injection of a variety of antigenic materials including Bacillus Calmette-Guérin (BCG) (Clark *et al.*, 1976) and *Corynebacterium parvum* (Clark *et al.*, 1976, 1977) may result in immunity to some rodent plasmodia and babesia but not to others, or to cattle babesia (Brocklesby and Purnell, 1977). Simultaneous elimination of both parasites in mixed infection may also occur (Cox, 1978). While the soluble mediator of the intraerythrocytic killing has not been identified, its existence is considered necessary to explain the immunity to plasmodia which occurs after injections of BCG and other heterologous antigenic materials. It is never said, but it must be assumed, that crisis forms occurring during plasmodial infection result from antigenic stimulation with plasmodial antigens by mechanisms similar to those which occur in animals protected by the injection of heterologous antigens. The soluble mediators of parasite killing, like the mediators of macrophage activation, are thus induced as a consequence of specific immunological stimulation, but their action, like the action of the activated macrophage, is not specified in an immunological sense. Interferon is a soluble factor which is induced by *P. berghei* (Huang *et al.*, 1968) and which has been shown to protect mice from the consequences of *P. berghei* infections (Jahiel *et al.*, 1968; Van Dijck *et al.* 1970; Gobert *et al.*, 1972). Interferon is, however, probably not the soluble factor causing intraerythrocytic parasite death in mice treated with BCG or *C. parvum* (Allison and Clark, 1977).

A role for lipopolysaccharide in the release of soluble nonantibody mediators of killing of intraerythrocyte plasmodia has also been proposed (Clark, 1978). This proposal is at present an unsupported hypothesis.

In addition to the soluble mediators of intraerythrocytic killing of plasmodia which appear to contribute to the control of plasmodia at least during the crisis, there have been suggestions that during the crisis some cell-associated mechanisms of parasite killing may occur. Interferon is a potent stimulator of natural killer cell activity (Welsh, 1978; Djeu et al., 1979). Thus interferon interacts with cellular mechanisms which have been suggested to participate in the destruction of susceptible cells.

Splenic lymphocytes from mice with malaria have been reported to lyse erythrocytes of malarious mice in the presence of antibody (Coleman et al., 1975), and spleen cells from monkeys in the crisis of P. Knowlesi malaria will lyse schizont-infected erythrocytes (Brown et al., 1970c) Roberts and Weidanz (1979) have reported that immunity to P. yoelii can be induced in B cell-deficient mice. Greenwood et al. (1977) have observed an increase in null cells and in K-cell activity in children with acute malaria. K-cell activity and augmented macrophage activity can occur in B cell-deficient animals and provide an immune system operative in the absence of B cells or antibody. Some splenic K-cell activity is antibody-mediated (McDonald and Phillips, 1978a). These activities of spleen cells from acutely infected animals probably represent some aspect of an inducible response. They develop after infection and do not presist after the crisis is over. The importance of interferon, other soluble nonantibody factors, antibody-dependent cytotoxicity by K cells, natural killer cells, and armed macrophages, except those armed by cytophilic antibody, in the control of plasmodia during and after the crisis is at the present time unclear.

III. SUMMARY AND HYPOTHESIS: PROBABLE MECHANISMS OF IMMUNITY TO PLASMODIA

The immune response to the asexual blood stages of plasmodia is almost certainly initiated by macrophages oriented toward the blood such as those of the spleen and bone marrow. The antigen which initiates this response is probably scavenged material released at the time of schizont rupture and probably consists of parasite materials not incorporated in the developed merozoites and may include imperfect and damaged merozoites. Normal serum opsonins may aid this ingestion. As much of this scavenged parasite material is not part of the parasite's defense against the host, much of the early response does not appear to bear much relationship to the development of immunity. It may, however, facilitate the clearance of parasite debris from the blood.

Some antigenic materials, probably merozoite capsular materials, not readily phagocytized in the absense of specific antibody are probably carried into the macrophages along with the scavenged parasite debris. It is probably this capsular material which initiates the protective immune response.

If, as is likely, the immune response to plasmodial components is comparable to the response to other more completely studied antigenic materials, the macrophage presents the antigen to the lymphocytes to initiate the chain of events which results in the developed immune response.

Cell transfer studies in inbred rodents and *in vivo* and *in vitro* studies of antiplasmodial antibody indicate that much of the protective immune response to plasmodia is mediated by antibody secreted by fully differentiated B cells. These B cells, however, can only differentiate with the collaboration of T cells. Once the B cells are differentiated the T cells do not, however, appear to have a direct role in parasite killing. The protective antibody secreted by the differentiated B cells, mainly IgG, is either cytophilic, binding to macrophages or opsonic, binding to the parasites. In both cases enhancement of parasite recognition and phagocytosis by the macrophages occurs. Complement does not appear to contribute to parasite destruction. In the immune or premune animal this antibody-mediated phagocytosis of merozoites during their brief extracellular period is probably the major means of parasite control. The probability of phagocytosis of extracellular merozoites is probably increased because antibody-coated merozoites are inhibited in their ability to penetrate red cells. Antibody appears to interfere with host cell penetration by relatively nonspecific means, e.g., inhibition of merozoite dispersion from schizonts (Green *et al.* 1980), merozoite agglutination and development of a cumbersome physical coat on the merozoite, rather than by specific blockage of merozoite receptors for the host cell.

In addition to the antibody phagocyte-mediated immunity which occurs in the immune or premune animal there appear to be other mechanisms of host defense against plasmodia which occur during the crisis stage of infection. These mechanisms are immunological in that they are induced by antigenic materials, but they do not have immunological specificity in the sense of an antigen–antibody reaction. These mechanisms include reticuloendothelial, particularly macrophage, activation, attendant splenic hypertrophy, and the production of increased amounts of autoantibodies to modified or enzymatically exposed host erythrocyte membrane materials. The macrophage activation and the increase in the amount of opsonic autoantibodies jointly enhance phagocytic clearance of erythrocytes which may have damaged membranes. The types of membrane lesions recognized by this activated phagocyte–autoantibody system may include those induced by parasite penetration or by absorption of parasite or host origin enzymes or antigen–antibody complexes which are not cleared as fast as they are produced in the period before the crisis. Such erythrocyte destruction coincidently destroys parasites. Further mechanisms of plasmodial control which occur during the crisis include a mechanism for killing of parasites inside the erythrocytes. Lymphokines and monokines, including intereferon, are probably involved in this parasite-killing mechanism. Cell-mediated parasite destruction mechanisms other than those carried out by macrophages either alone or in association with antibody have been proposed. These include direct destruction of parasites or parasitized erythrocytes by T cells, by natural killer cells, and by null cells (K cells), either alone or in association with antibody (antibody-dependent, cell-mediated cytoxicity). Evidence for these cell-mediated mechanisms of destruction of parasites and parasitized erythrocytes is very weak.

The physical filtering out of parasitized erythrocytes or the pitting of parasites from erythrocytes in the spleen may occur. Such filtering by the spleen is a normal splenic mechanism for the removal of abnormal red cells. It is not an induced immunological mechanism and, as it does not seem to very effective in the early precrisis period, it probably is not very important later in the infection either.

While the host is engaged in attempting to eliminate the plasmodia from its blood, the plasmodia are attempting to evade the host's defenses. The parasites hide from the antibody-mediated phagocytic defense by growing inside the erythrocytes for most of their life cycle and by surrounding themselves with an antiphagocytic capsule for the brief trip to a new host erythrocyte. The parasites may also release antigenic materials to occupy and confuse the immunological defense. The plasmodia also reproduce rapidly and thus compensate for their losses to the host defense mechanisms, and they may change the nature of their capsule to evade the response the host has mounted. It is not impossible that during the early stages of infection, when there is relatively unrestrained parasite reproduction, disruption of the host's homeostatic mechanism by the large parasite population may cause problems for the parasites we well as the host. During the crisis the host destroys many erythrocytes, and the parasites directly destroy many also. Erythrocyte production is increased to attempt to compensate for erythrocyte loss. The final outcome of the infection, recovery (with either elimination of the parasite or accommodation to it), chronic illness, or death, is determined by the interaction of all of the various host defense mechanisms and the parasite's mechanisms of survival. The purpose of the clinician is to shift the balance in favor of the host, and the purpose of the scientist is to provide the clinician with information permitting an intelligent choice of means for doing this. In this chapter we have attempted to arrange the information available on the host defense against the asexual blood stages of plasmodia into a general hypothesis. As new information is accumulated, our understanding of the mechanisms of action of the host defense against plasmodia will improve and the deficiencies in this hypothesis will be recognized and corrected. It is our hope, however, that the scheme for the action of host defenses against plasmodia we have offered will stimulate other scientists to undertake research in host–parasite interaction in malaria.

REFERENCE

Abele, D. C., Tobie, J. E., Hill, G. J., Contacos, P. G., and Evans, C. B. (1965). Alterations in serum proteins and IgG antibody production during the course of induced malarial infections in man. *Am. J. Trop. Med. Hyg.* **14,** 191–197.

Aikawa, M., and Sprinz, H. (1971). Erythrophagocytosis in the bone marrow of canary infected with malaria: Electron microscopic observations. *Lab. Invest.* **24,** 45–54.

Aikawa, M., Miller, L. H., Johnson, J., and Rabbage, J. (1978). Erythrocyte entry by malarial parasites: A moving junction between erythrocyte and parasite. *J. Cell Biol.* **77,** 72–82.

Allen, C., Saba, T. M., and Molnar, J. (1973). Isolation, purification and characterization of opsonic protein. *RES, J. Reticuloendothel. Soc.* **13,** 410–423.

Allison, A. C., and Clark, I. A. (1977). Specific and nonspecific immunity to haemoprotozoa. *Am. J. Trop. Med. Hyg.* **26,** 216–221.

Alvarez, D. A. (1952). Phagocytosis and destruction of *Plasmodium gallinaceum* by cells of the reticuloendothelial system. *Am. J. Hyg.* **56,** 31–38.

Areekul, S. (1973). Rigidity of red cells during malaria infection. *J. Med. Assoc. Thailand* **56,** 163–167.

Atkinson, J. P., Glew, R. H., Neva, F. A., and Frank, M. M. (1975). Serum complement and immunity in experimental simian malaria. II. Preferential activation of early components and failure of depletion of late components to inhibit protective immunity. *J. Infect. Dis.* **131,** 26–33.

Bannister, L. H. (1977). Structural aspects of *Plasmodium* relevant to vaccination against malaria. *Trans. R. Soc. Trop. Med. Hyg.* **71,** 275–276.

Barnwell, J. W., and Desowitz, R. S. (1977). Studies on parasitic crisis in malaria. I. Signs of inpending crisis in *Plasmodium berghei* infections of the white rat. *Ann. Trop. Med. Parasitol.* **71,** 429–433.

Bautista, C. R., and Kreier, J. P. (1979). Effect of immune serum on the growth of *Babesia microti* in hamster erythrocytes in short term culture. *Infect. Immun.* **25,** 470–472.

Blumenstock, F., Saba, T. M. Weber, P., and Cho, E. (1976). Purification and biochemical characterization of a macrophage stimulating alpha-2-globulin opsonic protein. *J. Reticuloendothel. Soc.* **19,** 157–172.

Box, E. D., and Gringrich, W. D. (1958). Acquired immunity to *Plasmodium berghei* in the white mouse. *J. Infect. Dis.* **103,** 291–300.

Briggs, N. T., Wellde, B. T., and Sadun, E. H. (1966). Effects of rat antiserum on the course of *Plasmodium berghei* infection in mice. *Mil. Med.* **131,** 1243–1249.

Briggs, N. T., Wellde, B. T., and Sadun, E. H. (1968). Variants of *Plasmodium berghei* resistant to passive transfer of immune serum. *Exp. Parasitol.* **22,** 338–345.

Brocklesby, D. W., and Purnell, R. E. (1977). Failure of BCG to protect calves against *Babesia divergens* infection. *Nature (London)* **265,** 343.

Brooks, C. B., and Kreier, J. P. (1978). Role of surface coat on *in vitro* attachment and phagocytosis of *Plasmodium berghei* by peritoneal macrophages. *Infect. Immun.* **20,** 927–835.

Brown, I. N., and Phillips, R. S. (1974). Immunity to *Plasmodium berghei* in rats: Passive serum transfer and role of the spleen. *Infect. Immun.* **10,** 1213–1218.

Brown, I. N., Brown, K. N., and Hills, L. A. (1968). Immunity to malaria: The antibody response to antigenic variation by *Plasmodium knowlesi*. *Immunology* **14,** 127–138.

Brown, K. N. (1971). Protective immunity to malaria provides a model in the survival of cells in an immunologically hostile environment. *Nature (London)* **230,** 163–167.

Brown, K. N., and Brown, I. N. (1965). Immunity to malaria: Antigenic variation in chronic infections of *Plasmodium knowlesi*. *Nature (London)* **208,** 1286–1288.

Brown, K. N., Brown, I. N., and Hills, L. A. (1970a). Immunity to malaria. I. Protection against

Plasmodium knowlesi shown by monkeys sensitized with drug suppressed infections or by dead parasites in Freund's adjuvant. *Exp. Parasitol.* **28,** 304-317.

Brown, K. N., Brown, I. N., Trigg, P. I., Phillips, R. S., and Hills, L. A. (1970b). Immunity to malaria. II. Serological response of monkeys sensitized by drug suppressed infection or by dead parasitized cells in Freund's complete adjuvant. *Exp. Parasitol.* **28,** 318-338.

Brown, K. N., Brown, I. N., Phillips, R. S., Trigg, P. I., Hills, L. A., Wollencraft, R. A., and Dunonde, D. C. (1970c). Immunity to malaria: Studies with *Plasmodium knowlesi. Trans. R. Soc. Trop. Med. Hyg.* **64,** 3-5.

Brown, K. N., Hills, L. A., and Jarra, W. (1976a) Preliminary studies on artifical immunization of rats against *Plasmodium berghei* and adoptive transfer of this immunity by splenic T and B cells. *Bull. W.H.O.* **54,** 149-154.

Brown, K. N., Jarra, W., and Hills, L. A. (1976b). T cells and protective immunity to *Plasmodium berghei* in rats. *Infect. Immun.* **14,** 858-871.

Butcher, G. A., and Cohen, S. (1972). Antigenic variation and protective immunity in *Plasmodium knowlesi* malaria. *Immunology* **23,** 503-521.

Butcher, G. A., Mitchell, G. H., and Cohen, S. (1978). Antibody mediated mechanisms of immunity to malaria induced by vaccination with *Plasmodium knowlesi* merozoites. *Immunology* **34,** 77-86.

Callow, L. L. (1977). Vaccination against bovine babesiosis. *Adv. Exp. Biol. Med.* **93,** 121-149.

Cantrell, W., Elko, E. E., and Hopff, B. M. (1970). *Plasmodium berghei:* Phagocytic hyperactivity of infected birds. *Exp. Parasitol.* **28,** 291-297.

Carter, R., and Diggs, C. L. (1977). Plasmodia of rodents. *In* "Parasitic Protozoa" (J. P. Kreier, ed.), Vol. 3, pp. 353-405. Academic Press, New York.

Causse-Vaills, C., Orfila, J., and Fabiani, M. G. (1960). Fractionment électrophorétique des protéines et pouvoir protecteur du serum du rat blanc immunise contra *Plasmodium berghei. Ann. Inst. Pasteur, Paris* pp. 232-242.

Chow, J. S., and Kreier, J. P. (1972). *Plasmodium berghei:* Adherence and phagocytosis by rat macrophages *in vitro. Exp. Parasitol.* **31,** 13-18.

Clark, I. A. (1978). Does endotoxin cause both the disease and parasite death in acute malaria and babesiosis. *Lancet* **2,** 75-77.

Clark, I. A., and Allison, A. C. (1974). *Babesia microti* and *Plasmodium yoelii* infections in nude mice. *Nature (London)* **252,** 328-329.

Clark, I. A., Allison, A. C., and Cox, F. E. G. (1976). Protection of mice against *Babesia* and *Plasmodium* with BCG. *Nature (London)* **259,** 309-311.

Clark, I. A., Cox, F. E. G., and Allison, A. C. (1977). Protection of mice against *Babesia* spp. and *Plasmodium* spp. with killed *Corynebacterium parvum. Parasitology* **74,** 9-18.

Coatney, G. R. (1976). Relapse in malaria—An enigma. *J. Parasitol.* **62,** 3-9.

Coggeshall, L. T. (1940). The occurrence of malaria antibodies in human serum following induced infection with *Plasmodium knowlesi. J. Exp. Med.* **72,** 21-31.

Coggeshall, L. T., and Eaton, M. D. (1938). The complement fixation reaction in monkey malaria. *J. Exp. Med.* **67,** 871-872.

Coggeshall, L. T., and Kumm, H. W. (1937). Demonstration of passive immunity in experimental monkey malaria. *J. Exp. Med.* **66,** 177-190.

Coggeshall, L. T., and Kumm, H. W. (1938). Effect of repeated superinfection upon the potency of immune serum of monkeys harboring chronic infections of *Plasmodium knowlesi. J. Exp. Med.* **68,** 17-27.

Cohen, B. E., Rosenthal, A. S., and Paul, W. E. (1973). Antigen-macrophage Interaction. II. Relative roles of cytophilic antibody and other membrane sites. *J. Immunol.* **111,** 820-827.

Cohen, S. (1976). Survival of parasites in the immunized host. *In* "Immunology of Parasitic Infections" (S. Cohen and E. H. Sadun, eds.), pp. 35-46. Blackwell, Oxford.

Cohen, S. (1977). Mechanisms of malarial immunity. *Trans. R. Soc. Trop. Med. Hyg.* **7**, 283–286.

Cohen, S., and Butcher, G. A. (1971). Serum antibody in acquired malarial immunity. *Trans. R. Soc. Trop. Med. Hyg.* **65**, 125–135.

Cohen, S., McGregor, I. A., and Carrington, S. P. (1961). Gamma globulin and acquired immunity to human malaria. *Nature (London)* **192**, 733–737.

Cohen, S., Butcher, G. A., and Mitchell, G. H. (1972). *In vitro* studies of malarial antibody. *Proc. Helminthol. Soc. Wash.* **39**, 231–237.

Cohen, S., Butcher, G. A., and Mitchell, G. H. (1974). Mechanisms of immunity to malaria. *Bull. W. H. O.* **50**, 251–257.

Cohen, S., Butcher, G. A., and Mitchell, G. H. (1977). Immunization against erythrocytic forms of malaria parasites. *Adv. Exp. Med. Biol.* **93**, 89–112.

Coleman, R. M., Rencicca, N. J., Stout, J. P., Brissette, W. H., and Smith, D. M. (1975). Splenic mediated erythrocyte cytotoxicity in malaria. *Immunology* **29**, 49–54.

Coleman, R. M., Bruce, A., and Roncicca, N. J. (1976). Malaria: Macrophage migration inhibition factor (MIF). *J. Parasitol.* **62**, 137–138.

Collins, W. E., and Skinner, J. C. (1972). The indirect fluorescent antibody test for malaria. *Am. J. Trop. Med. Hyg.* **21**, 690–695.

Collins, W. E., Jeffrey, G. M., and Skinner, J. C. (1964). Fluorescent antibody studies in human malaria. III. Development of antibodies to *Plasmodium falciparum* in semi-immune patients. *Am. J. Trop. Med. Hyg.* **13**, 777–782.

Collins, W. E., Skinner, J. C., Contacos, P. G., and Guinn, E. (1967). Fluorescent antibody studies on simian malaria. II. Development of antibodies to *Plasmodium cynomolgi. Am. J. Trop. Med. Hyg.* **16**, 267–272.

Collins, W. E., Contacos, P. G., Harrison, A. J., Stanfill, P. S., and Skinner, J. C. (1977). Attempts to immunize monkeys against *Plasmodium knowlesi* by using heat stable serum soluble antigens. *Am. J. Trop. Med. Hyg.* **26**, 373–376.

Cooper, N. R., and Fogel, B. J. (1966). Complement in acute experimental malaria. II. Alterations in the components of complement. *Mil. Med.* **131**, 1180–1190.

Corwin, R. M., Cox, H. W., Ludford, C. G., and McNett, S. L. (1970). Relapse mechanisms in malaria: Emergence of varient strains of *Plasmodium lophurae* from serum antigen-immunized ducks. *J. Parasitol.* **56**, 431–438.

Cox, F. E. G. (1974a). Antibody manipulation by malaria parasite. *Nature (London)* **250**, 12.

Cox, F. E. G. (1974b). Vaccination against malaria. *Nature (London)* **252**, 268.

Cox, F. E. G. (1978). Heterologous immunity between piroplasms and malaria parasites: The simultaneous elimination of *Plasmodium vinkei* and *Babesia microti* from the blood of doubly infected mice. *Parasitology* **76**, 55–60.

Cox, F. E. G., Nicol, T., and Bilbey, D. L. J. (1963a). Reticuloendothelial activity in *Haemamoeba* [*Plasmodium gallinacea* (sic)] infections. *J. Protozool.* **10**, 107–109.

Cox, F. E. G., Bilbey, D. L. J., and Nicol, T. (1963b). Reticuloendothelial activity in mice infected with *Plasmodium vinckei. J. Protozool.* **11**, 229–236.

Cox, H. W. (1959). A study of relapse *Plasmodium berghei* infections isolated from white mice. *J. Immunol.* **82**, 209–214.

Curtain, C. C., Gorman, J. G., and Kidson, C. (1965). Malaria antibody and gamma-globulin levels in Melanesian children in New Guinea. *Trans. R. Soc. Trop. Med. Hyg.* **59**, 42–45.

D'Antonio, L. E., Alger, N. E., and Mathot, C. (1969). Temporal relation between a serum electroabsorbing fraction and the course of acute *Plasmodium berghei* malaria in rats. *Am. J. Trop. Med. Hyg.* **18**, 866–871.

Davis, B. D. (1948). Complement fixation with soluble antigens of *Plasmodium knowlesi* and *Plasmodium lophurae. J. Immunol.* **58**, 269–281.

Desowitz, R. S. (1970). African trypanosomes. *In* "Immunity to Parasitic Animals" (G. J. Jackson, R. Herman, and I. Singer, eds.), Vol. 2, pp. 551–596. Appleton Century-Crofts, New York.

Desowitz, R. S. (1973). Some factors influencing the induction, maintenance and degree of naturally transmitted protective immunity to malaria (*Plasmodium berghei*). *Trans. R. Soc. Trop. Med. Hyg.* **67**, 238–244.

Desowitz, R. S., and Saave, J. J. (1965). The application of the haemagglutination test to the study of the immunity to malaria in protected and unprotected population groups in Australian New Guinea. *Bull. W. H. O.* **32**, 149–159.

Diggs, C. L., and Osler, A. G. (1969a). Humoral immunity in rodent malaria. I. Estimation of parasitemia by electronic particle counting. *J. Immunol.* **102**, 292–297.

Diggs, C. L., and Osler, A. G. (1969b). Humoral immunity in rodent malaria. II. Inhibition of parasitemia by serum antibody. *J. Immunol.* **102**, 298–305.

Diggs, C. L., and Osler, A. G. (1975). Humoral immunity in rodent malaria. III. Studies on the site of antibody action. *J. Immunol.* **114**, 1243–1247.

Diggs, C. L., Wellde, B. T., Anderson, J. S., Luzzatto, L., Weber, R. M., and Rodriguez, E., Jr. (1972a). The protective effect of African human immunoglobulin G in *Aotus trivirgatus* infected with Asian *Plasmodium falciparum. Proc. Helminthol. Soc. Wash.* **39**, 449–456.

Diggs, C. L., Shin, H., Briggs, N. J., Laudenslayer, K., and Weber, R. (1972b). Antibody mediated immunity to *Plasmodium berghei* independent of the third component of complement. *Proc. Helminthol. Soc. Wash.* **39**, 456–459.

DiLuzio, N. R., McNamee, R., Miller, E. F., and Pisano, J. C. (1972). Macrophage recognition-factor depletion after administration of particulate agents and leukemic cells. *RES, J. Reticuloendothel. Soc.* **12**, 314–323.

Djen, J. Y., Heinbaugh, J. A., Holden, H. T., and Herberman, R. B. (1979). Augmentation of mouse natural killer cell activity by interferon and interferon inducers. *J. Immunol.* **122**, 175–181.

Dooris, G. M., and McGhee, R. B. (1975). *Plasmodium gallinaceum:* Avian immunological tolerance to serum antigens. *Exp. Parasitol.* **37**, 105–107.

Dulaney, A. D., and Stratman-Thomas, W. K. (1940). Complement fixation in human malaria. I. Results obtained with various antigens. *J. Immunol.* **39**, 247–255.

Dvorak, J. A., Miller, L. H., Whitehause, W. C., and Shirosihi, T. (1975). Invasion of erythrocytes by malaria parasites. *Science* **187**, 748–750.

Eaton, M. D. (1939). The soluble malarial antigens in the serum of monkeys infected with *Plasmodium knowlesi. J. Exp. Med.* **69**, 517–532.

Eling, W. (1978a). Fading of malarial immunity in mice. *Tropenmed Parasitol.* **29**, 77–84.

Eling, W. (1978b). Survival of parasites in mice immunized against *Plasmodium berghei. Tropenmed. Parasitol.* **29**, 204–209.

Eling, W. (1978c). Malaria immunity and premunition in a *Plasmodium berghei* mouse model. *Isr. J. Med. Sci.* **14**, 542–553.

Elko, E. E., and Cantrell, W. (1970). Nonspecific phagocytic activity in rats infected with *Plasmodium berghei* and treated with aminodiaquine or chloroquine. *Am. J. Trop. Med. Hyg.* **19**, 899–904.

El-Nahal, H. S. (1966). Fluorescent antibody studies on infections with *Plasmodium gallinaceum:* Effect of splenectory during latency on parasitemia and antibody titer. *J. Parasitol.* **52**, 570–572.

Fife, E. H., Jr. (1971). Advances in methodology for immune diagnosis of parasitic diseases. *Exp. Parasitol.* **30**, 132–163.

Fife, E. H., Jr. (1972). Current state of serological tests used to detect blood parasite infections. *Exp. Parasitol.* **31**, 136–152.

Finerty, J. F., Evans, C. B., and Hyde, C. L. (1972). *Plasmodium berghei* and *Eperythrozoon coccoides:* Antibody and immunoglobulin synthesis in germfree and conventional mice simultaneously infected. *Exp. Parasitol.* **34**, 76–84.

Fogel, B. J., von Doenhoff, A. E., Jr., Cooper, N. R., and Fife, E. H., Jr. (1966). Complement in experimental malaria. I. Total hemolytic activity. *Mil. Med.* **131**, 1173–1179.

Frankenberg, S., Greenblatt, C. L., Golenser, J., and Spira, D. T. (1977). *Plasmodium berghei:* Relationship between mitosis and erythropoiesis in spleen cells of infected rats. *Exp. Parasitol.* **43**, 362–369.

Freeman, R. R. (1978). T cell function during fatal and self limiting malarial infection of mice. *J. Cell. Immunol.* **41**, 373–379.

Freeman, R. R., and Parrish, C. R. (1978). Polyclonal B-cell activation during rodent malarial infections. *Clin. Exp. Immunol.* **32**, 41–45.

Gautam, O. P., Kreier, J. P., and Kreier, R. C. (1970). Antibody coating on erythrocytes of chickens infected with *Plasmodium gallinaceum. Indian J. Med. Res.* **58**, 529–543.

Gingrich, W. D. (1941). Immunity in avian malaria. *J. Infect. Dis.* **68**, 37–45.

Glew, R. H., Atkinson, J. P., Frank, M. M., Collins, W. E., and Neva, F. A. (1975). Serum complement and immunity in experimental simian malaria. I. Cyclical alteration in C4 related to schizont rupture. *J. Infect. Dis.* **131**, 17–25.

Goberman, V., and Zuckerman, A. (1966). Dynamics of the formation of antiplasmodial precipitins in rats infected with *Plasmodium berghei. J. Protozool.* **13**, 34.

Gobert, G., Poindron, P., Germain, A., and Savel, J. (1972). Recherche sur le mécanisme d'action d'un inducteur viral de l'interféron dans la protection de la souris contre l'infestation massive par des formes endoerythrocytaires de *Plasmodium berghei. C. R. Hebd. Seances Acad. Sci., Ser. D* **274**, 1226–1229.

Goble, F. C., and Singer, I. (1960). The reticuloendothelial system in experimental malaria and trypanosomiasis. *Ann. N.Y. Acad. Sci.* **88**, 149–171.

Golenser, J., Spira, D. T., and Zuckerman, A. (1975). Neutralizing antibody in rodent malaria. *Trans. R. Soc. Trop. Med. Hyg.* **69**, 251–258.

Götze, O., and Müller-Eberhard, H. J. (1976). The alternate pathway of complement activation. *Adv. Immunol.* **24**, 1–35.

Gravely, S. M., and Kreier, J. P. (1976). Adoptive transfer of immunity to *Plasmodium berghei* with immune T and B lymphocytes. *Infect. Immun.* **14**, 184–190.

Gravely, S. M., Hamburger, J., and Kreier, J. P. (1976). T and B cell population changes in young and in adult rats infected with *Plasmodium berghei. Infect. Immun.* **14**, 178–183.

Green, T. J. (1978). Studies on the nature of the immune response to *Plasmodium berghei* in the rat. Doctoral Dissertation, Ohio State University, Columbus.

Green, T. J., Morhardt, M., and Brackett, R. G. (1980). Serum inhibition of merozoite dispersal from *Plasmodium falciparum* schizonts: an indicator of immune status (submitted).

Green, T. J., and Kreier, J. P. (1978). Demonstration of the role of cytophilic antibody in resistance to malaria parasites (*Plasmodium berghei*) in rats. *Infect. Immun.* **19**, 138–145.

Greenwood, B. M. (1974). Immune depression in malaria and trypanosomiasis. *In* "Parasites in the Immunized Host: Mechanism of Survival" (R. Porter and J. Knight, eds.), Ciba Found. Symp. No. 25 (New Ser.), pp. 136–159. Elsevier, Amsterdam.

Greenwood, B. M., and Brueton, M. J. (1974). Complement activation in children with acute malaria. *Clin. Exp. Immunol.* **18**, 267–272.

Greenwood, B. M., and Vick, R. M. (1975). Evidence for a malaria mitogen in human malaria. *Nature (London)* **257**, 592–594.

Greenwood, B. M., Brown, J. C., DeJesus, D. G., and Holborow, E. J. (1971). Immunosuppression in murine malaria. II. The effect on reticuloendothelial and germinal centre functions. *Clin. Exp. Immunol.* **9**, 345–354.

Greenwood, B. M., Aduloju, A. J., and Stratton, D. (1977). Lymphocyte changes in acute malaria. *Trans. R. Soc. Trop. Med. Hyg.* **71**, 408–410.

Greenwood, B. M., Stratton, D., Williamson, W. A., and Mohammed, I. (1978). A study of the role of immunological factors in the pathogenesis of the anaemia of acute malaria. *Trans. R. Soc. Trop. Med. Hyg.* **72**, 378–385.

Grothaus, D. G., and Kreier, J. P. (1980). The isolation of a soluble component of *Plasmodium berghei* which induces immunity in rats. IAI **28**, 245–253.

Guckian, J. C., Christensen, W. D., and Fine, D. P. (1978). Trypan blue inhibits complement-mediated phagocytosis by human polymorphonuclear leukocytes. *J. Immunol.* **120**, 1580–1586.

Hamburger, J., and Kreier, J. P. (1975). Antibody mediated elimination of malaria parasites *in vivo*. *Infect. Immun.* **12**, 339–345.

Hamburger, J., and Kreier, J. P. (1976). *Plasmodium berghei:* Use of free blood stage parasites to demonstrate protective humoral activity in the serum of recovered rats. *Exp. Parasitol.* **40**, 158–169.

Herman, R. (1977). *Plasmodium chabaudi:* Host lymphocyte-macrophage interaction *in vitro*. *Exp. Parasitol.* **42**, 211–220.

Heumann, A., Stiffel, C., Monjour, L., Bucci, A., and Biozzi, G. (1979). Correlation between genetic regulation of antibody responsiveness and protective immunity induced by *Plasmodium berghei* vaccination. *Infect. Immun.* **24**, 829–836.

Hobart, M. J., and McConnell, I. (1978). "The Immune system: A Course on the Molecular and Cellular Basis of Immunity," p. 149. Blackwell, Oxford.

Homewood, C. A., and Neame, K. D. (1974). Malaria and the permeability of the host erythrocyte. *Nature (London)* **252**, 718–719.

Houba, V., Faulk, W. P., and Malola, Y. G. (1974). Heterophilic antibodies in relation to malarial infection: Population and experimental studies. *Clin. Exp. Immunol.* **18**, 89–93.

Huang, K.-Y., Schultz, W. W., and Gordon, F. B. (1968). Interferon induced by *Plasmodium berghei*. *Science* **162**, 123–124.

Ingram, R. L., Otken, L. B., Jr., and Jumper, J. R. (1961). Staining of malarial parasites by the fluorescent antibody technique. *Proc. Soc. Exp. Biol. Med.* **106**, 52–54.

Jahiel, R. I., Vilcek, J., Nussenzweig, R., and Vanderberg, J. (1968). Interferon inducers protect mice against *Plasmodium berghei* malaria. *Science* **161**, 802–803.

Jayawardena, A. N., Targett, C.-A. T., Carter, R. L., Leuchars, E., and Davies, A. J. S. (1977). The immunological response of CBA mice to *P. yoelii*. *Immunology* **32**, 849–859.

Jerusalem, C. (1965). Histo- und biometrische Untersuchungen zur Frage der Autohaemaggression bei Infektion mit *Plasmodium berghei*. *Ann. Soc. Belge Med. Trop.* **45**, 405–416.

Jerusalem, C., Weiss, M. L., and Poels, L. (1971). Immunological enhancement in malaria infection (*Plasmodium berghei*). *J. Immunol.* **107**, 260–268.

Katz, D. H., and Benacerraf, B. (1972). The regulating influence of activated T cells on B cell responses to antigen. *Adv. Immunol.* **15**, 1–94.

Kay, M. M. B. (1975). Mechanism of removal of senescent cells by human macrophages *in situ*. *Proc. Natl. Acad. Sci. U.S.A.* **72**, 3521–3525.

Kilejian, A. (1976). Does histidine-rich protein from *Plasmodium lophurae* have a function in merozoite penetration? *J. Protozool.* **23**, 272–277.

Kilejian, A. (1978). Histidine rich protein as a model malaria vaccine. *Science* **201**, 922–924.

Kitchen, A. G., and DiLuzio, N. R. (1971). Influence of *Plasmodium berghei* infections on phagocytic and humoral recognition factor activity. *J. Reticuloendothel. Soc.* **9**, 237–247.

Kortmann, H. F., Lelijveld, J., Ross, J. P. J., and Lohn, L. F. (1971). A capillary agglutination test for malaria. *Bull. W.H.O.* **45**, 839–844.

Krahenbuhl, J. L., Rosenberg, L. T., and Remington, J. S. (1973). The role of thymus derived lymphocytes in the *in vitro* activation of macrophages to kill *Listeria monocytogenes*. *J. Immunol.* **111**, 992–995.

Kreier, J. P. (1969). Mechanisms of erythrocyte destruction in chickens infected with *Plasmodium gallinaceum*. *Mil. Med.* **134**, 1203–1219.

Kreier, J. P. (1977). The isolation and fractionation of malaria infected cells. *Bull. W. H. O.* **55**, 317–331.

Kreier, J. P., and Dilley, D. A. (1969). *Plasmodium berghei:* Nucleic acid agglutinating antibodies in rats. *Exp. Parasitol.* **26**, 175–180.

Kreier, J. P., and Leste, J. (1967). Relationship of parasitemia to erythrocyte destruction in *Plasmodium berghei* infected rats. *Exp. Parasitol.* **21**, 78–83.

Kreier, J. P., and Leste, J. (1968). Parasitemia and erythrocyte destruction in *Plasmodium berghei* infected rats. II. Effect of infected host globulin. *Exp. Parasitol.* **23**, 198–204.

Kreier, J. P., and Ristic, M. (1964). Detection of a *Plasmodium berghei* antibody complex formed *in vivo*. *Am. J. Trop. Med. Hyg.* **13**, 6–10.

Kreier, J. P., Pearson, G. L., and Stilwell, D. (1965). A capillary agglutination test using *Plasmodium gallinacium* parasites freed from erythrocytes. *Am. J. Trop. Med. Hyg.* **14**, 529–532.

Kreier, J. P., Shapiro, H., Dilley, D., Szilvassy, I. P., and Ristic, M. (1966). Autoimmune reactions in rats with *Plasmodium berghei* infection. *Exp. Parasitol.* **19**, 155–162.

Kreier, J. P., Hamburger, J., Seed, T. M., Saul, K., and Green, T. J. (1976). *Plasmodium berghei:* Characteristics of a selected population of small free blood stage parasites. *Tropenmed. Parasitol.* **27**, 82–88.

Kretschmar, W., and Jerusalem, C. (1963). Milz und Malaria: Der Infections-verlauf (*Plasmodium berghei*) in splenikomierter NMRI Mausen und seine Deutung anhand der histopathologischen Veranderungen der Milz nicht splenektimierter Mause. *Z. Tropenmed. Parasitol.* **14**, 279–310.

Krettli, A. J., and Nussenzweig, R. (1974). Depletion of T and B lymphocytes during malarial infections. *Cell. Immunol.* **3**, 440–446.

Krettli, A. J., Nussenzweig, V., and Nussenzweig, R. (1976). Complement alterations in rodent malaria. *Am. J. Trop. Med. Hyg.* **25**, 34–41.

Ladda, R. L. (1969). New insights into the fine structure of rodent malarial parasites. *Mil. Med.* **134**, 825–865.

Loose, L. D., and DiLuzio, N. R. (1976). A temporal relationship between reticuloendothelial system phagocytic alterations and antibody responses in mice infected with *Plasmodium berghei* (NYW-2 Stark). *Am. J. Trop. Med. Hyg.* **25**, 221–228.

Loose, L. D., Trejo, R., and DiLuzio, N. R. (1971). Impaired endotoxin detoxification as a factor in enhanced endotoxin sensitivity of malaria infected mice. *Proc. Soc. Exp. Biol. Med.* **137**, 794–797.

Loose, L. D., Cook, J. A., and DiLuzio, N. R. (1972). Malarial immunosuppression—A macrophage mediated defect. *Proc. Helminthol. Soc. Wash.* **39**, 484–491.

Loose, L. D., Breitenbach, R. P., and Barrett, J. T. (1973a). Suppression of the avian reticuloendothelial system and enhancement of a *Plasmodium lophurae* infection in diethylstilbestrol treated chickens. *Comp. Biochem. Physiol. A* **45**, 587–593.

Loose, L. D., Breitenbach, R. P., and Barrett, J. T. (1973b). Effect of reticuloendothelial system alteration on *Plasmodium lophurae* infection and haemagglutinin function in the chicken. *Microbios* **7**, 45–51.

Lourie, S. H., and Dunn, M. A. (1972). The effect of protective sera on the course of *Plasmodium berghei* in immunosuppressed rats. *Proc. Helminthol. Soc. Wash.* **39**, 470–476.

Lucia, H. L., and Nussenzweig, R. S. (1969). *Plasmodium chabaudi* and *Plasmodium vinckei:* Phagocytic activity of the mouse reticuloendothelial system. *Exp. Parasitol.* **25**, 319–323.

Lunn, J. S., Chin, W., Contacos, P. G., and Coatney, G. R. (1966). Changes in antibody titers and serum fractions during the course of prolonged infections with vivax or with falciparum malaria. *Am. J. Trop. Med. Hyg.* **15**, 3–10.

Lustig, H. J., Nussenzweig, V., and Nussenzweig, R. S. (1977). Erythrocyte membrane associated globulins during malaria infection in mice. *J. Immunol.* **119**, 210-216.

McDonald, V., and Phillips, R. S. (1978a). Increase in nonspecific antibody mediated cytotoxicity in malarious mice. *Clin. Exp. Immunol.* **34**, 159-163.

McDonald, V., and Phillips, R. S. (1978b). *Plasmodium chabaudi* in mice: Adoptive transfer of immunity with enriched population of spleen T and B lymphocytes. *Immunology* **34**, 821-830.

McGregor, I. A. (1972). Immunology of malarial infection and its possible consequences. *Br. Med. Bull.* **28**, 22-27.

McGregor, I. A., Carrington, S. P., and Cohen, S. (1963). Treatment of East African *Plasmodium falciparum* malaria with West African human gamma globulin. *Trans. R. Soc. Trop. Med. Hyg.* **57**, 170-175.

McGregor, I. A., Hall, P. J., Williams, K., and Hardy, M. W. (1966). Demonstration of circulating antigens of *Plasmodium falciparum* by gel diffusion techniques. *Nature (London)* **210**, 1384-1386.

McGregor, I. A., Turner, M. W., Williams, K., and Hall, P. (1968). Soluble antigens in the blood of African patients with serum *Plasmodium* falciparum malaria. *Lancet* **1**, 881-884.

Mackaness, G. B. (1969). The influence of immunologically committed lymphoid cells on macrophage activation *in vivo*. *J. Exp. Med.* **129**, 973-992.

Mantovani, B., Rabinovitch, M., and Nussenzweig, V. (1972). Phagocytosis of immune complexes by macrophages. Different roles of the macrophage receptor sites for complement (C3) and for immunoglobulins (IgG). *J. Exp. Med.* **135**, 780-792.

Mason, S. J., Aikawa, M., Shiroishi, T., and Miller, L. H. (1977). Further evidence for the parasitic origins of the surface coat on malaria merozoites. *Am. J. Trop. Med. Hyg.* **26**, 195-197.

Matthews, H. M., Fried, J. A., and Kagan, I. C. (1975). The indirect haemagglutination of antigens prepared from *Plasmodium falciparum* and *Plasmodium vivax*. *Am. J. Trop. Med. Hyg.* **24**, 417-422.

Meuwissen, J. H. P. T., Leuwenberg, A. D. E. M., and Molenkamp, G. E. (1972). Studies on various aspects of the indirect haemagglutination test for malaria. *Bull. W. H. O.* **46**, 771-782.

Miller, L. H. (1977). Current prospects and problem for a malaria vaccine. *J. Infect. Dis.* **135**, 855-864.

Miller, L. H., Cooper, G. W., Chien, S., and Freemount, H. N. (1972). Surface charge on *Plasmodium knowlesi* and *P. coatneyi*-infected red cells of *Macaca mulatta*. *Exp. Parasitol.* **32**, 86-95.

Miller, L. H., Dvorak, J. A., Shiroishi, T., and Durocher, J. R. (1973a). Influence of erythrocyte membrane components on malaria merozoite invasion. *J. Exp. Med.* **138**, 1597-1601.

Miller, L. H., Powers, K. G., Finerty, J., and Vanderberg, J. P. (1973b). Difference in surface change between host cells and malarial parasites. *J. Parasitol.* **59**, 925-927.

Miller, L. H., Mason, S. J., Dvorak, J. A., McGinniss, and Rothman, I. K. (1975a). Erythrocyte receptors for (*Plasmodium knowlesi*) malaria: Duffy blood group determinants. *Science* **189**, 561-563.

Miller, L. H., Aikawa, M., and Dvorak, J. A. (1975b). Malaria (*Plasmodium knowlesi*) merozoites: Immunity and the surface coat. *J. Immunol.* **114**, 1237-1242.

Miller, L. H., McAuliffe, F., and Mason, S. J. (1977a). Erythrocyte receptors for malaria parasites. *Am. J. Trop. Med. Hyg.* **26**, 204-208.

Miller, L. H., Powers, K. G., and Shiroishi, T. (1977b). *Plasmodium knowlesi:* Functional immunity and antimerozoite antibodies in rhesus monkeys after repeated infection. *Exp. Parasitol.* **41**, 105-111.

Mitchell, G. H., Butcher, G. A., and Cohen S. (1975). Merozoite vaccination against *Plasmodium knowlesi* malaria. *Immunology* **29**, 397-407.

Mosier, D. E. (1976). The role of macrophage in the specific determination of immunogenicity and tolerogenicity. *In* "Immunology of the Macrophage" (D. S. Nelson, ed.), Chapter 2, pp. 35-44. Academic Press, New York.

Mungyerova, G., and Jerusalem, C. (1966). Reaktionen von Miltzellen *in vitro* bei der experimentellen Malaria-infektron (*Plasmodium berghei*). *Z. Zellforsch. Mikrosk. Anat.* **71**, 364-386.

Neame, K. D., and Homewood, C. A. (1975). Alterations in the permeability of mouse erythrocytes infected with the malaria parasite, *Plasmodium berghei. Int. J. Parasitol.* **5**, 537-540.

Nelson, D. S. (1976). Nonspecific immunoregulation by macrophages and their products. *In* "Immunobiology of the Macrophage" (D. S. Nelson, ed.), Chapter 9, pp. 235-257. Academic Press, New York.

North, R. J. (1973). Cellular mediators of anti listeria immunity as an enlarged population of short lived replicating T cells. *J. Exp. Med.* **138**, 342-355.

Palmer, T. T. (1978). *Plasmodium berghei* infection in pregnant rats: Effects on antibody response and course of infection in offspring. *J. Parasitol.* **64**, 493-496.

Pearsall, N. N., and Weiser, R. S. (1970). "The Macrophage." Lea & Febiger, Philadelphia, Pennsylvania.

Phillips, R. S. (1970). *Plasmodium berghei:* Passive transfer of immunity by antiserum and cells. *Exp. Parasitol.* **27**, 479-495.

Phillips, R. S., and Jones, V. E. (1972). Immunity to *Plasmodium berghei* in rats: Maximum levels of protective antibody activity are associated with eradication of the infection. *Parasitology* **64**, 117-127.

Phillips, R. S., Wolstencroft, R. A., Brown, I. N., Brown, K. N., and Dumonde, D. C. (1970). Immunity to malaria. III. Possible occurrence of a cell-mediated immunity to *Plasmodium knowlesi* in chronically infected and Freund's complete adjuvent-sensitized monkeys. *Exp. Parasitol.* **28**, 339-355.

Phillips, R. S., Trigg, P. I., Scott-Finnigan, T. J., and Bartholomew, R. K. (1972). Culture of *Plasmodium falciparum in vitro:* A subculture technique used for demonstrating antiplasmodial activity in serum from some Gambians resident in an endemic malarious area. *Parasitology* **65**, 525-535.

Pierce, C. W., and Kapp, J. A. (1976). The role of the macrophage in antibody responses. *In* "Immunobiology of the Macrophage" (D. S. Nelson, ed.), Chapter 1, pp. 1-33. Academic Press, New York.

Playfair, J. H. L. (1978). Effective and ineffective immune responses to parasites: Evidence from experimental models. *Curr. Top. Microbiol. Immunol.* **80**, 37-64.

Playfair, J. H. L., Desouza, J. B., and Cattrell, B. J. (1977). Reactivity and cross reactivity of mouse helper T cells to malaria parasites. *Immunology* **32**, 681-687.

Poels, L. G. (1977). *Plasmodium berghei:* Polyribosome profiles in the spleens of infected mice. *Exp. Parasitol.* **41**, 83-88.

Poels, L. G., and Van Niekerk, C. C. (1977). *Plasmodium berghei:* Immunosuppression and hyperimmunoglobulinemia. *Exp. Parasitol.* **42**, 235-247.

Powell, R. D., McNamara, J., and Rieckmann, K. H. (1972). Clinical aspects of acquisition of immunity to falciparum malaria. *Proc. Helminthol. Soc. Wash.* **39**, 51-66.

Raff, M. C., and Cantor, H. I. (1971). Subpopulations of thymus cells and thymus derived lymphocytes. *In* "Progress in Immunology" (D. B. Amos, ed.), p. 83. Academic Press, New York.

Rank, R. G., and Weidanz, W. P. (1976). Nonsterilizing immunity in avian malaria: An antibody independent phenomenon. *Proc. Soc. Exp. Biol. Med.* **151**, 257-259.

Ree, G. H. (1976). Complement and malaria. *Ann. Trop. Med. Parasitol.* **70**, 247-248.

Roberts, D. W., and Weidanz, W. P. (1978). Splenomegaly, enhanced phagocytosis and anemia are thymus dependent responses to malaria. *Infect. Immun.* **20**, 728-731.

Roberts, D. W., and Weidanz, W. P. (1979). T-cell immunity to malaria in the B-cell deficient mouse. *Am. J. Trop. Med. Hyg.* **28**, 1-3.

Roberts, D. W., Rank, R. G., Weidanz, W. P., and Finerty, J. F. (1977). Prevention of recrudescent malaria in nude mice by thymus grafting or by treatment with hyperimmune serum. *Infect. Immun.* **16**, 821–826.

Rosenberg, E. B., Strickland, E. T., Yang, S.-L., and Whalen, C. E. (1973). IgGm antibodies to red cells and autoimmune anemia in patients with malaria. *Am. J. Trop. Med. Hyg.* **22**, 146–152.

Rosenberg, Y. J. (1978). Autoimmune and polyclonal B cell responses during murine malaria. *Nature (London)* **274**, 170–171.

Rosenstreich, D. L., and Oppenheimer, J. J. (1976). The role of macrophages in the activation of T and B lymphocytes *in vitro*. *In* "Immunobiology of the Macrophage" (D. S. Nelson, ed), Chapter 7, pp. 162–234. Academic Press, New York.

Sadun, E. H., Williams, J. S., and Martin, L. K. (1966). Serum biochemical changes in malarial infections in a man, chimpanzees and mice. *Mil. Med.* **131**, 1094–1106.

Saul, K., and Kreier, J. P. (1977). *Plasmodium berghei:* Immunization of rats with antigens from a population of free parasites rich in merozoites. *Tropenmed. Parasitol.* **28**, 302–318.

Schindler, R. (1966). Further investigations on resistance and immunity in mice against infection with *Plasmodium berghei*. *Bull. Soc. Pathol. Exot.* **59**, 585–593.

Schindler, R., and Dennig, H. K. (1962). Über eine Methode zum Nachweis von Antikorper gegen intraerythrozytare Protozoan. *Berl. Muench. Tieraerztl. Wochenschr.* **75**, 111–112.

Schmidt, L. H. (1978a). *Plasmodium falciparum* and *Plasmodium vivax* infection in the owl monkey (*Aotus trivirgatus*). I. Course of untreated infections. *Am. J. Trop. Med. Hyg.* **27**, 671–702.

Schmidt, L. H. (1978b). *Plasmodium falciparum* and *Plasmodium vivax* infections in the owl monkey (*Aotus trivirgatus*) II. Responses to chloroquinine, quinine and pyrimethionine. *Am. J. Trop. Med. Hyg.* **27**, 703–717.

Schnitzer, B., Sodeman, T., Mead, M. L., and Contacos, P. G. (1972). Pitting function of the spleen in malaria: Ultrastructural observations. *Science* **177**, 175–177.

Seed, T. M., and Kreier, J. P. (1969). Autoimmune reactions in chickens with *Plasmodium gallinaceum* infection: The isolation and characterization of a lipid from trypsinized erythrocytes which reacts with serum from acutely infected chickens. *Mil. Med.* **134**, 1220–1227.

Seed, T. M., and Kreier, J. P. (1976). Surface properties of extracellular malaria parasites: Electrophretic and lectin-binding characteristics. *Infect. Immun.* **14**, 1339–1347.

Seed, T. M., and Manwell, R. D. (1977). Plasmodia of birds. *In* "Parasitic Protozoa" (J. P. Kreier, ed.), Vol. 3, pp. 311–357. Academic Press, New York.

Seed, T. M., Aikawa, M., Sterlinl, C., and Rabbage, J. (1974). Surface properties of extracellular malaria parasites: Morphological and cytochemical study. *Infect. Immun.* **9**, 750–761.

Seitz, H. M. (1975). The *Plasmodium berghei* infection in isogenic F_1 (C57B1 × DBA)-mice. I. The course of the infection and immunization experiments. *Tropenmed. Parasitol.* **26**, 417–425.

Seitz, H. M. (1976). The *Plasmodium berghei* infection in isogenic F_1 (C57B1 × DBA) mice. II. Antibodies and antigen in the serum. *Tropenmed. Parasitol.* **27**, 33–43.

Seitz, H. M., Weibler, E. E., and Claviez, M. (1977). Lichtmikroskopische und rastelectronmikroskopische Befund zur phagozytose *Plasmodium berghei*-infezierter roter Blutkorperchen durch Mausemakrophages. *Tropenmed. Parasitol.* **28**, 481–490.

Sergent, E., Parrot, L., and Donatien, A. (1924). Une question de terminologie immuniser et premunizer. *Bull. Soc. Pathol. Exot.* **17**, 37–38.

Sergent, E., Sergent, E. T., and Catanei, A. (1934). Un type de maladie a prémunition: Le paludisine des passeraux a *Plasmodium relictum*. *Ann. Inst. Pasteur, Paris* **53**, 101–119.

Sergent, E., Donatien, A., Parrot, L., and Lestoguard, F. (1945). Etudes sur les piroplasmoses bovines. *Inst. Pasteur Alger.* p. 816.

Sheagren, J. N., Tobie, J. E., Fox, L. M., and Wolff, S. M. (1970). Reticuloendothelial system phagocytic function in naturally acquired human malaria. *J. Lab. Clin. Med.* **75**, 481–487.

Singer, I. (1954a). The effect of splenectomy or phenylhydrazine on infections with *Plasmodium berghei* in the white mouse. *J. Infect. Dis.* **94,** 159–163.

Singer, I. (1954b). The cellular reactions to infections with *Plasmodium berghei* in the white mouse. *J. Infect. Dis.* **94,** 241–261.

Spira, D., and Zuckerman, A. (1965). The effect of splenectomy on anemia in the malarious rat. *Prog. Protozool., Int. Cont. Protozool., 2nd, 1965* Int. Congr. Ser. No. 91, p. 169 (abstr.).

Spitalny, G. L., Revera-Ortez, C., and Nussenzweig, R. S. (1976). *Plasmodium berghei:* The spleen in sporozoite-induced immunity to mouse malaria. *Exp. Parasitol.* **40,** 179–188.

Stechschulte, D. J. (1969). Cell mediated immunity in rats infected with *Plasmodium berghei. Mil. Med.* **134,** 1147–1152.

Stechschulte, D. J., Briggs, N. T., and Wellde, B. T. (1969). Characterization of protective antibodies produced in *Plasmodium berghei* infected rats. *Mil. Med.* **134,** 1140–1146.

Sterzl, J., and Nordin, A. (1971). The common cell precursor for cells producing different immunoglobulins. *In* "Cell Interactions and Receptor Antibodies in Immune Responses" (O. Mäkelä, A. Cross, and T. Kosunen, eds.), pp. 213–230. Academic Press, New York.

Strickland, G. T. (1978). Lymphocyte mitogenic factor in sera from patients with falciparum malaria. *Tropenmed. Parasitol.* **29,** 198–203.

Strossel, T. P. (1976). The mechanisms of phagocytosis. *J. Reticuloendothel. Soc.* **19,** 237–245.

Stuart, A. E. (1970). Phylogeny of mononuclear phagocytes. *In* "Mononuclear Phagocytes" (R. Van Furth, ed.), pp. 316–334. Davis, Philadelphia, Pennsylvania.

Stutz, D. R., Ferris, D. H., and Voss, E. W., Jr. (1972a). Enhanced susceptibility of bursectomized chickens to *Plasmodium gallinaceum:* Comparison of three bursectomy methods. *Proc. Helminthol. Soc. Wash.* **39,** 460–464.

Stutz, D. R., Ferris, D. H., and Voss, E. E., Jr. (1972b). Passive serum transfer experiments in bursectomized chickens infected with *Plasmodium gallinaceum. Proc. Helminthol. Soc. Wash.* **39,** 464–470.

Swann, I. A., and Kreier, J. P. (1973). *Plasmodium gallinaceum:* Mechanisms of anemia in infected chickens. *Exp. Parasitol.* **33,** 79–88.

Taliaferro, W. H., and Taliaferro, L. G. (1944). The effect of immunity on the asexual reproduction of *Plasmodium brasilianum. J. Infect. Dis.* **75,** 1–32.

Taliaferro, W. H., and Taliaferro, L. G. (1947). Asexual reproduction of *Plasmodium cynomolgi* in rhesus monkeys. *J. Infect. Dis.* **80,** 78–104.

Terry, R. J. (1977). Immunodepression in parasite infections. INSERM **72,** 161–178.

Thompson, P. E. (1944). Changes associated with acquired immunity during initial infections in saurian malaria. *J. Infect. Dis.* **75,** 138–149.

Tobie, J. E., and Coatney, G. R. (1964). The antibody response in volunteers with cynomolgi malaria infections. *Am. J. Trop. Med. Hyg.* **13,** 786–789.

Tobie, J. E., Wolff, S. M., and Jeffrey, G. M. (1966a). Immune response of man to inoculation with *Plasmodium cynomolgi* and challenge with *P. vivax. Lancet* **2,** 300–303.

Tobie, J. E., Abele, D. C., Hill, G. J., II, Contacos, P. G., and Evans, C. B. (1966b). Fluorescent antibody studies of the immune response in sporozoite induced and blood-induced vivax malaria and the relationship of antibody production to parasitemia. *Am. J. Trop. Med. Hyg.* **15,** 676–683.

Todorovic, R., Ferris, D., and Ristic, M. (1967). Roles of the spleen in acute plasmodial and babesial infections in rats. *Exp. Parasitol.* **21,** 354–372.

Trubowitz, S., and Masek, B. (1968). *Plasmodium falciparum:* Phagocytosis by polymorphonuclear leukocytes. *Science* **162,** 273–274.

Umanue, E. R. (1972). The regulatory role of macrophages in antigenic stimulation. *Adv. Immunol.* **15,** 95–165.

Van Dijck, P. J., Claesen, M., and De Somer, P. (1970). Effect of polyacrylic acid on experimental malaria and trypanosomiasis in mice. *Ann. Trop. Med. Parasitol.* **64**, 5–9.

Voller, A., and Rossan, R. N. (1969). Immunological studies on simian malaria. III. Immunity to challenge and antigenic variation in *P. knowlesi*. *Trans. R. Soc. Trop. Med. Hyg.* **63**, 507–523.

Voller, A., Huldt, G., Thors, C., and Engvall, E. (1975). New serological test for malaria antibodies. *Br. Med. J.* **22**, 659–661.

Warren, H. S., and Weidanz, W. P. (1976). Malarial immunodepression *in vitro:* Adherent spleen cells are functionally defective as accessory cells in the response to horse erythrocytes. *Eur. J. Immunol.* **6**, 818–819.

Wedderburn, N. (1974). Immunodepression produced by malarial infections in mice. *In* "Parasites in the Immunized Host: Mechanism of Survival" (R. Porter and J. Knight, eds.), Ciba Found. Symp. No. 25 (New Ser.), pp. 123–135. Elsevier, Amsterdam.

Weidanz, W. P., and Rank, R. G. (1975). Regional immunosuppression induced by *Plasmodium berghei yoelii* infection in mice. *Infect. Immun.* **11**, 211–212.

Weiss, M. C., and Zuckerman, A. (1968). Precipitins in mice immunized with attenuated strains of malaria parasites. *Isr. J. Med. Sci.* **4**, 1265–1267.

Weiss, M. C., and Zuckerman, A. (1971). *Plasmodium berghei:* Precipitins in rats infected with attenuated strains made hyperimmune to virulent strains or vaccinated with extracts of virulent strains. *Exp. Parasitol.* **29**, 80–85.

Wellde, B. T., Diggs, C. L., Rodriguez, E., Jr., Briggs, N. T., Wehen, R. M., and von Doenhoff, A. E., Jr. (1972). Requirements for induction of immunity to *Plasmodium berghei* malaria by irradiated parasitized erythrocytes. *Proc. Helminthol. Soc. Wash.* **39**, 529–538.

Wells, R. A., and Diggs, C. L. (1976). Protective activity in sera from mice immunized against *Plasmodium berghei*. *J. Parasitol.* **62**, 638–639.

Welsh, R. M., Jr. (1978). Mouse natural killer cells: Induction, specificity and function. *J. Immunol.* **121**, 1631–1635.

Williams, A. I. O., Rosen, F. S., and Heff, R. (1975). Role of complement components in the susceptibility to *Plasmodium berghei* infection among inbred strains of mice. *Ann. Trop. Med. Parasitol.* **69**, 179–184.

Williamson, W. A., and Greenwood, B. M. (1978). Impairment of the immune response to vaccination after acute malaria. *Lancet* **1**, 1328–1329.

Wilson, R. J. M. (1974). Soluble antigens as blocking antigen. *In* "Parasites in the Immunized Host: Mechanism of Survival" (R. Porter and J. Knight, eds.), Ciba Found. Symp. No. 25 (New Ser.), pp. 185–203. Elsevier, Amsterdam.

Wilson, R. J. M., and Bartholomew, R. K. (1975). The release of antigens by *Plasmodium falciparum*. *Parasitology* **71**, 183–192.

Wilson, R. J. M., and Phillips, R. S. (1976). Method to test inhibitory antibodies in human sera to wild populations of *Plasmodium falciparum*. *Nature (London)* **263**, 132–134.

Wilson, R. J. M., McGregor, I. A., and Hall, P. J. (1975). Persistence and recurrence of S-antigens in *Plasmodium falciparum* infections in man. *Trans. Royal Soc. Trop. Med. Hyg.* **69**, 460–467.

Winkelstein, J. A., Smith, M. R., and Shin, H. S. (1975). The role of C3 as an opsonin in the early stages of infection. *Proc. Soc. Exp. Biol. Med.* **149**, 397–401.

Wyler, D. J. (1978). "Cellular Aspects of Immunoregulation in Malaria," NMRI/USAID/WHO Conference on Biology of Malaria. NMRI, Bethesda, Maryland. *Bull. W.H.O.* **57** (Suppl. 1), 239–243 (1979).

Wyler, D. J., and Brown, J. (1977). Malaria antigen-specific T cell responsiveness during infection with *Plasmodium falciparum*. *Clin. Exp. Immunol.* **29**, 401–407.

Wyler, D. J., and Gallin, J. I. (1977). Spleen derived mononuclear cell chemotactic factor in malaria infections: A possible maximum for splenic macrophage accumulation. *J. Immunol.* **118,** 478–484.

Wyler, D. J., Miller, L. H., and Schmidt, L. H. (1977). Spleen function in quarten malaria (due to *Plasmodium inui*): Evidence for both protective and suppressing roles in host defense. *J. Infect. Dis.* **135,** 86–93.

Zuckerman, A. (1945). *In vitro* opsonic tests with *Plasmodium gallinaceum* and *Plasmodium lophurae*. *J. Infect. Dis.* **77,** 28–59.

Zuckerman, A. (1970). Dynamics of the passive transfer of protection and antiplasmodial precipitin in their litters by mother rats hyperimmune to *Plasmodium berghei*. *Isr. J. Med. Sci.* **6,** 461.

Zuckerman, A., and Yoeli, M. (1954). Age and sex as factors influencing *Plasmodium berghei* infections in intact and splenectomized rats. *J. Infect. Dis.* **94,** 225–236.

Zuckerman, A., Goberman, V., Ron, N., Spira, D., Hamburger, J., and Berg, R. (1969a). Antiplasmodial precipitins demonstrated by double diffusion in agar gel in the serum of rats infected with *Plasmodium berghei*. *Exp. Parasitol.* **24,** 299–312.

Zuckerman, A., Abzug, S., and Burg, R. (1969b). Anemia in rats with equivalent splenomegalies induced by methyl cellulose and *Plasmodium berghei*. *Mil. Med.* **134,** 1084–1099.

Zuckerman, A., Spira, D., and Shore, A. (1969c). Partial protection and precipitins passively transferred to their litters by mother rats infected or susceptible with *Plasmodium berghei*. *Mil. Med.* **134,** 1249–1257.

Immunization against Sporozoites

A. H. Cochrane, R. S. Nussenzweig, and E. H. Nardin

I. INTRODUCTION

The sporozoite stage of malaria parasites has been used in vaccination attempts involving a variety of hosts ranging from birds and rodents to primates including humans. The repeated administration of attenuated sporozoites has completely protected a variable percentage of these immunized hosts against an otherwise severe or even lethal malarial infection. For the various mammalian hosts, data are available on sporozoite immunization and protection against two different malarial species. Thus, mice have been immunized and protected with x-irradiated sporozoites of *Plasmodium berghei* and *P. chabaudi;* a relatively small number of rhesus monkeys have been immunized with γ-attenuated sporozoites of either *P. cynomolgi* or *P. knowlesi;* and finally a small number of

Malaria, Vol. 3
Copyright © 1980 by Academic Press, Inc.
All rights of reproduction in any form reserved.
ISBN 0-12-426103-5

humans have been successfully immunized by the bites of x-irradiated *P. vivax-* or *P. falciparum*-infected mosquitoes.

However, the concept that sporozoites of mammalian malaria induce a protective immune response is a relatively novel one which is, in fact, contrary to the previously held view that sporozoites and exoerythrocytic stages do not induce an immune response. This erroneous concept was based on the observations that (1) sporozoites are a short-lived stage within mammalian hosts, (2) sporozoites and exoerythrocytic stages do not induce detectable antibodies to erythrocytic stages, and (3) animals immune to blood stages of the parasite develop numerous exoerythrocytic forms following sporozoite challenge.

All these observations are basically correct, but what was not realized then was that sporozoites, as well as other developmental stages of plasmodia, induce a strictly stage-specific immune response. The protection resulting from sporozoite immunization is only effective against sporozoite challenge, and the antibody response to sporozoites is directed toward stage-specific sporozoite surface antigen(s).

In reviewing the data on sporozoite immunization, we have presented them in a manner we feel will facilitate a comparison of the findings in the various host species. This, we believe, makes apparent the many analogies and also some of the peculiarities of sporozoite–host interaction in the various systems, and also shows rather clearly the areas where further research is needed.

II. IMMUNIZATION OF RODENTS AGAINST SPOROZOITE-INDUCED MALARIA

A series of publications (Mulligan *et al.*, 1941; Russell and Mohan 1942; Russell *et al.*, 1942) which reported the successful immunization of birds with ultraviolet-irradiated sporozoites, undoubtedly provided the basis for immunization of rodents using sporozoites as the immunogen. However, considerable differences were known to exist between the exoerythrocytic cycles of avian and mammalian malarias. The finding that exoerythrocytic forms of *P. berghei,* a rodent malaria, developed within hepatocytes established the close relationship between rodent and primate malarias (Yoeli *et al.*, 1966). Standardization of the conditions for the reproducible cyclic transmission of *P. berghei* (Yoeli *et al.*, 1965) made it feasible to obtain large numbers of sporozoites and to characterize the protective response of rodents to sporozoite immunization.

A variety of parasite preparations, routes, and schedules of immunization have been used to determine optimal conditions for obtaining protection in rodents against sporozoite-induced malaria. Experimental approaches have utilized immunization with radiation-attenuated, viable, and inactivated or disrupted sporozoites. The rodent model has permitted examination of the roles of nonspecific factors in resistance to sporozoite-induced infections and adjuvants in attempts to obtain immunopotentiation of the specific antisporozoite responses. Successful immunization of rodents against sporozoites has also made it possible to characterize the various manifestations of the immune response to this parasite stage and to establish methods for monitoring these responses, particularly with regard to antisporozoite antibody formation. The rodent model has also permitted definition of the relative roles of both the humoral and cellular components of the sporozoite-induced immune response, although the effector mechanisms of the protection still remain to be clarified.

A. Antigen Preparations Used for Immunization of Rodents

1. Immunization with Radiation-Attenuated Sporozoites

a. **Dose Dependency of the Protective Immune Response.** The initial observation of sporozoite-induced protection in a rodent malaria system was made in experiments in which A/J mice were immunized by the administration of a single intravenous dose of x-irradiated sporozoites of the NK65 strain of *P. berghei* (Nussenzweig *et al.*, 1967). The percentage of animals protected against an otherwise lethal sporozoite challenge, although appreciable, varied considerably from experiment to experiment. Increasing the number of immunizing doses to three or more resulted in greater than 90% protection against challenge (Nussenzweig *et al.*, 1969a). Protection remained unaltered for up to 2 months after the last immunizing dose and then declined progressively. More recently, it was observed that preincubation of sporozoites in normal mouse serum reduced both the size and the number of immunizing doses required to establish a solid immunity (Orjih and Nussenzweig, 1980).

The experiments of Beaudoin *et al.* (1976) confirmed and extended these earlier observations on sporozoite-induced immunity in rodent malaria by demonstrating that NIH/NMRI albino mice were protected following the repeated administration of irradiated sporozoites of the ANKA strain of *P. berghei*. The number of NIH/NMRI mice protected against sporozoite challenge following a single immunizing dose of irradiated sporozoites was dependent both on the size of the immunizing dose as well as the time interval between immunization and challenge (Pacheco and Beaudoin, 1978; Pacheco *et al.*, 1979).

The duration of protection in mice immunized with irradiated sporozoites of *P. berghei* was prolonged by challenge with viable sporozoites. Repeated intravenous challenge of immunized mice at approximately monthly intervals extended the period of protection from 3 to 12 months (A. U. Orjih, unpublished).

b. Effect of Irradiation on Sporozoite Infectivity and Immunogenicity. The effect of x-irradiation on the infectivity and subsequent development of the sporozoites of *P. berghei* into tissue stages was studied by Vanderberg *et al.* (1968a). The number of sporozoites capable of developing into recognizable exoerythrocytic forms was found to vary inversely with the amount of radiation. At low levels of radiation, i.e., 4 krads, there was a reduction both in the size and number of exoerythrocytic forms that developed following inoculation of the irradiated sporozoites. Detectable tissue stages occurred very rarely when the sporozoites were irradiated at 8–10 krads, and these sporozoites failed to produce patent infections in the large majority of animals. Sporozoites irradiated with more than 10 krads consistently failed to develop into recognizable exoerythrocytic forms and did not produce patent infections.

Exposure of sporozoites to considerably higher doses of irradiation, i.e., 50 krads, did not abolish their immunogenicity, since multiple immunization with these parasites still resulted in complete protection of A/J mice (Nussenzweig *et al.*, 1969a).

c. Effectiveness of Different Routes of Immunization. Mice immunized by the repeated bites of x-irradiated *P. berghei*-infected mosquitoes developed total resistance to challenge similar to that of mice immunized intravenously (Vanderberg *et al.*, 1970). However, the repeated intraperitoneal, intramuscular, intracutaneous, or per os administration of x-irradiated sporozoites of *P. berghei* failed to induce high and reproducible levels of protection against intravenous challenge (Spitalny and Nussenzweig, 1972). This was interpreted as indicating that the mice immunized by these routes may have developed a localized rather than a systemic immune response which failed to protect them against intravenous challenge.

2. Immunization with Viable Sporozoites

Immunization of rats with nonattenuated sporozoites of *P. berghei* induced a protective response to a subsequent sporozoite challenge (Verhave, 1975). In these experiments, viable sporozoites were administered to the animals either by intravenous injection or by the bites of infected mosquitoes. Addition of chloroquine to the drinking water of the experimental animals suppressed the erythrocytic phase of the infection. The number of exoerythrocytic forms developing after challenge was used to evaluate the degree of protection. Results were somewhat variable but, in general, three or four immunizing doses were sufficient to reduce the number of exoerythrocytic forms to undetectable levels. Animals challenged 1 year following the last immunizing dose still showed a considerable reduction in the number of developing liver stages.

Similar observations were made by Beaudoin *et al.* (1975, 1977) who immunized NIH/NMRI mice against the ANKA strain of *P. berghei* using viable sporozoites as the immunogen. During the course of immunization the animals were placed on a suppressive regimen of chloroquine and, prior to challenge, a curative dose of primaquine was given to eliminate exoerythrocytic stages. All mice resisted sporozoite challenge but succumbed to challenge with infected red blood cells. The authors concluded that unaltered infective sporozoites were immunogenic and stimulated a degree of protection against sporozoite challenge comparable to that obtained by immunization with irradiated sporozoites.

3. Immunization with Inactivated or Disrupted Sporozoites

Thus far, effective and consistent protection against sporozoites of *P. berghei* has only been achieved by using either intact irradiated or viable sporozoites as the immunogen. Various attempts to use inactivated or disrupted sporozoites for immunization have either failed completely to induce protection or have only been successful in a relatively low and variable percentage of animals. Alger *et al.* (1972) and Spitalny and Nussenzweig (1972) reported a variable degree of protection in mice following their repeated injection with heat-inactivated sporozoites. Similarly, a variable percentage of mice was protected following immunization with noninfective metabolically inactivated sporozoites which had been treated with iodoacetamide (A. H. Cochrane, unpublished).

Protection of mice immunized with either irradiated or nonirradiated Formalin-fixed sporozoites of *P. berghei* has been reported (Beaudoin *et al.*, 1975). However, our observations indicate that mice immunized with either Formalin-treated or lyophilized sporozoites of *P. berghei* showed minimal or no protection upon challenge even though they consistently produced circumsporozoite precipitation (CSP) antibodies (A. H. Cochrane, unpublished). Similarly, animals immunized with sporozoites disrupted by repeated freezing and thawing, or by sonication, showed minimal or no protection (Spitalny and Nussenzweig, 1972). In addition, immunization using various sporozoite fractions obtained by homogenization followed by differential centrifugation also failed to elicit a protective immune response.

4. Immunopotentiation of Sporozoite-Induced Immunity

Adjuvants have only been used in a few instances to attempt to potentiate the immune response of rodents to sporozoites. Administration of *Corynebacterium parvum*, a potent stimulant of the mononuclear phagocyte system, prior to a single intravenous injection of irradiated sporozoites protected a significant number of A/J mice against challenge with *P. berghei* sporozoites (E. H. Nardin and R. S. Nussenzweig, unpublished). Most of these animals failed to develop parasitemia, and in those which did, the prepatent period was considerably increased. Control animals receiving a single injection of either *C. parvum* or irradiated sporozoites alone were only minimally protected.

The administration of Bacillus Calmette-Guérin (BCG) to NIH/NMRI mice, in conjunction with irradiated sporozoites of the ANKA strain of *P. berghei,* was observed to have a synergistic effect under certain experimental conditions. Increased protection against challenge with sporozoites was found only when the two immunogens were administered on the same day and when the mice were challenged within 3 days after immunization (Smrkovski and Beaudoin, 1978; Smrkovski and Strickland, 1978). However, mice treated with BCG and irradiated sporozoites were unable to resist rechallenge, whereas mice immunized with sporozoites in the absence of BCG were totally resistant to rechallenge.

B. Properties of Sporozoite-Induced Immunity in Rodents

1. Development of Sterile Immunity

A basic difference in the protective response induced by immunization with sporozoites versus blood stages of rodent malarias is the extent of protection. Animals successfully immunized with sporozoites acquire a sterile immunity, i.e., no patent or subpatent parasitemia occurs upon challenge. The total absence of parasite development in immunized and protected animals was documented by the failure of patency to occur upon subinoculation of large blood volumes from immunized animals into normal recipients or upon splenectomy of the immunized animals (Nussenzweig *et al.,* 1969b; Beaudoin *et al.,* 1976). In addition, actively immunized and protected mice failed to develop exoerythrocytic forms when challenged with viable sporozoites of *P. berghei* (Nussenzweig *et al.,* 1972b). In contrast, protection induced by immunization with blood stages is usually partial. Upon challenge, immunized animals frequently presented a very mild, short-lived infection (Corradetti *et al.,* 1966; Wellde and Sadun, 1967).

2. Specificity of Sporozoite-Induced Protection

The range of protection in sporozoite-immunized mice is broader than in animals immunized with blood stages. Thus, animals immunized with blood forms are usually only protected against the plasmodial species used for immunization and remain fully susceptible to challenge with other rodent malaria species. In contrast, the protective response induced in mice following immunization with sporozoites is characterized by cross-protection against challenge with sporozoites of other species of rodent malaria. Mice immunized against *P. berghei* sporozoites not only resisted challenge with sporozoites of this species but were also extensively protected against challenge with sporozoites of *P. vinckei* and *P. chabaudi* (Nussenzweig *et al.,* 1972a). This cross-protection was accompanied by serological cross-reactivity (Nussenzweig *et al.,* 1969a) and suggested a close antigenic relationship among the sporozoites of rodent malarias. Cross-protection against sporozoites of different plasmodial species is unique, however, to the rodent system. It contrasts sharply with what has been observed in immunization with sporozoites of simian (R. W. Gwadz, unpublished results) and human malarias (Clyde *et al.*, 1973b) where protection is limited to the plasmodial species used for immunization.

In rodent malarias, sporozoite-induced protection is furthermore strictly stage-specific. Thus, mice immunized and protected against sporozoites of *P. berghei* were fully susceptible to infection induced by *P. berghei*-infected red blood cells and developed a course of parasitemia similar to that of control animals (Nussenzweig *et al.*, 1969b). Similarly, NIH/NMRI albino mice protected against challenge with sporozoites of the ANKA strain of *P. berghei* were fully susceptible to infection by blood stages of this parasite (Beaudoin *et al.*, 1976).

C. Characterization of Sporozoite Antigens of Rodent Malaria

1. Development of Sporozoite Antigenicity

Sporozoites of rodent malaria acquire or express the antigen(s) responsible for inducing a protective immune response only at a late stage in their morphogenesis, when the sporozoites invade the mosquitoes' salivary glands. Studies based on serological assays demonstrated that salivary gland parasites expressed a "mature" sporozoite antigen which was first detected on oocyst sporozoites and which increased as the sporozoites matured in the salivary glands (Vanderberg *et al.*, 1972). In contrast to the total protection induced by immunization with salivary gland sporozoites, immunization with oocyst sporozoites induced only a minimal degree of protection. The acquisition of immunogenicity coincided with the development of sporozoite infectivity. Salivary gland sporozoites, in fact, showed more than a 10,000-fold increase in infectivity over that of oocyst sporozoites (Vanderberg, 1975).

2. Localization of Sporozoite Antigen(s)

Ultrastructural observations on sporozoites of both rodent and simian malaria, following incubation with their respective antisera, demonstrated the interaction of antibodies with the outer surface membrane of the parasites (Cochrane *et al.*, 1976). Both transmission electron microscopy (TEM) and scanning electron microscopy (SEM) of sporozoites incubated in immune sera showed a very prominent surface deposition of fine fibrillar material (Figs. 1 and 2). This deposition occurred along most of the sporozoite surface, except for the anterior end which frequently appeared to be relatively free of the precipitate. Incubation of immune serum-treated sporozoites of *P. berghei* with hemocyanin-conjugated anti-mouse IgG indicated that the fibrillar coat resulted from the interaction of immunoglobulin with the sporozoite surface. No coat formation was observed on sporozoites incubated in normal serum (Figs. 1 and 2).

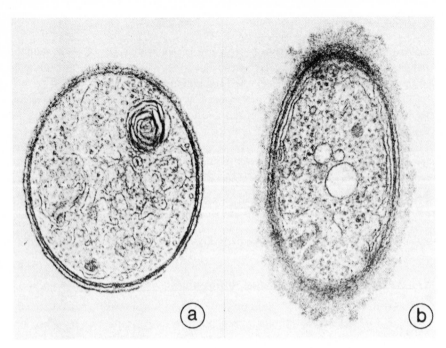

FIG. 1. Electron micrographs of sporozoites of *P. berghei*. ×50,000. Effects of incubation in immune serum. (a) Sporozoite incubated in serum of a normal mouse (30 minutes at 37°C). (b) Sporozoite incubated in serum of an immunized mouse. A prominent coat of fine, fibrillar material covers the entire surface of the parasite. [With permission from "Rodent Malaria," Academic Press Inc. (London) Ltd., 1978.]

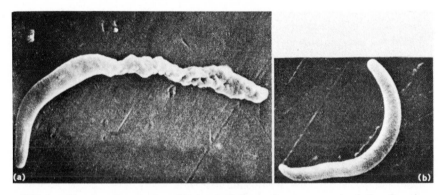

FIG. 2. Alteration of sporozoites of *P. berghei* following immune serum incubation. Scanning electron micrographs. ×9000. (a) Sporozoite incubated in immune serum. The body of the parasite appears smooth. The irregular configuration of the CSP reaction extends a considerable distance posteriorly. (b) Sporozoite incubated in normal serum. Note the smooth surface of the parasite. The anterior end of the sporozoite is narrow and can be clearly distinguished from the rounder posterior end. [With permission from "Rodent Malaria," Academic Press Inc. (London) Ltd., 1978.]

Metabolically inactive parasites, such as Formalin-treated sporozoites and sporozoites kept on ice during their incubation with immune serum, also developed prominent surface coats. Thus, the antibody responsible for coat formation is directed against preformed antigen(s) present on the parasite's surface membrane, and the reaction is independent of the secretion of antigen(s) initiated by antibody–parasite interaction.

Recent freeze-fracture studies of Aikawa *et al.* (1979) on the surface membrane of malarial sporozoites have demonstrated the redistribution of intramembranous particles (IMPs) on the P face of the outer membrane after incubation of the parasite with immune serum. The IMPs of the intermediate and inner pellicular membranes did not show any detectable alteration in their distribution and number, indicating that antisporozoite antibodies altered only the structural arrangement of the plasma membrane. Sporozoites incubated with immune serum also developed an outer layer of particle aggregates which appeared to correspond to the electron-dense surface coat seen by thin-section TEM.

3. Identification of Sporozoite Antigen(s)

In an initial attempt to identify sporozoite surface membrane antigens, partially purified sporozoites were radiolabeled by lactoperoxidase-mediated iodination (Gwadz *et al.*, 1979). The parasites were then disrupted in a French pressure cell, and the soluble fraction submitted to sodium dodecyl sulfate polyacrylamide gel electrophoresis (SDS PAGE) followed by autoradiography. A small number of labeled proteins were present in this extract. Immunoprecipitation with specific antisera to *P. berghei* sporozoites detected primarily one of these membrane components having a molecular weight of ca. 41,000.

D. Manifestations of Sporozoite-Induced Immunity in Rodents

1. Humoral Antisporozoite Immunity

The protective mechanism(s) operating in sporozoite-immunized rodents is as yet not fully understood. However, it is certain that protection is at least, in part, antibody-mediated. Antisporozoite antibodies have been shown, both *in vivo* and *in vitro,* to alter sporozoite infectivity and to interact with sporozoite antigens.

a. Effect of Antibodies on Sporozoite Infectivity

i. Passive Transfer of Immunity.   Transfer of large amounts of immune serum to normal mice, just prior to their inoculation with viable sporozoites of *P. berghei,* resulted in a rapid clearance of infective parasites from the peripheral circulation, similar to that observed in actively immunized animals (Nussenzweig *et al.*, 1972b). In addition, there was a significant decrease in the number of exoerythrocytic forms developing in the livers of these recipients of immune serum as compared to those of normal serum recipients. However, in contrast to mice actively immunized with irradiated sporozoites, the infections in immune serum recipients were never totally suppressed and were invariably lethal. These observations suggest that, in actively sporozoite-immunized rodents, there is, in addition to a humoral factor, an as yet undefined mechanism of resistance which is nontransferable by immune serum alone.

ii. Sporozoite Neutralization Activity.   Incubation of sporozoites of *P. berghei* for 45 minutes at room temperature in immune serum resulted in a considerable loss of their infectivity as detected by inoculation of the parasites into normal recipients (Nussenzweig *et al.*, 1969a). This sporozoite-neutralizing activity (SNA) was detected in the serum of mice which received two immunizing doses and increased in titer with further immunization. Complement was not required for SNA (Spitalny, 1973), and this activity was stage-specific and did not affect other developmental stages of the same strain of parasites (Vanderberg *et al.*, 1972).

The exact mechanism of the *in vitro* serum-mediated loss of sporozoite infec-

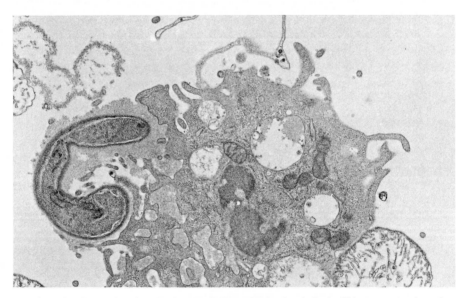

FIG. 3. Sporozoite of *P. berghei* attached to and being interiorized within a mouse peritoneal macrophage after a 30-minute incubation at 37°C. The parasite, which was preincubated with immune mouse serum, shows a prominent surface coat. Material similar in appearance to the surface coat is in macrophage vacuoles. ×15,000. (With permission from harry D. Danforth, Masamichi Aikawa, Alan H. Cochrane and R. S. Nussenzweig.)

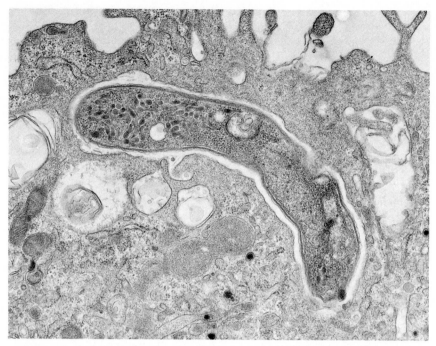

FIG. 4. Intracellular sporozoite of *P. berghei* after a 30-minute incubation at 37°C with mouse peritoneal macrophage. The parasite, which was preincubated in normal mouse serum, shows no ultrastructural degeneration and is enclosed in a membrane-bound parasitophorous vacuole within the macrophage. ×25,000. (with permission from Harry D. Danforth, Masamichi Aikawa, Alan H. Cochrane and R. S. Russenzweig.)

tivity and its role in sporozoite-induced protection *in vivo* remain to be clarified. In this connection, a recent study by Danforth *et al.* (1980) indicated that the incubation of sporozoites with antibody facilitated their uptake and ultimate "digestion" by phagocytic cells *in vitro*. Ultrastructural observations on sporozoites of *P. berghei* incubated in immune serum and then exposed to peritoneal mouse macrophages showed parasites covered by a thick surface coat being interiorized (Fig. 3). Within a short time period, most of the intracellular parasites appeared to have undergone degeneration. Sporozoites incubated in normal serum were also rapidly interiorized, in part as a result of active penetration into the macrophages. However, these intracellular parasites appeared to be unaltered (Fig. 4) and to cause deterioration of the macrophages.

b. Sporozoite–Antibody Interactions

i. Circumsporozoite Precipitation Reaction. The first observation on the interaction between viable sporozoites and antisporozoite antibodies was made by

Russell *et al.* (1941). The sera of birds, immunized by repeated administration of *P. gallinaceum* sporozoites attenuated by ultraviolet radiation, agglutinated sporozoites at high serum dilutions. However, sera from nonimmunized fowls or from birds with blood-induced infections failed to agglutinate sporozoites at these same serum dilutions.

In 1969, Vanderberg and others found that rodent malarial sporozoites developed a terminal, threadlike precipitate following *in vitro* interaction with immune serum. This reaction was designated the circumsporozoite precipitation (CSP) reaction (Fig. 5). The CSP reaction can be clearly seen by phase-contrast microscopy after 10 or more minutes of incubation of parasites with immune serum at either room temperature or at 37°C. Ultrastructural observations using SEM (Cochrane *et al.*, 1976) (Fig. 2) have shown the CSP reaction to consist of a terminal prolongation of the surface coat.

The CSP reaction was complement-independent (Vanderberg *et al.*, 1969; Spitalny, 1973) and did not occur at 4°C or with Formalin-treated sporozoites (Cochrane *et al.*, 1976). Frozen and thawed sporozoites, when incubated with immune serum, developed a peculiar CSP reaction consisting of a granulated deposit along most of the parasite's surface (Vanderberg *et al.*, 1969). The CSP reaction is apparently not an *in vitro* artifact, since it has been observed on sporozoites recovered from the peripheral circulation of immunized mice (A. H. Cochrane, unpublished).

The antibodies detected by the CSP reaction are produced by mice and rats immunized by the intravenous inoculation of irradiated sporozoites of *P. berghei* or by the bites of infected irradiated mosquitoes (Vanderberg *et al.*, 1970). Animals injected intravenously with viable *P. berghei* sporozoites also produced CSP antibodies (Spitalny and Nussenzweig, 1973). The CSP antibody response in rats given a single inoculum of irradiated sporozoites was detectable for a

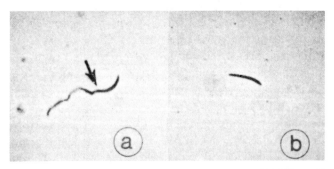

FIG. 5. Phase-contrast microscopy of sporozoites of *P. berghei.* × 1000. Effects of incubation in immune serum. (a) Sporozoite incubated in immune mouse serum for 30 minutes at 37°C. Note the very long threadlike precipitate (positive CSP reaction) to the left of the arrow. (b) Sporozoite incubated in normal mouse serum. [With permission from "Rodent Malaria," Academic Press Inc. (London) Ltd., 1978.]

longer period of time than in rats injected with viable sporozoites. Viable sporozoites were shown to enhance the CSP antibody response in mice immunized with irradiated sporozoites (Vanderberg *et al.*, 1969).

ii. Indirect Immunofluorescent Antibody Test. Immunoglobulin deposits on malarial sporozoites incubated with immune serum are also detectable by immunofluorescence. The initial immunofluorescent studies were carried out by Corradetti *et al.* (1964) using air-dried sporozoites of avian malaria. The immunofluorescent antibody (IFA) technique has also been applied to the study of the antisporozoite antibody response in immunized rodents (McNamara, 1976; Golenser *et al.*, 1977). The level and persistence of sporozoite-specific antibodies in mice and rats immunized with *P. berghei* sporozoites was dependent upon the route of inoculation and the number of immunizing doses administered.

Antisporozoite antibodies were detected by the IFA test in the serum of NIH/NMRI mice 3 days after a single immunizing dose of *P. berghei* (ANKA strain) sporozoites (Bawden *et al.*, 1978). The antibody response peaked on days 4 and 5 and declined rapidly thereafter. Similarly, Orjih and Nussenzweig (1979), using the IFA test, detected antisporozoite antibodies in mice 2 days after their inoculation with irradiated sporozoites. The sensitivity of this technique allowed the detection of an anamnestic antibody response in mice following the bite of a single infected mosquito (Bawden *et al.*, 1979; McConnell *et al.*, 1978).

Orjih and Nussenzweig (1979), using the IFA test, demonstrated suppression of the antibody response to sporozoites of *P. berghei* by acute blood stage infections. The duration of the primary response and the capacity to mount a secondary response during an ongoing infection were particularly affected. However, when the antisporozoite immunity was solidly established and the animals were protected against sporozoite challenge, a subsequent blood-induced infection did not reduce the antibody response to the sporozoite antigen.

c. Specificity of Antisporozoite Antibodies

i. Stage Specificity. The antisporozoite antibodies detected by the CSP assay are strictly stage-specific. The sera of animals immunized with sporozoites of *P. berghei* had no detectable effect on the asexual blood stages, gametocytes, ookinetes, or exoerythrocytic forms of the same parasite strain (Vanderberg *et al.*, 1972; Vanderberg, 1973).

While stage-specific antigens have been demonstrated by the CSP assay, evidence obtained primarily by immunofluorescence indicates that antigens common to all stages of the malaria parasite also occur. The observations of Danforth *et al.* (1978) indicated that the exoerythrocytic forms of *P. berghei*, developing in the livers of parasitized rats, shared antigens common to both sporozoites and erythrocytic stages. Exoerythrocytic forms found in rat livers, fixed less than 30 hours after the injection of *P. berghei* sporozoites, fluoresced with antisera directed against either sporozoites or infected red blood cells. As the liver stages became more mature, there was a loss of the sporozoite-specific antigen(s), and positive reactions were obtained only with anti-infected red blood cell antisera.

Numerous workers have shown cross-reactions between sporozoites and blood stage parasites in both avian (Ingram *et al.*, 1961; Sodeman and Jeffery, 1964) and rodent malaria systems (Golenser *et al.*, 1977) by using air-dried parasites and the IFA test. However, Nardin and Nussenzweig (1978) demonstrated that only stage-specific antigens were localized on the surface membrane of malarial sporozoites. Viable or glutaraldehyde-fixed sporozoites of *P. berghei* fluoresced only when incubated with antisporozoite antisera. In contrast, air-dried and frozen sporozoites of *P. berghei* reacted with both antisporozoite antisera and sera of mice repeatedly infected with or immunized against blood stages of *P. berghei*. Alteration of the sporozoite's surface membrane by air-drying and freezing presumably exposes internal antigens common to both developmental stages of the parasite.

The stage specificity of antisporozoite immunofluorescent antibodies was also demonstrated by adsorption experiments (Golenser *et al.*, 1978). In sera containing antibodies directed against both sporozoites and blood stage parasites, adsorption with large numbers of sporozoites completely removed the antisporozoite antibodies but not the anti-blood stage immunofluorescent activity.

Bawden *et al.* (1978) reported on the development of a sporozoite stage-specific IFA inhibition test. The assay was based on inhibition of the reaction between sporozoites of *P. berghei* and highly specific rabbit antisporozoite antiserum by antibodies present in the sera of sporozoite-immunized rodents. With this test, it was possible to distinguish between antisporozoite antibodies and antibodies directed against blood stage antigens or mosquito debris.

ii. Species Specificity. Antibodies detected by the CSP reaction strongly cross-react with sporozoites of heterologous species of murine malaria parasites. Thus the serum of mice immunized with x-irradiated sporozoites of *P. berghei* produced a positive CSP reaction with sporozoites of *P. vinckei* and *P. chabaudi*, and the reverse was also true (Vanderberg *et al.*, 1969; Nussenzweig *et al.*, 1972a). In addition, sporozoites of *P. vinckei* lost their infectivity when incubated with antisera directed against sporozoites of *P. berghei* (Nussenzweig *et al.*, 1969a). Protection against sporozoite challenge paralleled these serological findings (Nussenzweig *et al.*, 1969b).

The anti-*P. berghei* sporozoite antisera, however, did not produce CSP reactions when incubated with sporozoites of simian (*P. cynomolgi*) or avian (*P. gallinaceum*) malaria (Vanderberg *et al.*, 1969). Consistent with this species specificity of antisporozoite antibodies, the IFA assay also failed to detect serological cross-reactions between viable or glutaraldehyde-fixed *P. berghei* sporozoites and antisera directed against sporozoites of simian (*P. cynomolgi* and *P. knowlesi*) and human (*P. vivax* and *P. falciparum*) malaria (Nardin and Nussenzweig, 1979a).

d. Relationship of Antisporozoite Antibodies to Protection. The stage- and species-specific protection observed in sporozoite-immunized animals corre- lates well with the specificity of antisporozoite antibodies as detected by both the CSP and IFA assays.

Although the presence of antisporozoite antibodies is very often associated with protective immunity, humoral and protective antisporozoite responses can be dissociated under a variety of experimental conditions. Thus, immunization of mice with homogenized, sonicated, or otherwise disrupted sporozoites of *P. berghei* (Spitalny and Nussenzweig, 1972) or with lyophilized sporozoites (A. H. Cochrane, unpublished) induced CSP antibody formation in the absence of significant protection.

On the other hand, a protective response may be present in the absence of detectable CSP activity. After the administration of a single, relatively large dose of irradiated sporozoites of *P. berghei,* a variable percentage of mice developed a sterile immunity at a time (i.e., 7 days after immunization) when CSP an- tibodies were not yet detectable in their sera (Spitalny and Nussenzweig, 1973). In addition, mice immunized after splenectomy developed a significant degree of protection against sporozoite challenge in the absence of detectable levels of CSP antibodies (Spitalny *et al.,* 1976).

Chen *et al.* (1977) demonstrated that B-cell immunocompetence was not an absolute requirement for the induction of sporozoite-induced immunity in mice, suggesting a major role for T cells in the acquisition of protective immunity. A considerable proportion of mice injected from birth on with goat antiserum to mouse μ chain (μ-suppressed) became protected against sporozoite challenge after receiving several immunizing doses of irradiated *P. berghei* sporozoites. Neither CSP antibodies nor SNA could be demonstrated in the serum of the immunized and protected animals.

2. Cell-Mediated Responses in Sporozoite-Immunized Rodents

Very few studies have focused on the role of cell-mediated responses in sporozoite-immunized animals. In fact, a reliable *in vitro* or *in vivo* test for measuring cell-mediated responses to sporozoites, and their correlation with protection, still remains to be established.

a. Role of the Thymus. The development of protection, as well as anti- sporozoite antibodies, is thymus-dependent. Thus, mice which were thymec- tomized, x-irradiated, and bone marrow-reconstituted, as well as congenitally athymic nude (*nu/nu*) mice, failed to develop a protective immune response following the repeated administration of irradiated sporozoites of *P. berghei* (Spitalny *et al.*, 1977). Sera of these T cell-deficient mice failed to show any detectable SNA, and CSP antibodies were detected in only some of the animals in low titers. Reconstitution of the animals with thymocytes, prior to immunization, restored both the capacity to develop a protective immune response as well as antisporozoite antibodies.

b. Adoptive Transfer of Immunity Mediated by Cells.   Recent studies have shown that the protection of sporozoite-immunized mice could be transferred by immune spleen cells to sublethally irradiated normal recipients (Verhave *et al.*, 1978). The immune spleen cell transfer had to be followed by a single immunization of the recipients with irradiated sporozoites, which per se failed to induce significant protection. *In vitro* treatment of immune spleen cells with an anti-θ serum abolished their capacity to transfer protection against sporozoite challenge, indicating again that T cells play an essential role in sporozoite-induced protection.

3. Nonspecific Protection against Sporozoite-Induced Malaria

Nussenzweig (1967) found that pretreatment of mice with heat-inactivated *C. parvum* significantly increased their resistance to subsequent challenge with sporozoites of *P. berghei*. A certain percentage of mice completely failed to develop parasitemias, and in others the length of the prepatent period was considerably increased. The repeated administration of Freund's complete adjuvant (FCA) also resulted in increased resistance of the mice to sporozoite-induced infections.

One dose of 10^7 viable units of *Mycobacterium bovis* (strain BCG) administered intravenously protected a significant number of Swiss mice from an initial challenge with sporozoites of the ANKA strain of *P. berghei* (Smrkovski and Beaudoin, 1978). However, the observed nonspecific protection induced by the BCG treatment was not as long-lasting as that resulting from immunization with a single dose of irradiated sporozoites (Smrkovski and Strickland, 1978). *Mycobacterium bovis*-treated animals surviving the initial challenge were not protected against a second challenge, whereas sporozoite-immunized animals were fully resistant to a second sporozoite inoculation. Increasing the number of doses of BCG did not increase the nonspecific resistance to rechallenge.

Three interferon inducers, Newcastle disease virus, statolon, and a double-stranded copolymer of polyriboinosinic acid and polyribocytidylic acid [poly (I:C)] protected mice either totally or partially against *P. berghei* sporozoite challenge (Jahiel *et al.*, 1968a,b, 1969, 1970). The data indicated that the stage most sensitive to the protective effect of the interferon inducers occurred late in exoerythrocytic development.

Alger *et al.* (1972) reported that the repeated intraperitoneal injection of mice with noninfected salivary gland tissue conferred protection on some of the animals against intraperitoneal inoculation of viable sporozoites of *P. berghei*. As suggested by the authors, this protection could have been due to nonspecifically stimulated cells in the peritoneal cavity, which might have interfered with development of the sporozoites used for challenge. However, other studies have clearly demonstrated that mosquito material does not induce resistance to sporozoite-induced infections. The administration of noninfected irradiated salivary glands, injected according to the same schedule and in amounts equivalent to those of sporozoite-infected glands, failed to protect A/J mice against challenge with *P. berghei* sporozoites (Nussenzweig *et al.*, 1967, 1969b; Spitalny and Nussenzweig, 1972). Likewise, Beaudoin *et al.* (1976) were not able to protect NIH/NMRI mice by immunizing them with triturated noninfected mosquito thoraxes.

III. IMMUNIZATION OF SIMIAN HOSTS AGAINST SPOROZOITE-INDUCED MALARIA

Attempts to vaccinate simian hosts against sporozoite-induced malaria have been aimed at clarifying the extent to which the findings on sporozoite-induced immunity in rodents reflect a general phenomenon applicable also to plasmodia–primate systems. Because of limitations on the availability of rhesus monkeys, vaccination attempts, initiated in 1972, have been restricted to methods which have proved successful in rodents, specifically, the use of irradiated sporozoites administered either intravenously or by the bites of infected irradiated mosquitoes.

In the rhesus monkey, immunization studies have utilized *P. cynomolgi* and *P. knowlesi* because of the numerous analogies these parasites have with certain species of human malaria. Monkeys infected with *P. cynomolgi* develop a mild, benign infection, not unlike that of *P. vivax* in humans, while monkeys infected with *P. knowlesi* develop a severe, fulminating infection, similar to that of *P. falciparum* in young children and adults when they are first exposed to the parasite. In addition, *P. knowlesi* has been used to obtain much of the information concerning immunization with merozoites (Cohen *et al.*, 1977) and gametes (Gwadz and Green, 1978) and thus allows a comparison of vaccination results in rhesus monkeys using different developmental stages of the same parasite. Because of their analogies with the human malarias, these simian malaria systems, it is hoped, will produce findings directly applicable to vaccination attempts in humans.

A. Antigen Preparations Used for Immunization of Simian Hosts

Optimal conditions for simian immunization against sporozoite-induced malaria including best dosage, route, and schedule for immunization, have yet to be established. All successful immunizations have used irradiated sporozoites administered either intravenously or by the bites of irradiated infected mosquitoes.

1. Intravenous Immunization

In the initial study on sporozoite-induced immunity in a simian malaria system, two juvenile rhesus monkeys (*Macaca mulatta*) were inoculated intravenously with x-irradiated sporozoites of *P. cynomolgi* (Collins and Contacos, 1972). Over a period of 146 days, each of these animals received a total of approximately 1.25×10^5 sporozoites divided into five immunizing doses. When challenged by the bites of infected mosquitoes, these immunized monkeys showed only a slight delay in patency. Their parasitemias, once initiated, followed the same course as that of the single control animal.

The most extensive study on the immunization of rhesus monkeys against sporozoites of *P. cynomolgi* was that of Chen (1974). A total of 12 rhesus monkeys was immunized intravenously with irradiated sporozoites of *P. cynomolgi*, using different schedules of administration and various doses of immunogen. Monkeys were challenged when high titers of CSP antibodies or SNA were detected in their sera. Sporozoite challenge was administered by the intravenous inoculation of $1–2 \times 10^4$ infective sporozoites, the dose found to be sufficient consistently to induce infection in control animals.

Extensive or total protection of rhesus monkeys against sporozoite challenge was obtained only after a period of immunization of several months and the intravenous administration of multiple large immunizing doses. The two animals which were totally protected against challenge received a total of 4.0×10^7 and 1.7×10^8 sporozoites over a period of 9½ and 13½ months, respectively. However, the remaining 10 rhesus monkeys receiving comparable numbers of sporozoites failed to resist intravenous challenge.

More recently, sporozoites of *P. knowlesi* have been used to immunize rhesus monkeys (Gwadz *et al.*, 1979). Four young adult rhesus monkeys were immunized by the multiple intravenous injection of a total of $3–4 \times 10^8$ γ-irradiated sporozoites of *P. knowlesi*. Three of these animals and their respective controls were challenged by the bites of infected mosquitoes. Two of these monkeys had developed sterile immunity and were completely resistant to challenge. The third animal was partially protected, since its prepatent period was considerably prolonged. Of the two protected animals, one was resistant to a second and also to a third challenge administered 3 months after the last immunizing dose.

However, the remaining 10 rhesus monkeys receiving comarable numbers of

2. Immunization by Bite

Ward and Hayes (1972) immunized three rhesus monkeys against sporozoites of *P. cynomolgi* by the bites of x-irradiated infected mosquitoes. Three immunizing doses of irradiated sporozoites were administered over a period of 42 days. When the immunized animals were challenged by the bites of infected mosquitoes, there was no significant delay in patency, and parasitemia followed that of control animals.

Chen (1974) found that multiple exposure, at short intervals, to the bites of irradiated *P. cynomolgi*-infected mosquitoes appeared to be a promising immunization procedure. Although rhesus monkeys immunized by this technique were never totally protected, they did show a significantly prolonged prepatent period.

3. Immunopotentiation of Sporozoite-Induced Immunity

In an attempt to amplify the antisporozoite protective response, viable or irradiated *P. knowlesi* sporozoites were emulsified in FCA and injected intramuscularly into six rhesus monkeys (Gwadz *et al.*, 1979). Three animals received a single immunizing dose of 5.0×10^7 sporozoites, and three others were each given two immunizing doses totaling 1.2×10^8 sporozoites. The animals showed no detectable degree of protection when challenged with sporozoites 1 month after the last immunizing dose.

These results are in sharp contrast to the protective immunity obtained following intramuscular immunization of rhesus monkeys using *P. knowlesi* merozoites (Cohen *et al.*, 1977). Similarly, rhesus monkeys immunized with *P. knowlesi* gametes emulsified in FCA developed high levels of transmission-blocking immunity. These findings indicate that the protective immune response in rhesus monkeys varies according to the life stage of the parasite used as immunogen.

Based on the adjuvant activity of *C. parvum* in rodents, a single rhesus monkey was pretreated with *C. parvum* prior to immunization with irradiated sporozoites of *P. cynomolgi* (Chen, 1974). Upon challenge, the adjuvant-pretreated immunized monkey exhibited a significantly prolonged prepatent period when compared to a nonimmunized control animal.

B. Properties of Sporozoite-Induced Immunity in Simian Hosts

Rhesus monkeys, successfully immunized against sporozoites, developed a sterile immunity. No parasitemia was detected in daily blood smears taken for extended periods following sporozoite challenge.

Protection in the sporozoite-immunized rhesus monkey has also been observed to be species-specific. A single monkey immunized by the repeated intravenous administration of irradiated sporozoites of *P. knowlesi* developed parasitemia following challenge with sporozoites of *P. cynomolgi*. This occurred at a time when the monkey had repeatedly resisted challenge with sporozoites of *P. knowlesi* (R. W. Gwadz, unpublished).

In addition, the protective immune response of rhesus monkeys was found to be stage-specific and thus failed to alter the course of the blood stage infection. This was clearly observed in partially protected sporozoite-immunized animals, which upon sporozoite challenge developed parasitemia after a prolonged prepatent period. Once initiated, the course of the erythrocytic phase of the infection of these animals was indistinguishable from that of controls (Chen, 1974; R. S. Nussenzweig, unpublished).

C. Characterization of Sporozoite Antigens of Simian Malaria

1. Development of Sporozoite Antigenicity

Sporozoites of *P. cynomolgi* were observed to undergo a process of progressive antigenic maturation (Chen, 1974), similar to the earlier described antigenic maturation of *P. berghei* (Vanderberg *et al.*, 1972). This was reflected in a gradual increase in infectivity and immunogenicity of the *P. cynomolgi* sporozoites as they migrated from the midgut to the salivary glands of the mosquitoes.

The infectivity of *P. cynomolgi* sporozoites was determined by inoculating rhesus monkeys intravenously with sporozoite populations recovered from mosquito midguts, abdominal and thoracic hemocoels, and salivary glands. Midgut sporozoites consistently failed to induce patent infections in monkeys. Thoracic and abdominal hemocoel sporozoites were infective, but the prepatent periods of recipient animals were invariably longer than those of monkeys receiving salivary gland sporozoites.

The development of sporozoite infectivity correlates with the acquisition of specific salivary gland sporozoite antigen(s). The immunogenicity of the different sporozoite preparations was determined by inoculating them into rats which were then monitored for CSP antibodies. The presence of stage-specific antigen(s) was also demonstrated by determining the CSP reactivity of the different sporozoite preparations by incubating them with antisera of known specificity.

Midgut sporozoites completely failed to induce CSP antibody formation when used as immunogen and were totally nonreactive when incubated with antisera raised against salivary gland sporozoites. Salivary gland sporozoites were most efficient in inducing CSP antibody formation and were most reactive when tested with antisera raised against midgut, abdominal, and thoracic hemocoel sporozoites.

The capacity of the sporozoites to induce antibody formation increased with length of stay within the salivary glands. Salivary gland sporozoites obtained on day 10 following mosquito infection were poorly reactive when tested against known antisera. Maximal levels of CSP reactivity were noted using salivary gland sporozoites obtained 21–25 days after mosquito infection.

The occurrence of antigenic maturation was corroborated when the antigen–antibody reactions were monitored by indirect immunofluorescence and electron microscopy. In contrast to reactions using salivary gland sporozoites, only weak immunofluorescence was observed when 11-day *P. knowlesi* oocyst sporozoites were incubated with antisera raised against salivary gland sporozoites (Nardin *et al.*, 1979a). This observation is consistent with ultrastructural studies on *P. cynomolgi* oocyst sporozoites which demonstrated a weakly developed surface coat upon interaction with antisera raised against salivary gland sporozoites (Cochrane *et al.*, 1976). When 20- to 25-day salivary gland sporozoites were tested with the same antisera, prominent electron-dense surface coats were observed on the parasites.

2. Localization of Sporozoite Antigen(s)

Electron microscopy (Cochrane *et al.*, 1976) and freeze-fracture studies (Aikawa *et al.*, 1979) on sporozoites of *P. cynomolgi* have indicated that the outer surface membrane of the parasite is the site of interaction with antibody. These studies have been discussed in some detail in Section II,C. Antibodies reacting with antigens on the surface of viable and glutaraldehyde-fixed sporozoites of *P. cynomolgi* and *P. knowlesi* have also been detected using the IFA test (Nardin and Nussenzweig, 1978; Nardin *et al.*, 1979a).

3. Identification of Sporozoite Antigen(s)

Partially purified, labeled sporozoites were disrupted by French pressure cell treatment and centrifuged. The supernatant, which contained about 80% of the labeled material, was designated sporozoite extract and submitted to SDS-PAGE. An aliquot of this extract was immunoprecipitated with an anti-*P. knowlesi* serum obtained from a sporozoite-immunized and protected monkey. As a control, other aliquots of the extract were immunoprecipitated with anti-*P. cynomolgi* and anti-*P. berghei* sera, as well as normal monkey serum. The corresponding immune complexes were removed by *Staphylococcus aureus*, eluted, and also electrophoresed on SDS PAGE. Autoradiography of the gels revealed the presence of at least 10 bands in the extract, corresponding to labeled surface protein. Only one of these was immunoprecipitated specifically by the anti-*P. knowlesi* serum and not by the other antisera. The molecular weight of this protein was close to 100,000, quite different from that of the *P. berghei*-specific surface protein (MW ca. 41,000) (Gwadz *et al.*, 1979).

The surface antigen of sporozoites does not appear to be a glycoprotein. When viable *P. knowlesi* sporozoites were reacted with either fluorescein-conjugated concanavalin A, wheat germ agglutinin, or soybean agglutinin, the parasites failed to fluoresce (Nardin *et al.*, 1979a). The absence of a carbohydrate moiety on the surface of sporozoites was also supported by their failure to be retained on lectin-conjugated Sepharose columns (Yoshida *et al.*, 1980).

D. Manifestations of Sporozoite-Induced Immunity in Simian Hosts

1. Humoral Antisporozoite Immunity

Consistent with the findings in rodents, sporozoite-immunized rhesus monkeys develop antisporozoite antibodies. *In vitro* incubation with these antisporozoite antibodies alters both the morphology and infectivity of simian malarial sporozoites.

a. Effect of Antibodies on Sporozoite Infectivity. Incubation of *P. cynomolgi* sporozoites with immune serum obtained from a rhesus monkey totally protected against *P. cynomolgi* sporozoite challenge, resulted in a total loss of parasite infectivity (Chen, 1974). This SNA was detectable in serum samples obtained approximately 2 months before and 1 month following challenge. Sera from partially protected monkeys had lower levels of neutralizing activity. Recipients of sporozoites incubated with immune serum from a partially protected rhesus monkey became patent, but their prepatent periods were considerably greater than those of controls.

Rhesus monkeys immunized with irradiated sporozoites of *P. knowlesi* also developed SNA (Gwadz *et al.*, 1979). Sera obtained from protected rhesus monkeys either partially or completely abolished sporozoite infectivity. This was demonstrated by the inoculation of serum-incubated sporozoites into recipients, which either failed completely to develop an infection or did so after a considerably prolonged prepatent period. Immune serum from a nonprotected rhesus had no detectable SNA.

b. Sporozoite–Antibody Interactions. Ultrastructural observations on sporozoites of *P. cynomolgi* incubated with specific antisera have demonstrated that the CSP reaction consists of a posterior prolongation of the surface coat formed by antigen–antibody interaction (Cochrane *et al.*, 1976). The fixation of sporozoites with formaldehyde eliminated CSP reactivity but did not inhibit surface coat formation.

The development of CSP antibodies has been used to monitor the immune response of rhesus monkeys immunized with sporozoites of either *P. cynomolgi* (Chen, 1974) or *P. knowlesi* (Gwadz *et al.*, 1979). In both studies, considerable variability was observed in the CSP antibody response of individual animals, even in the case of monkeys subjected to similar schedules of immunization. The CSP titers fluctuated considerably between immunizing injections and remained at relatively low levels during the initial months of immunization. In most animals, however, high levels of CSP antibodies were detectable 1½–3 months after they had received several immunizing doses. A more rapid appearance of high CSP titers was noted in monkeys which had undergone multiple exposures, at short intervals, to the bites of irradiated *P. cynomolgi*-infected mosquitoes (Chen, 1974).

c. Specificity of Antisporozoite Antibodies

i. Species Specificity and Strain Cross-Reactivity. Species-specific antisera can be produced in rats by immunization with salivary gland sporozoites of a variety of different simian and human malaria species (Nussenzweig *et al.*, 1973). Studies based on the CSP reaction were conducted to determine if sporozoites of various simian malarial species were closely related among themselves or antigenically related to sporozoites of some human malarial species (Nussenzweig and Chen, 1974a,b; Chen *et al.*, 1976). Since CSP cross-reactivity and cross-protection against various rodent malarial species had been observed in mice immunized with sporozoites of *P. berghei* or *P. chabaudi* (Nussenzweig *et al.*, 1972a), it was hoped that simian malarias would provide a potential source of sporozoites for human vaccination trials. However, no CSP cross-reactivity was detected between sporozoites of six different species of simian malaria and two species of human malaria. Even sporozoites of *P. fieldi* and *P. simiovale,* two simian malarial species considered to be closely related, failed to cross-react.

Positive CSP reactions were detected only when antisera were incubated with sporozoites of the homologous species. Sporozoites of diverse geographic strains of the same malaria species, however, cross-reacted intensely in the CSP assay, indicating the presence of shared antigenic determinants. This was documented for the Cambodian, Ceylonensis, and B strains of *P. cynomolgi* (Chen *et al.*, 1976).

Findings obtained by using the IFA reaction corroborated the species specificity of the antisporozoite antibodies (Nardin *et al.*, 1979a). Viable, air-dried, and glutaraldehyde-fixed sporozoite preparations of both *P. cynomolgi* and *P. knowlesi* reacted only with species-specific antisporozoite antisera and failed to cross-react with *P. berghei, P. vivax,* and *P. falciparum* antisporozoite antisera.

In the same study, an apparent exception to the extensive cross-reactions among the strains of a homologous species was noted. With the use of both the CSP reaction and the IFA test, the antigenic relationship between sporozoites of the H (Malaya) and P (Philippine) strains of *P. knowlesi* was studied. No CSP reactions occurred when H-strain sporozoites were tested with antisera directed against P-strain sporozoites, and vice versa. However, some degree of cross-reactivity between the two strains was detected using immunofluorescence. Weak but clearly positive IFA reactions were detected when either glutaraldehyde-treated or air-dried and frozen sporozoites were used as antigen, indicating a sharing of common antigen(s) between the two strains. Consistent with these findings, strain-dependent cross-resistance was noted in rhesus monkeys immunized with semipurified gametes of the H and P strains of *P. knowlesi* (Gwadz and Green, 1978).

ii. Stage Specificity. The stage specificity of sporozoite surface antigens was determined by using antisera obtained from animals exposed exclusively to sporozoites, merozoites, or the various erythrocytic stages and incubating them first with viable sporozoites and then with fluorescein-conjugated antisera (Nardin *et al.,* 1979a). Viable *P. knowlesi* sporozoites reacted only with antisporozoite antiserum and failed to react with antibodies directed against blood stages of *P. knowlesi.* When the integrity of the sporozoites' surface membrane was disrupted by air-drying and freezing, cross-reactions with antisera raised against *P. knowlesi* merozoites or *P. knowlesi*-infected red blood cells and gametes were detected, presumably resulting from the exposure of internal common antigens. Glutaraldehyde fixation maintained the integrity of the sporozoite membrane and eliminated cross-reactions with antibodies against blood stage parasites while preserving reactions with antisporozoite antibodies.

2. Relationship of Antisporozoite Antibodies to Protection

A close correlation between the level of antisporozoite antibodies and protection against challenge has frequently been observed in sporozoite-immunized rhesus monkeys. High levels of CSP antibodies and SNA were detected in a sporozoite-immunized rhesus monkey which had repeatedly resisted *P. cynomolgi* sporozoite challenge (Chen, 1974). A number of nonprotected immunized animals had considerably lower levels of both CSP antibodies and SNA. However, resistance to sporozoite challenge was observed in a *P. cynomolgi* sporozoite-immunized rhesus which had low CSP levels and no detectable SNA.

The study of Gwadz *et al.* (1979) on *P. knowlesi* sporozoite-induced immunity in rhesus monkeys indicated a strong correlation between the level of antisporozoite antibodies and protection against challenge. Protection in two rhesus monkeys was consistently associated with high CSP titers and SNA at the time of challenge. The single animal not protected following the intravenous inoculation of irradiated sporozoites failed repeatedly throughout the immunization schedule to produce significant levels of CSP antibodies or SNA. The absence or a low level of antisporozoite antibodies was also associated with lack of protection in six animals immunized by the intramuscular inoculation of *P. knowlesi* sporozoites emulsified in FCA. Recent unpublished observations (R. S. Nussenzweig and A. H. Cochrane) on a number of *P. knowlesi* sporozoite-immunized rhesus monkeys have further demonstrated the association of high levels of antisporozoite antibodies with protection against challenge, and low levels of antisporozoite antibodies with an absence of protection.

3. Antisporozoite Humoral Response in Naturally Infected Monkeys

Both the CSP assay and the IFA test have been used to demonstrate the presence of antisporozoite antibodies in naturally infected simian hosts. Sera of squirrel monkeys (*Saimiri sciureus*) recently imported from areas of South America endemic for *P. brasilianum* gave positive CSP reactions, while the sera of laboratory-born squirrel monkeys were consistently negative (Nussenzweig *et al.*, 1970). More recently, Nardin *et al.* (1979a), using the IFA test, detected antisporozoite antibodies against *P. knowlesi* in the sera of *M. irus* recently imported from Malaysia, an area endemic for numerous simian malarias.

IV. IMMUNIZATION OF HUMANS AGAINST SPOROZOITE-INDUCED MALARIA

The first attempt to immunize humans against sporozoites was carried out as early as 1936 by Boyd and Kitchen. Four volunteers were exposed one to three times to the bites of a total of 15–50 mosquitoes containing degenerated, noninfective sporozoites of *P. vivax*. When challenged by the bites of infective mosquitoes, all of the immunized hosts developed clinical attacks of vivax malaria after a prepatent period similar to that of nonimmune controls. The authors reached the conclusion that "the small volume of [sporozoites] normally introduced and the short duration of the period of which they retain their identity as sporozoites may be insufficient for them to produce any immune response in the body."

Clyde *et al.* (1973a,b, 1975), McCarthy and Clyde (1977), and Rieckmann *et al.* (1974, 1979) reported several successful attempts to immunize human volunteers by exposing them to the bites of infected, irradiated mosquitoes. This method of immunization was based on earlier experiments done in rodents which had become protected as a result of repeated exposure to the bites of *P. berghei*-infected irradiated *Anopheles stephensi* (Vanderberg *et al.*, 1970). Although attempts to vaccinate humans using this technique were performed on a relatively small number of volunteers, the results clearly demonstrated the feasibility of protecting humans against the infection induced by sporozoites of *P. falciparum* and *P. vivax*. These studies also defined a number of the characteristics of this sporozoite-induced protection, namely, the need for multiple immunizing doses, the stage and species specificity of the protection, and its relation to anti-sporozoite antibodies.

A. Antigen Preparation Used for Immunization of Humans

Radiation-attenuated sporozoites introduced by mosquito bite have, with one exception (Bray, 1976), been the only type of immonogen and route of administration used for immunization purposes in humans. This is due to the fact that irradiated intact sporozoites have, so far, been the most effective immunogen in both rodent and simian systems. Furthermore, immunization by bite, besides being effective in the various host–parasite systems, appears to be the most acceptable route of immunization, since it introduces the least amount of contaminating mosquito material into the host. Also, this route mimics the natural exposure to the bites of infected mosquitoes experienced by individuals living in malaria endemic areas.

Immunization by the bite of infected irradiated mosquitoes was first successfully applied in the immunoprophylaxis of human malaria by Clyde *et al.* (1973a). A total of 6 of 13 volunteers have now been protected against sporozoite challenge following immunization by multiple exposures to the bites of *P. falciparum*-infected irradiated mosquitoes over a period of time ranging from 3 to 10 months (Clyde *et al.*, 1973a,b, 1975; Rieckmann *et al.*, 1974, 1979). A minimum of six to eight exposures to a total of 379–440 irradiated mosquitoes was used to induce immunity in 3 of the 6 volunteers protected against falciparum malaria (Clyde *et al.*, 1973a; Rieckmann *et al.*, 1974, 1979). The remaining 3 successfully immunized volunteers were exposed more frequently to larger numbers of irradiated infected mosquitoes in order to induce protection (Clyde *et al.*, 1975; Rieckmann *et al.* 1979). Exposure to less than 200 mosquitoes over the same period of time failed to protect 4 volunteers (Rieckmann *et al.*, 1979). These results suggest that multiple exposures to a critical amount of antigen may be essential for the induction of a protective immune response to sporozoites.

The requirement for numerous exposures to large numbers of infected irradiated mosquitoes was also corroborated by the findings on immunization against *P. vivax* sporozoites. Two out of five volunteers were protected against *P. vivax* sporozoite challenge following immunization by the bites of irradiated vivax-infected mosquitoes (Clyde *et al.*, 1975; McCarthy and Clyde, 1977; Rieckmann *et al.*, 1979). The two successfully immunized volunteers were exposed 7–10 times to a total of 539–1979 *P. vivax*-infected mosquitoes (Clyde *et al.*, 1975; McCarthy and Clyde, 1977).

Attempts have been made to quantitate the number of sporozoites injected by the bite of an infected mosquito. While it has not been possible to determine the exact number, studies on *P. falciparum*-infected mosquitoes (Shute, 1945) and *P. berghei*-infected mosquitoes (Vanderberg, 1977) have shown that only a small number of sporozoites are inoculated into the host during a blood meal. It has been suggested that the number of sporozoites exiting through the proboscis of the mosquito is restricted by the size and chitinization of the salivary gland duct (Sterling *et al.*, 1973). The problem of estimating the number of sporozoites released during mosquito feeds makes it difficult to determine an optimal sporozoite inoculum for immunizing humans.

A single attempt to immunize with irradiated *P. falciparum* sporozoites administered intramuscularly did not protect the vaccinated hosts (Bray, 1976). Two volunteers living in a hyperendemic area of West Africa were injected twice with a total of 1×10^6 irradiated *P. falciparum* sporozoites. After natural exposure to the bites of infected mosquitoes, high parasitemia developed in both the immunized hosts and nonimmunized controls.

B. Properties of Sporozoite-Induced Immunity in Humans

1. Development of Sterile Immunity

Multiple exposures to the bites of malaria-infected irradiated mosquitoes resulted in sterile immunity in all sporozoite-immunized volunteers who resisted challenge. Daily examination of blood films after challenge completely failed to reveal parasites, and no symptoms suggestive of malaria were observed in the immune hosts. Nonprotected immunized volunteers developed patent parasitemias 1 day later than nonimmunized controls (Clyde *et al.*, 1973a).

2. Specificity of Sporozoite-Induced Protection

Sporozoite-induced immunity in humans was found to be species-specific and thus did not protect immunized volunteers against challenge with sporozoites of different human malarial species. At a time when total protection against falciparum sporozoite challenge was demonstrable, no resistance to challenge with sporozoites of *P. vivax* was detected in a falciparum-immunized host (Clyde *et al.*, 1973b). The falciparum-immunized volunteer who became patent as a result of challenge with *P. vivax* sporozoites exhibited a prepatent period similar to that of a nonimmune control. Similarly, a sporozoite-immunized host, protected against *P. vivax*, developed patent parasitemia following mosquito-borne challenge with *P. falciparum* (Clyde *et al.*, 1975).

While resistance in sporozoite-immunized volunteers was strictly species-specific, extensive protection against the various geographic isolates and strains of a given species was noted. Immunization with sporozoites of a strain of *P. falciparum* isolated from Burma induced protection against sporozoite challenge by falciparum strains isolated from Malaysia, Panama, and the Philippines

(Clyde *et al.*, 1973b). Similarly, cross-resistance was observed in vivax-immunized volunteers who were protected against challenge with a Central American strain of *P. vivax* after immunization with a Southeast Asian strain (Clyde *et al.*, 1975; McCarthy and Clyde, 1977).

Cross-protection was also noted between strains of *P. falciparum* that varied in drug susceptibility. A volunteer immunized with various chloroquine-resistant strains of *P. falciparum* totally resisted challenge with sporozoites of these strains as well as a chloroquine-sensitive strain (Clyde *et al.*, 1975). The reverse was also observed, i.e., immunization with a chloroquine-sensitive falciparum strain protected against challenge with a chloroquine-resistant strain (Rieckmann *et al.*, 1979).

Sporozoite-induced immunity was found to be strictly stage-specific and did not provide any protection against blood stage parasites. Thus, a sporozoite-immunized volunteer, who had totally resisted two challenges with *P. falciparum* sporozoites, developed a typical attack of malaria following the intravenous injection of blood containing erythrocytic stages of *P. falciparum* (Clyde *et al.*, 1973a).

C. Characterization of Sporozoite Antigens of Human Malaria

Consistent with findings in rodent and simian malarias, sporozoites of *P. falciparum* appear to require a period of antigenic maturation. Sporozoites collected from the salivary glands at an early stage (10 days after the infective blood meal) failed to produce a positive CSP reaction when incubated with known immune sera (E. H. Nardin, unpublished). After the parasites had been localized for several days in the salivary glands, the majority of sporozoites gave a clearly positive CSP reaction when incubated with the same antisera.

It was further observed that stage-specific sporozoite antigens were localized on the surface membrane of sporozoites of *P. falciparum* and *P. vivax* (Nardin and Nussenzweig, 1978; Nardin *et al.*, 1979a). These antigens were detected by incubating viable or glutaraldehyde-fixed sporozoites with the respective stage-specific antisera followed by incubation with fluorescein-conjugated antihuman immunoglobulin.

Characterization of sporozoite surface antigen(s) of rodent and simian malarias has been pursued by surface labeling followed by immunoprecipitation (Gwadz *et al.*, 1979). The feasibility of applying this methodology to human malaria hinges on the availability of sufficient quantities of sporozoites. Up to the present time, studies on vivax and falciparum sporozoites have been limited by the requirement for volunteers or naturally infected gametocyte carriers as a source of mosquito infections. *Plasmodium falciparum* infections in monkeys fail to produce gametocytes that are consistently highly infective for mosquitoes. In addition, although the *in vitro* system for continuous cultivation of *P. falciparum* (Trager and Jensen, 1976) supports the development of sexual forms, these gametocytes still fail to become mature and infective for mosquitoes under present culture conditions (Jensen, 1979).

D. Manifestations of Sporozoite-Induced Immunity in Humans

1. Humoral Antisporozoite Immunity

In the past, failure to detect an antisporozoite response in individuals exposed to the bites of malaria-infected mosquitoes led to the belief that the sporozoite stage of the malaria parasite was nonimmunogenic. Subsequently, however, studies on sporozoite-immunized rodent and simian hosts clearly demonstrated that sporozoites introduced by the bites of infected mosquitoes were capable of inducing an antibody response. Consistent with these findings, species- and stage-specific antisporozoite antibodies have been detected in the sera of sporozoite-immunized volunteers by using both the CSP assay and the IFA test.

a. Species Specificity and Strain Cross-Reactivity of Antisporozoite Antibodies. The sera of volunteers immunized by multiple exposures to the bites of infected irradiated mosquitoes gave positive CSP reactions when tested against the homologous species of sporozoites (Clyde *et al.,* 1973a,b, 1975; McCarthy and Clyde, 1977). The species specificity of the antisporozoite antibodies was clearly shown when the serum of a falciparum-immunized volunteer failed to give a CSP reaction when incubated with *P. vivax* sporozoites (Clyde *et al.,* 1973b).

Studies using indirect immunofluorescence also detected species-specific antisporozoite antibodies in the sera of hosts immunized with sporozoites of either *P. vivax* or *P. falciparum*. Viable *P. vivax* sporozoites did not fluoresce after incubation in serum obtained from a *P. falciparum*-immunized volunteer possessing high IFA titers against *P. falciparum* sporozoites (Nardin *et al.,* 1979a). The vivax sporozoites also failed to react with antisera raised against sporozoites of various species of rodent and simian malaria. Similarly, sporozoites of *P. falciparum* failed to fluoresce when incubated with antisera raised against sporozoites of *P. knowlesi* and *P. vivax* (Nardin and Nussenzweig, 1978).

Studies based on the CSP assay used the sera of rodents immunized with sporozoites of simian and human malaria to show that species-specific antigens were shared by various strains of the same malaria species (Nussenzweig and Chen, 1974a,b; Chen *et al.,* 1976). Extensive CSP cross-reactions between sporozoites of different strains were also observed in the sera of sporozoite-immunized human volunteers. Serum samples, obtained from a volunteer immunized with sporozoites of the Burma strain of *P. falciparum,* gave CSP reactions when incubated with sporozoites of the Burma strain as well as strains from Malaysia, Panama, and the Solomon Islands (Clyde *et al.,* 1973b). Similarly, the serum of a volunteer immunized with *P. vivax* sporozoites reacted equally well with vivax sporozoites of strains from New Guinea or El Salvador (Clyde *et al.,* 1975; McCarthy and Clyde, 1977). Cross-reactivity detected by the CSP reaction also occurred between chloroquine-resistant and chloroquine-sensitive strains of *P. falciparum* (Clyde *et al.,* 1973b, 1975).

The sharing of species-specific antigens by sporozoites of different geographic isolates was also demonstrated by the IFA test. The serum of a volunteer immunized and protected against challenge with a drug-resistant strain of *P. falciparum* had a high IFA titer (1:4096) when tested with sporozoites of a drug-sensitive West African strain (Nardin and Nussenzweig, 1978). Similarly, serum of an immunized volunteer, protected against sporozoites of *P. vivax* strains isolated from New Guinea and El Salvador, gave a 1:256 IFA titer when tested against *P. vivax* sporozoites obtained from an infection acquired in India (Nardin *et al.,* 1979a).

b. Stage Specificity of Antisporozoite Antibodies.   The stage specificity of the CSP antibodies has been clearly documented in the rodent–*P. berghei* model (Vanderberg *et al.,* 1972; Vanderberg, 1973). Similarly, the CSP reactions observed in the sera of immunized volunteers were dependent on the presence of antibodies specific for the sporozoite stage of the parasite. No CSP reactions were detected when sporozoites were incubated in sera obtained from individuals with high levels of immunity to erythrocytic stages of the parasite (McCarthy and Clyde, 1977).

Stage-specific antisporozoite antibodies were also detected by using indirect immunofluorescence. The serum of a volunteer, who had resisted sporozoite challenge after immunization by the bites of over 1000 irradiated falciparum-infected mosquitoes, had a negligible IFA titer against *P. falciparum*-infected red blood cells (Clyde *et al.,* 1973a). Similarly, another serum sample of the same volunteer gave a CSP titer of 1:40 and an IFA titer of 1:4096 when tested against viable falciparum sporozoites but failed to produce a significant immunofluorescent reaction with blood stages of *P. falciparum* (Nardin and Nussenzweig, 1978). Shortly after this volunteer had developed parasitemia following challenge with *P. falciparum*-infected blood, his IFA titer against blood stage parasites rose to 1:1024, while his titer against sporozoites remained unchanged. Repeated absorption of the serum with *P. falciparum*-infected red blood cells removed the antierythrocytic stage antibodies but did not affect the IFA reaction with falciparum sporozoites.

2. Relationship of Antisporozoite Antibodies to Protection

The stage and species specificity of the antisporozoite antibodies detected by immunofluorescence and the CSP assay correlate well with the specificity of protection in sporozoite-immunized volunteers. Resistance to challenge, not only with sporozoites of the strain used for immunization but also with various other isolates of the same malarial species, is reflected in serological cross-reactivity. Conversely, susceptibility to challenge with sporozoites of a different plasmodial species or with blood stages is paralleled by the absence of serological cross-reactions with heterologous species and stages of malaria parasites.

Based on the close correlation between the stage and species specificity of protection and the presence of antisporozoite antibodies in all successfully immunized volunteers, Clyde, McCarthy, and co-workers suggested that the ability to resist sporozoite challenge could be predicted by the individual's antisporozoite antibody response. They noted that a volunteer immunized with *P. vivax* sporozoites withstood challenge when the CSP titers were at their highest level (McCarthy and Clyde, 1977). Five months after the last immunizing dose, at a time when the CSP reaction with vivax sporozoites was no longer detectable, the volunteer developed malaria following the bites of *P. vivax*-infected mosquitoes. However, the challenge with viable sporozoites was shown to increase both the CSP response as well as protection and enabled the immunized host to resist two subsequent sporozoite challenges.

Similarly, in a volunteer immunized with *P. vivax* and *P. falciparum* sporozoites, the ability to resist challenge with either species of parasite was correlated with the presence of the respective species-specific CSP antibodies (Clyde *et al.*, 1975). The initial immunization by the bites of irradiated *P. falciparum*-infected mosquitoes induced resistance and CSP antibodies to *P. falciparum* sporozoites. Over the next 4 months, additional immunization with *P. vivax*-infected irradiated mosquitoes produced protection and a humoral response to vivax sporozoites. In the presence of serological reactivity with *P. vivax* sporozoites, and in the absence of any residual CSP activity with *P. falciparum,* the volunteer resisted vivax challenge but was not protected against the bites of *P. falciparum*-infected mosquitoes.

3. Humoral Antisporozoite Response in Naturally Infected Humans

As early as 1940, Sinton suggested that antisporozoite immunity might be responsible for the resistance to sporozoite challenge of patients who had undergone multiple exposures to the bites of nonattenuated *P. ovale*-infected mosquitoes. This raises the important question of the role of antisporozoite immunity in the development of resistance to malaria observed in individuals living in endemic areas.

Initial attempts to detect sporozoite agglutinating, neutralizing, or CSP reactions in the sera of adult Gambians and Liberians living in West Africa were not successful (Bray, 1978). However, tests for CSP antibodies and SNA are not sufficiently sensitive to ensure the detection of low levels of antisporozoite antibodies. These tests are limited by the requirement for viable sporozoites.

The need for a rapid, practical serological assay for antisporozoite antibodies has been met by a recently developed IFA test which uses either glutaraldehyde-fixed or viable sporozoites (Nardin and Nussenzweig, 1978; Nardin et al., 1979a). Various experimental approaches, summarized in Sections II,D and III, D, have demonstrated the sensitivity and stage specificity of the indirect immunofluorescent assay when reactions are limited to surface antigens of the sporozoite.

Recently, indirect immunofluorescence and the CSP assay were used to examine the sera of residents of the Gambia, West Africa (Nardin and Nussenzweig, 1978; Nardin et al., 1979b). Sera of villagers, living in an area in which P. falciparum is endemic, were found to have significant levels of antibodies against the sporozoite stage of the parasite. The level of antisporozoite activity was shown to increase gradually with age. Positive CSP reactions and high IFA titers (1:512) against P. falciparum sporozoites were observed in a large percentage of adult Gambians. In contrast, little or no CSP activity and low (1:8) IFA titers were noted in the majority of children in the 10- to 15-year-old age group. The species specificity of the reaction was demonstrated by the failure of fixed or viable P. falciparum sporozoites to react with antisera raised against sporozoites of P. knowlesi or P. vivax. The sporozoites also failed to react with normal serum obtained from an individual living in a nonendemic area.

In several of the adult Gambians studied, high titers of anti-P. falciparum sporozoite antibodies were detected in the absence of both parasitemia and a significant antibody response against P. falciparum-infected red blood cells. As in the experimentally immunized hosts, these antisporozoite antibodies may function in the removal of infective sporozoites and the prevention of subsequent patent infections.

V. CONCLUSIONS

1. Intact irradiated or viable sporozoites are highly immunogenic and confer complete protection against sporozoite-induced malaria infections without the need for immunopotentiation. In contrast, immunization with the erythrocytic stages of plasmodia requires the use of FCA in order to induce protection.

2. Successful vaccination of rodents, monkeys, and humans against sporozoites is characterized by the development of sterile immunity, i.e., sporozoite-immunized hosts fail to develop parasitemia following challenge.

Animals immunized with blood stages, however, frequently develop low levels of parasitemia after challenge.

3. At present, the most effective sporozoite antigen preparations are intact sporozoites, either irradiated or viable, administered intravenously or by the bites of infected mosquitoes. In rodents, protection can be obtained by immunization with a single dose of irradiated sporozoites. However, multiple administration of relatively large numbers of sporozoites is required to induce protective immunity in rhesus monkeys and humans.

4. Sporozoite-induced immunity is strictly stage-specific. Immunized hosts, while totally resistant to sporozoite challenge, remain fully susceptible to challenge with blood stages of the malaria parasite.

5. In sporozoite-vaccinated rhesus monkeys and humans, protection, as well as antisporozoite antibodies, is strictly species-specific. Immunized primates are protected only against challenge with sporozoites of the plasmodial species used for immunization. However, these immunized hosts are fully resistant to challenge with sporozoites of various strains of the homologous species. This protection is accompanied by the development of species-specific antisporozoite antibodies which cross-react with sporozoites of the various strains of a given plasmodial species.

6. Sporozoites of rodent malaria appear to be more closely related than primate malarias. Protection induced by immunization with sporozoites of *P. berghei* is effective against challenge with sporozoites of *P. chabaudi* and *P. vinckei;* the reverse cross-protection also occurs. Antisporozoite antibodies raised against *P. berghei* cross-react with sporozoites of these rodent malarial species.

7. Both cell-mediated and humoral immune responses play a role in sporozoite-induced immunity. In rodents, the transfer of immune spleen cells confers protection and, in addition, μ-suppressed mice have been successfully immunized. Antisporozoite antibodies are also functional. Sporozoites lose their infectivity following incubation with immune serum from sporozoite-immunized simian or rodent hosts. The passive transfer of rodent immune serum decreases both the circulation time and the number of sporozoites which develop into exoerythrocytic stages.

8. Sporozoites of rodent, simian, and human malaria undergo a process of maturation as they migrate from the mosquito midgut to the salivary gland. The development of salivary gland sporozoite surface antigen(s) is associated with the acquisition of sporozoite infectivity and immunogenicity.

9. The antisporozoite antibodies which develop in the sporozoite-immunized hosts are directed primarily, if not exclusively, against sporozoite surface antigen(s). Surface labeling of intact sporozoites of rodent and simian malaria has detected a single species-specific protein-containing surface antigen.

VI. PERSPECTIVES

The development of a sporozoite vaccine for malaria, which would protect humans by establishing a sterile immunity, has been successful in its first experimental phase. The feasibility of inducing protection in humans by multiple immunizations with attentuated sporozoites has been documented both for *P. falciparum* (Clyde *et al.*, 1973a, 1975; Rieckmann *et al.*, 1974, 1979) and *P. vivax* (Clyde *et al.*, 1975; McCarthy and Clyde, 1977).

Recent seroepidemiological findings indicate that individuals living in areas of high malaria endemicity develop an antisporozoite humoral response after many years of exposure to the bites of infected mosquitoes (Nardin *et al.*, 1979b). These observations support the view that sporozoite vaccination should primarily be aimed at younger individuals who are particularly susceptible to severe malaria infections. The continued exposure to infected mosquitoes would, hopefully, maintain and prolong the protection resulting from the vaccination procedure.

Thus, the development of a sporozoite vaccine for the immunization of individuals living in malaria endemic areas constitutes a realistic, although not an immediate, goal. It is certain that a great number of scientific and technical problems will have to be solved in order to obtain an effective, potent, stable vaccine. Other, possibly less difficult, problems relate to the storage and preservation of sporozoites or the protective antigen. Undoubtedly, the most important problem is that of providing an adequate source of large amounts of antigen. Sporozoites obtained from laboratory-bred infected mosquitoes, although providing sufficient antigen for all the experimental work on sporozoite immunization thus far, obviously are not a suitable antigen source for mass production of a malarial vaccine.

The production of sporozoites *in vitro*, using cultures initiated with gametocytes obtained from the *in vitro* system of Trager and Jensen (1976), represents one potentially fruitful approach in solving the problem of antigen source. However, most of the experimental conditions for *in vitro* growth of the sporogonic stages of the mammalian malaria parasite still remain to be developed. This area of research is difficult and is under study by very few investigators, and therefore the possibility of success in the near future is not very likely.

Another potentially useful approach to the problem of antigen source is the identification and purification of the protective sporozoite antigens, which might lead to their synthesis for vaccination purposes. Research toward this goal has been initiated with both rodent and simian malaria sporozoites and has led to the partial characterization of a specific protein-containing surface antigen of sporozoites of *P. berghei* and *P. knowlesi* (Gwadz *et al.*, 1979).

Recently, a hybrid cell line, formed by the fusion of spleen cells of sporozoite-immunized mice with a mouse plasmacytoma, was found to secrete antisporozoite antibodies *in vitro* (Yoshida *et al.*, 1980). This hybridoma secretes large amounts of monospecific antibodies directed against the *P. berghei* sporozoite surface antigen which previously was characterized on acrylamide gel (MW ± 44,000). Hybridoma-inoculated animals develop very high CSP and IFA titers of antisporozoite antibodies, 50–100 times greater than those we have observed in sporozoite-immunized mice. These antibodies are directed against a functional, protective antigen, since mice inoculated with the hybrid cells are protected against sporozoite challenge. Passive transfer of antibodies from these hybridoma-inoculated mice to control animals also confers resistance to sporozoite challenge (Potocnjak *et al.*, 1980).

These monospecific antibodies, which can be obtained from hybridomas in practically unlimited amounts, provide a powerful tool for purification of the corresponding sporozoite antigen. Antigenic and biochemical characterization of the purified antigen would hopefully lead to its synthesis for the development of a vaccine. This methodology, once developed in rodent and simian malaria systems, would be applicable to human malaria sporozoites, where it would hopefully solve the problem of an antigen source for vaccination.

Another rather important aspect of a future sporozoite vaccine relates to amplification of the protective effect through immunopotentiation. This is an area which has been explored only minimally and which, in fact, might also provide further insight into the effector mechanism(s) of sporozoite-induced immunity.

In conclusion, recent findings appear to indicate that we now have the necessary powerful tools which should provide the means for clarifying the mechanism of sporozoite-induced immunity and for isolating the protective antigens. Under these conditions, the various obstacles to the development of a sporozoite vaccine for malaria appear to be surmountable, hopefully in the not too remote future.

ACKNOWLEDGMENTS

We are grateful to Dr. Hannah Lustig Shear for critically reading the manuscript and to Ms. Sharon Hecht-Ponger for manuscript preparation.

REFERENCES

Aikawa, M., Cochrane, A. H., and Nussenzweig, R. S. (1979). A freeze fracture study of malarial sporozoites: Antibody induced changes of the pellicular membranes. *J. Protozool.* **26,** 273–279.

Alger, N., Harant, J., Willis, L., and Jorgensen, G. (1972). Sporozoite and normal salivary gland induced immunity in malaria. *Nature (London)* **238,** 341–343.

Bawden, M. P., Palmer, T. T., Beaudoin, R. L., and Leef, M. F. (1978). Development of a serologic test specific for malaria parasites. *Proc. Congr. Parasitol., 4th, 1978* Short Commun., Sect. E, pp. 113–114.

Bawden, M. P., Palmer, T. T., Leef, M. F., and Beaudoin, R. L. (1979). Malaria vaccination with irradiated sporozoites: Serologic evaluation of the antigen and antibody responses. *Bull. W.H.O.* **57,** Suppl. 1, 205–209.

Beaudoin, R. L., Strome, C. P. A., Palmer, T. T., and Bawden, M. P. (1975). Immunogenicity of sporozoites of the ANKA strain of *Plasmodium berghei berghei* following different treatments. *Am. Soc. Parasitol. Abstr.* **231,** 98–99.

Beaudoin, R. L., Strome, C. P. A., Tubergen, T. A., and Mitchell, F. (1976). *Plasmodium berghei berghei:* Irradiated sporozoites of the ANKA strain as immunizing antigens in mice. *Exp. Parasitol.* **39,** 438–443.

Beaudoin, R. L., Strome, C. P., Mitchell, F., and Tubergen, T. A. (1977). *Plasmodium berghei:* Immunization of mice against the ANKA strain using unaltered sporozoites as an antigen. *Exp. Parasitol.* **42,** 1–5.

Boyd, M. F., and Kitchen, S. F. (1936). Is the acquired heterologous immunity to *P. vivax* equally effective against sporozoites and trophozoites? *Am. J. Trop. Med.* **16,** 317–322.

Bray, R. S. (1976). Vaccination against *Plasmodium falciparum:* A negative result. *Trans. R. Soc. Trop. Med. Hyg.* **70,** 258.

Bray, R. S. (1978). Absence of circumsporozoite antibodies in areas of hyperendemic malaria. *J. Parasitol.* **64,** 410.

Chen, D. (1974). Aspects of host-parasite interactions in the rhesus-*P. cynomolgi-A. stephensi* system. Ph.D. Thesis, New York University School of Medicine (Microfilm No. 7SZ75-09, 647).

Chen, D. H., Nussenzweig, R. S., and Collins, W. E. (1976). Specificity of the circumsporozoite precipitation antigen(s) of human and simian malarias. *J. Parasitol.* **62,** 636–637.

Chen, D. H., Tigelaar, R. E., and Weinbaum, F. I. (1977). Immunity to sporozoite-induced malaria infection in mice. I. The effect of immunization of T and B cell-deficient mice. *J. Immunol.* **118,** 1322–1327.

Cochrane, A. H., Aikawa, M., Jeng, M., and Nussenzweig, R. S. (1976). Antibody-induced ultrastructural changes of malarial sporozoites. *J. Immunol.* **116,** 859–867.

Cohen, S., Butcher, G. A., Mitchell, G. H., Deans, J. A., and Langhorne, J. (1977). Acquired immunity and vaccination in malaria. *Am. J. Trop. Med. Hyg.* **26,** 223–232.

Clyde, D. F., Most, H., McCarthy, V., and Vanderberg, J. P. (1973a). Immunization of man against sporozoite induced falciparum malaria. *Am. J. Med. Sci.* **266,** 169–177.

Clyde, D. F., McCarthy, V. C., Miller, R. M., and Hornick R. B. (1973b). Specificity of protection of man immunized against sporozoite-induced falciparum malaria. *Am. J. Med. Sci.* **266,** 398–403.

Clyde, D. F., McCarthy, V., Miller, R. M., and Woodward, W. E. (1975). Immunization of man against falciparum and vivax malaria by use of attenuated sporozoites. *Am. J. Trop. Med. Hyg.* **24,** 397–401.

Collins, W. E., and Contacos, P. G. (1972). Immunization of monkeys against *Plasmodium cynomolgi* by X-irradiated sporozoites. *Nature New Biol.* **236,** 176–177.

Corradetti, A., Verolini, F., Sebastiani, A., Proietti, A., and Amati, L. (1964). Fluorescent antibody testing with sporozoites of Plasmodia. *Bull. W.H.O.* **30,** 747–750.

Corradetti, A., Verolini, F., and Bucci, A. (1966). Resistenze a *Plasmodium berghei* da parte di ratti albini precedentemente immunizzati con *P. berghei* irradiato. *Parasitologia* **8,** 133–145.

Danforth, H. D., Orjih, A. U., and Nussenzweig, R. S. (1978). Immunofluorescent staining of exoerythrocytic schizonts of *Plasmodium berghei* in fixed liver tissue with stage specific immune sera. *J. Parasitol.* **64,** 1123–1125.

Danforth, H., Aikawa, M., Cochrane, A., and Nussenzweig, R. S. (1980). Sporozoites of mammalian malaria: Attachment, interiorization and intracellular fate within macrophages. *J. Protozool.* (in press)

Golenser, J., Heeren, J., Verhave, J. P., Kaay, H. J. V. D., and Meuwissen, J. H. E. Th. (1977). Cross-reactivity with sporozoites, exoerythrocytic forms and blood schizonts of *Plasmodium berghei* in indirect fluorescent antibody tests with sera of rats immunized with sporozoites or infected blood. *Clin. Exp. Immunol.* **29,** 43–51.

Golenser, J., Verhave, J. P., DeValk, J., Heeren, J., and Meuwissen, J. H. E. Th. (1978). Studies on the role of antibodies against sporozoites in *Plasmodium berghei* malaria. *Isr. J. Med. Sci.* **14,** 606–610.

Gwadz, R. W., and Green, I. (1978). Malaria immunization in rhesus monkeys: A vaccine effective against both the sexual and asexual stages of *Plasmodium knowlesi. J. Exp. Med.* **148,** 1311–1323.

Gwadz, R. W., Cochrane, A. H., Nussenzweig, V., and Nussenzweig, R. S. (1979). Preliminary studies on vaccination of rhesus monkeys with irradiated sporozoites of *Plasmodium knowlesi* and characterization of surface antigens of these parasites. *Bull. W.H.O.* **57,** Suppl. 1, 165–173.

Ingram, R., Otken, L., and Jumper, J. (1961). Staining of malaria parasites by the fluorescent antibody technique. *Proc. Soc. Exp. Biol. Med.* **106,** 52–54.

Jahiel, R. I., Nussenzweig, R. S., Vanderberg, J., and Vilček, J. (1968a). Antimalarial effect of interferon inducers at different stages of development of *Plasmodium berghei* in the mouse. *Nature (London)* **220,** 710–711.

Jahiel, R. I., Vilček, J., Nussenzweig, R. S., and Vanderberg, J. (1968b). Interferon inducers protect mice against *Plasmodium berghei* malaria. *Science* **161,** 802–804.

Jahiel, R. I., Nussenzweig, R. S., Vilček, J., and Vanderberg, J. (1969). Protective effect of interferon inducers on *Plasmodium berghei* malaria. *Am. J. Trop. Med. Hyg.* **18,** 823–835.

Jahiel, R. I., Vilček, J., and Nussenzweig, R. S. (1970). Exogenous interferon protects mice against *Plasmodium berghei* malaria. *Nature (London)* **227,** 1350–1351.

Jensen, J. B. (1979). Observations on gametogenesis in *Plasmodium falciparum* from continuous culture. *J. Protozool.* **26,** 129–132.

McCarthy, V., and Clyde, D. F. (1977). *Plasmodium vivax:* Correlation of circumsporozoite precipitation (CSP) reaction with sporozoite-induced protective immunity in man. *Exp. Parasitol.* **41,** 167–171.

McConnell, E., Tubergen, T. A., Bawden, M. P., and Beaudoin, R. L. (1978). The effect of single bites of *Anopheles stephensi* mosquitoes infected with *Plasmodium berghei* on the level of sporozoite-specific IFAT antibody in white mice previously immunized with irradiated sporozoites. *Proc. Int. Congr. Parasitol., 4th, 1978* Short Commun., Sect. E, pp. 111–112.

McNamara, J. G. (1976). Application of the indirect fluorescent antibody technique for the detection of anti-malarial sporozoite antibodies. Master's Thesis, New York University Medical School.

Mulligan, H. W., Russell, P. F., and Mohan, B. N. (1941). Active immunization of fowls against *Plasmodium gallinaceum* by injections of killed homologous sporozoites. *J. Malar. Inst. India* **4,** 25–34.

Nardin, E. H., and Nussenzweig, R. S. (1978). Stage-specific antigens on the surface membrane of sporozoites of malaria parasites. *Nature (London)* **274,** 55–57.

Nardin, E. H., Nussenzweig, R. S., and Gwadz, R. (1979a). Characterization of sporozoite surface antigens by indirect immunofluorescence: Application of this technique to detect stage and species specific antimalarial antibodies. *Bull. W.H.O.* **57,** Suppl. 1, 211–217.

Nardin, E. H., Nussenzweig, R. S., McGregor, I. A., and Bryan, J. (1979b). Antisporozoite antibodies: Their frequent occurrence in individuals living in an area of hyperendemic malaria. *Science* 206, 597–599.

Nussenzweig, R. S. (1967). Increased nonspecific resistance to malaria produced by administration of killed *Corynebacterium parvum*. *Exp. Parasitol.* **21**, 224–231.

Nussenzweig, R. S., and Chen, D. (1974a). Some characteristics of the immune response to sporozoites of simian and human malaria. *Bull. P.A.H.O.* **8**, 198–204.

Nussenzweig, R. S., and Chen, D. (1974b). The antibody response to sporozoites of simian and human malaria parasites: Its stage and species specificity and strain cross-reactivity. *Bull. W.H.O.* **50**, 293–297.

Nussenzweig, R., Vanderberg, J., Most, H., and Orton, C. (1967). Protective immunity produced by the injection of X-irradiated sporozoites of *Plasmodium berghei*. *Nature (London)* **216**, 160–162.

Nussenzweig, R., Vanderberg, J., and Most, H. (1969a). Protective immunity produced by the injection of X-irradiated sporozoites of *Plasmodium berghei*. IV. Dose response, specificity and humoral immunity. *Mil. Med.* **134**, Suppl., 1176–1182.

Nussenzweig, R. S., Vanderberg, J. P., Most, H., and Orton, C. (1969b). Specificity of protective immunity produced by X-irradiated *Plasmodium berghei* sporozoites. *Nature (London)* **222**, 488–489.

Nussenzweig, R. S., Vanderberg, J., Most, H., and Orton, C. (1970). Immunity in simian malaria induced by irradiated sporozoites. *J. Parasitol.* **56** (Sect. II, 2nd Int. Congr.), Abstr. No. 459, p. 252.

Nussenzweig, R. S., Vanderberg, J. P., Spitalny, G., Rivera, C. I. O., Orton, C., and Most, H. (1972a). Sporozoite-induced immunity in mammalian malaria: A review. *Am. J. Trop. Med. Hyg.* **21**, 722–728.

Nussenzweig, R. S., Vanderberg, J. P., Sanabria, Y., and Most, H. (1972b). *Plasmodium berghei: Accelerated clearance of sporozoites from blood as part of immune mechanism in mice*. *Exp. Parasitol.* **31**, 88–97.

Nussenzweig, R. S., Montuori, W., Spitalny, G. L., and Chen, D. (1973). Antibodies against sporozoites of human and simian malaria produced in rats. *J. Immunol.* **110**, 600–601.

Orjih, A. U., and Nussenzweig, R. S. (1979). *Plasmodium berghei:* Suppression of antibody response to sporozoite stage by acute blood stage infection. *Clin. Exp. Immunol.* 38, 1–8.

Orjih, A. U., and Nussenzweig, R. S. (1980). Immunization against rodent malaria with cryopreserved irradiated sporozoites of *Plasmodium berghei*. *Am. J. Trop. Med. Hyg.* **29,** (in press).

Pacheco, N. D., and Beaudoin, R. L. (1978). Single dose immunization using irradiated sporozoites of *Plasmodium berghei*. *Proc. Congr. Parasitol.,* 4th, 1978, Short Commun., Sect. E, pp. 114–115.

Pacheco, N. D., McConnell, E., and Beaudoin, R. L. (1979). Duration of immunity following a single vaccination with irradiated sporozoites of *Plasmodium berghei*. *Bull. W.H.O.* **57**, Suppl. 1, 159–163.

Potocnjak, P., Yoshida, N., Nussenzweig, R. S., and Nussenzweig, V. (1980). Monovalent fragments (Fab) of monoclonal antibodies to a sporozoite surface antigen (Pb44) protect mice against malarial infection. *J. Exp. Med.* **151**, 1504–1513.

Rieckmann, K. H., Carson, P. E., Beaudoin, R. L., Cassells, J., and Sell, K. W. (1974). Sporozoite induced immunity in man against an Ethiopian strain of *Plasmodium falciparum*. *Trans. R. Soc. Trop. Med. Hyg.* **68**, 258–259.

Rieckmann, K. H., Beaudoin, R. L., Cassells, J., and Sell, K. (1979). Clinical studies with a sporozoite vaccine against falciparum malaria. *Bull. W.H.O.* **57**, Suppl. 1, 261–265.

Russell, P. F., and Mohan, B. N. (1942). The immunization of fowls against mosquito-borne *Plasmodium gallinaceum* by injections of serum and of inactivated homologous sporozoites. *J. Exp. Med.* **76**, 477–495.

Russell, P. F., Mulligan, H. W., and Mohan, B. N. (1941). Specific agglutinogenic properties of inactivated sporozoites of *Plasmodium gallinaceum*. *J. Malar. Inst. India* **4**, 15–24.

Russell, P. F., Mulligan, H. W., and Mohan, B. N. (1942). Active immunization of fowls against sporozoites but not trophozoites of *Plasmodium gallinaceum* by injection of homologous sporozoites. *J. Malar. Inst. India* **4**, 311–319.

Shute, P. G. (1945). An investigation into the number of sporozoites found in the salivary glands of *Anopheles* mosquitoes. *Trans. R. Soc. Trop. Med. Hyg.* **38**, 493–498.

Sinton, J. A. (1940). Studies on infections with *Plasmodium ovale*. IV. The efficacy and nature of immunity acquired as a result of infections induced by sporozoite inoculations as compared with those by trophozoite injections. *Trans. R. Soc. Trop. Med. Hyg.* **33**, 439–446.

Smrkovski, L. L., and Beaudoin, R. L. (1978). Suppression of irradiated sporozoite-induced protective immunity in rodent malaria by BCG. *Proc. Int. Congr. Parasitol., 4th, 1978* Short Commun., Sect. E, p. 113.

Smrkovski, L. L., and Strickland, G. T. (1978). Rodent malaria: BCG-induced protection and immunosuppression. *J. Immunol.* **121**, 1257–1261.

Sodeman, W. A., and Jeffery, G. M. (1964). Immunofluorescent staining of sporozoites of *Plasmodium gallinaceum*. *J. Parasitol.* **50**, 477–478.

Spitalny, G. L. (1973). Immunological aspects of sporozoite-induced resistance in rodent malaria. Ph.D. Thesis, New York University School of Medicine (Microfilm No. T12385).

Spitalny, G. L., and Nussenzweig, R. S. (1972). Effect of various routes of immunization and methods of parasite attenuation on the development of protection against sporozoite-induced rodent malaria. *Proc. Helminthol. Soc. Wash.* **39**, 506–514.

Spitalny, G. L., and Nussenzweig, R. S. (1973). *Plasmodium berghei:* Relationship between protective immunity and antisporozoite (CSP) antibody in mice. *Exp. Parasitol.* **33**, 168–178.

Spitalny, G. L., Rivera-Ortiz, C. I., and Nussenzweig, R. S. (1976). *Plasmodium berghei:* The spleen in sporozoite-induced immunity to mouse malaria. *Exp. Parasitol.* **40**, 179–188.

Spitalny, G. L., Verhave, J. P., Meuwissen, J. H. E. Th. and Nussenzweig, R. S. (1977). *Plasmodium berghei:* T cell dependence of sporozoite-induced immunity in rodents. *Exp. Parasitol.* **42**, 73–81.

Sterling, C., Aikawa, M., and Vanderberg, J. (1973). The passage of *Plasmodium berghei* sporozoites through the salivary glands of *Anopheles stephensi*. *J. Parasitol.* **59**, 593–605.

Trager, W., and Jensen, J. B. (1976). Human malaria parasites in continuous culture. *Science* **193**, 673–675.

Vanderberg, J. P. (1973). Inactivity of rodent malaria antisporozoite antibodies against exoerythrocytic forms. *Am. J. Trop. Med. Hyg.* **22**, 573–577.

Vanderberg, J. P. (1975). Development of infectivity by the *Plasmodium berghei* sporozoite. *J. Parasitol.* **61**, 43–50.

Vanderberg, J. P. (1977). *Plasmodium berghei:* Quantitation of sporozoites injected by mosquitoes feeding on a rodent host. *Exp. Parasitol.* **42**, 169–181.

Vanderberg, J. P., Nussenzweig, R. S., Most, H., and Orton, C. G. (1968). Protective immunity produced by the injection of X-irradiated sporozoites of *Plasmodium berghei*. II. Effects of radiation on sporozoites. *J. Parasitol.* **54**, 1175–1180.

Vanderberg, J. P., Nussenzweig, R., and Most, H. (1969). Protective immunity produced by injections of X-irradiated sporozoites of *Plasmodium berghei*. V. *In vitro* effects of immune serum on sporozoites. *Mil. Med.* **134**, Suppl., 1183–1190.

Vanderberg, J. P., Nussenzweig, R. S., and Most, H. (1970). Protective immunity produced by the bite of X-irradiated mosquitoes infected with *Plasmodium berghei*. *J. Parasitol. (Sect. II)* **56**, 350–351.

Vanderberg, J. P., Nussenzweig, R., Sanabria, Y., Nawrot, R., and Most, H. (1972). Stage specificity of antisporozoite antibodies in rodent malaria and its relationship to protective immunity. *Proc. Helminthol. Soc. Wash.* **39**, 514–525.

Verhave, J. P. (1975). Immunization with sporozoites: An experimental study of *Plasmodium berghei* malaria. Ph.D. Thesis, Katholiere Universiteit te Nijmegen, The Netherlands.

Verhave, J. P., Strickland, G. T., Jaffe, H. A., and Ahmed, A. (1978). Studies on the transfer of protective immunity with lymphoid cells from mice immune to malaria sporozoites. *J. Immunol.* **121,** 1031–1033.

Ward, R. A., and Hayes, D. E. (1972). Attempted immunization of rhesus monkeys against cynomolgi malaria with irradiated sporozoites. *Proc. Helminthol. Soc. Wash.* **39,** 525–529.

Wellde, B. T., and Sadun, E. H. (1967). Resistance produced in rats and mice by exposure to irradiated *Plasmodium berghei*. *Exp. Parasitol.* **21,** 310–324.

Yoeli, M., Vanderberg, J., Nawrot, R., and Most, H. (1965). Studies on sporozoite-induced infections of rodent malaria. II. *Anopheles stephensi* as an experimental vector of *Plasmodium berghei*. *Am. J. Trop. Med. Hyg.* **14,** 927–930.

Yoeli, M., Upmanis, R. S., Vanderberg, J., and Most, H. (1966). Life cycle and patterns of development of *Plasmodium berghei* in normal and experimental hosts. *Mil. Med.* **131,** 900–914.

Yoshida, N., Nussenzweig, R. S., Potocnjak, P., Nussenzweig, V., and Aikawa, M. (1980). Hybridoma produces protective antibodies directed against the sporozoite stage of malaria parasite. *Science* **207,** 71–73.

Immunization against Exoerythrocytic Stages of Malaria Parasites

Thomas W. Holbrook

I. INTRODUCTION

Of the various developmental stages of malaria parasites in vertebrate hosts the exoerythrocytic (EE) forms are the least understood. This relative gap in knowledge can be attributed in part to the relatively late demonstration of EE stages. Schaudinn's (1903) description of direct invasion of erythrocytes by sporozoites probably deterred attempts to find stages at other sites, although several investigators studying avian malaria described forms which were probably EE stages (Raffaele, 1934, 1936; Huff and Bloom, 1935; reviewed by Huff, 1969).

Before EE stages were demonstrated evidence for their existence evolved primarily from two observations. First, a "negative blood phase" followed sporozoite inoculation. Boyd and Stratman-Thomas (1934) showed that sub-inoculation of blood from a human recipient of *Plasmodium vivax* sporozoites was not infective for an uninfected recipient until at least 8 days later. Fairly

Malaria, Vol. 3

(1947) subinoculated blood from human subjects at intervals after infection with *P. falciparum* or *P. vivax* sporozoites. Within 0.5 hour after sporozoite inoculation subinoculated blood produced infections in recipients, but further subinoculations failed to produce infections until several days later (days 7 and 9 after sporozoite inoculation of *P. falciparum* and *P. vivax,* respectively). A period of noninfectivity of subinoculated blood also occurs in sporozoite-induced avian malaria (Warren and Coggeshall, 1937). Blood taken at 0.5 hour from a recipient of *P. cathemerium* sporozoites was infective for clean canary recipients but for the next 48 hours blood subinoculation produced no infection. A proportion of birds receiving blood taken at 72 hours from the sporozoite-injected canaries became infected. These results of studies on sporozoite-induced infections of mammals and birds strongly suggested that malaria parasites must undergo a developmental process at an exoerythrocytic site before the infection of red blood cells (RBCs) could occur.

The second factor which suggested the existence of EE stages in malaria was the differential activity of drugs used for treatment of blood- or sporozoite-induced *P. vivax* infections. While infections initiated with parasitized erythrocytes could be cured with quinine treatment, sporozoite-induced infections with this parasite often relapsed after quinine treatment (Yorke and Macfie, 1924). Davey (1946) discussed the implications of both lines of evidence leading to the conclusion that the development of EE stages must precede RBC invasion in sporozoite-induced human malaria.

James and Tate (1937) provided unequivocal evidence for the existence of EE stages in avian malaria. These forms were found in spleen, liver, kidneys, brain, and other organs of chicks inoculated with *P. gallinaceum* sporozoites. The authors also confirmed earlier speculation that EE forms were not affected by drugs active against RBC stages. Chickens receiving quinine for prophylaxis or for treatment of parasitemia died later with EE forms in organs.

Studies by Clay Huff and his colleagues form the basis for much of our knowledge of EE stages in avian hosts. Huff and Coulston (1944) demonstrated the successive development of two preerythrocytic developmental phases after the inoculation of *P. gallinaceum* sporozoites into wing skin of chicks. The first EE generation developed within cells of the lymphoid–macrophage series and produced merozoites in 36–48 hours, which invaded and matured within endothelial cells. These preerythrocytic generations were termed cryptozoites and metacryptozoites, respectively. The EE stages found in endothelial cells later during sporozoite-induced infection or after injection of parasitized red cells were called phanerozoites (Huff and Coulston, 1946). This pattern of EE development in avian malaria was characterized as the gallinaceum type as opposed to the elongatum type. The EE forms of *P. elongatum* and *P. huffi* develop within cells of the erythroid series rather than in lymphoid–macrophage elements or endothelium (Porter and Huff, 1940). All avian malaria parasites studied thus far, with these two exceptions, undergo gallinaceum-type EE development in susceptible hosts. Studies on immune responsiveness against EE forms in birds have been conducted exclusively using parasites with gallinaceum-type EE forms. Following the demonstration of preerythrocytic stages of *P. gallinaceum* (Huff and Coulston, 1944), Huff and Coulston (1946) cautioned against necessarily expecting to find EE forms of mammalian malaria parasites at the same sites, and their search for the EE stages of *P. vivax* after injection of sporozoites into the skin of human volunteers and monkeys was not successful. A search for the EE stages of *P. cynomolgi* in skin, bone marrow, spleen, and liver of rhesus monkeys also failed, but organs were examined no later than 72 hours after sporozoite injection (Huff and Coulston, 1947).

The initial demonstration of EE forms in mammalian malaria was accomplished a decade after the discovery of these stages in birds. Shortt and Garnham (1948a) found EE stages in the liver of monkeys injected with *P. cynomolgi* sporozoites 6–7 days earlier. These forms were not seen in other organs and were not infective by subinoculation of liver tissue into clean animals. Erythrocytic stages were first seen on the ninth day after sporozoite injection (Shortt *et al.*, 1948a).

The discovery that EE forms of *P. cynomolgi* developed in the liver soon led to the demonstration of EE forms of *P. vivax* in the liver of a human subject (Shortt *et al.*, 1948b) and to the eventual description of EE forms of *P. falciparum* (Shortt *et al.*, 1951), *P. ovale* (Garnham *et al.*, 1955), and *P. malariae* (Bray, 1960). The apparent *in vivo* specificity of EE stages of all mammalian plasmodia for parenchymal cells of the liver is suggested by the demonstration of these forms of rodent malaria parasites in this organ (Yoeli and Most, 1965).

The EE forms of avian and mammalian malarias differ in several basic respects (Table I). A unique feature of avian malaria is that EE stages can develop in a susceptible host following the injection of parasitized erythrocytes, while EE forms occur only in sporozoite-induced infections in mammals. That merozoites from avian erythrocytic stages can infect endothelial cells and develop as EE forms (i.e., the phanerozoites of Huff and Coulston, 1946) was shown by Coulston and Manwell (1941). Blood from a canary initially injected with a single parasitized red cell (*P. circumflexum*) produced demonstrable EE forms in subinoculated birds. In contrast, EE forms have never been seen in mammals inoculated with infected blood, and results of chemotherapeutic trials indicate that EE stages are found only in sporozoite-induced infections of mammals (Davey, 1946).

This apparent *in vivo* host cell specificity of mammalian EE stages (i.e., development only in hepatic parenchyma cells) contrasts sharply with the ability of avian EE forms to mature in a variety of host cells. The ability of avian EE stages to invade and develop within vascular endothelial cells in several organs and the capability of merozoites from phanerozoites to produce successive gener-

TABLE I

Comparison of Some Characteristics of Exoerythrocytic Stages of Malaria Parasites of Birds and Mammals

Characteristic	Birds	Mammals
Induction of EE forms in sporozoite-induced infection	Initial develop in lymphoid–macrophage elements and then in vascular endothelium	Development in hepatic parenchymal cells
Induction of EE forms in erythrocytic stage-induced infection	Development in vascular endothelium	Absent
Induction of EE forms in EE stage-induced infection	Development in vascular endothelium; parasitemia also results	Results in parasitemia only
Generations of EE stages	Multiple generations	Possibly a single pre-erythrocytic phase, but reinvasion of hepatic parenchymal cells by EE merozoites not disproved in some *Plasmodium* spp.
Pathology	May cause death in susceptible host	Limited to destruction of individual parenchymal cells
Cultivation *in vitro*	Yes	Yes, development presently incomplete

ations of EE stages often result in severe disease and death of the avian host. In contrast, pathological effects of mammalian EE stages seem to be limited to the cell within which the schizont resides and resultant compression of adjacent cells as the parasite increases in size (Shortt *et al.*, 1949, 1951; Hawking *et al.*, 1948; Bray, 1957a,b; Sodeman *et al.*, 1970).

The ease with which avian EE stages can be maintained in cell cultures was thought to be attributed, in part, to their less stringent host cell specificity as compared with mammalian EE forms. Avian EE stages can be established within cell cultures by initiation with infected tissue (Hegner and Wolfson, 1939; Rodhain *et al.*, 1940; Hawking, 1945; Dubin *et al.*, 1949, 1950; Huff *et al.*, 1960; Davis *et al.*, 1966; or by inoculation of cell monolayers with merozoites from EE forms in culture (Beaudoin *et al.*, 1974), with sporozoites (Dubin *et al.*, 1949, 1950), and possibly with erythrocytic forms (Meyer, 1947). An added feature of avian EE forms in culture is the ability of merozoites liberated into culture medium to invade other cells and continue development.

The development of a system for *in vitro* cultivation of the EE stages of mammalian malaria parasites would be a significant advance. Little is known of the events which occur during the brief period the mammalian malaria sporozoite is in the bloodstream, the mechanism by which hepatic parenchyma cells are entered, and the physiology of the developing EE trophozoite. A culture system could also be of benefit in chemotherapeutic studies. Early attempts to cultivate EE stages of mammalian plasmodia failed (Hawking *et al.*, 1948; Dubin *et al.*, 1950), but recent advances in methods for the cultivation of hepatocytes of mammals may provide a useful approach for *in vitro* studies of these forms. Beaudoin *et al.* (1974) reported that rodent liver cells in culture supported the multiplication of EE stages of the avian malaria parasite *P. fallax*, further demonstrating the relative flexibility in the ability of avian EE forms to develop within various types of cells and also that the rodent hepatocyte in culture can harbor an intracellular protozoan. Doby and Barker (1976) described forms resembling EE stages of *P. vivax* in cultures of human hepatocytes inoculated with sporozoites.

In a more recent study Strome *et al.* (1979) initiated development of EE forms of *P. berghei* by sporozoite inoculation of cells cultured from embryonic rat liver and brain and from turkey embryo brain. Nuclear division was evident within 24 hours after infection and by 48–56 hours parasites with more than 100 nuclei were seen. Complete EE stage maturation did not occur since individual merozoites were not produced. This important demonstration that the *in vivo* restriction of mammalian EE forms to hepatic parenchyma cells does not reflect a similar host cell specificity *in vitro* will no doubt stimulate needed studies of this phase of the infection course in mammalian malaria.

Using a different approach, Foley *et al.* (1978a) obtained infected cells by enzymatic digestion of livers after the inoculation of *P. berghei* sporozoites into rats. The EE stages produced patent infections in rats following *in vitro* cultivation of infected liver cells for up to 44 hours. The viability of parenchymal cells and the numbers of infective parasites decreased with increasing time in culture, but parasite infectivity was lost more rapidly than liver cell viability. Although the survival of parasites in cell cultures was proved by demonstrable infectivity, EE stages were not detected by microscopic examination of infected cell cultures, and these investigators were unable to determine whether the culture system supported EE form development. EE stages within parenchyma cells and free merozoites were seen, however, in suspension of cells obtained by enzymatic digestion of livers from rats injected with sporozoites 48 hours earlier (Foley *et al.*, 1978b).

Success in the use of sporozoites, merozoites from erythrocytic stages, and sexual forms in the immunization of experimental animals has stimulated a degree of enthusiasm for eventual vaccination against malaria parasites of humans (see this volume, Chapters 4, 6, and 7). Indeed, the introduction of sporozoites by irradiated mosquitoes confers protection against subsequent infection with this stage in human subjects (Clyde *et al.*, 1973, 1975; Rieckmann *et al.*, 1974; McCarthy and Clyde, 1977). The factors which presently prevent practical application of the methods for vaccination of human subjects have been discussed by Miller (1977a,b). Briefly, a source of sufficient numbers of sporozoites and the need for intravascular injection of irradiated parasites are limitations for use of that method. In addition, immunity elicited by sporozoite immunization must be absolute since no protection is conferred against erythrocytic stages. Application of merozoite vaccination may be limited by the present necessity for inclusion of complete Freund's adjuvant with dead parasites to induce resistance in monkeys against challenge. Use of gamete-enriched preparation from infected blood is a promising approach. The method blocks transmission by preventing parasite development in vectors and also provides a degree of protection against asexual parasites in rodents (Mendis and Targett, 1979) and monkeys (Gwadz and Green, 1978).

Avian and mammalian EE stages differ in several biological characteristics, but they share an important common feature relative to potential use for immunization. The development of EE forms invariably precedes the invasion of erythrocytes in sporozoite-induced infections, thus presenting a point at which the clinical disease associated with enythrocytic infection may be prevented or modified. The purpose of this discussion is to review studies on immune responsiveness to EE stages and to evaluate the potential use of these forms in immunization against malaria parasites.

II. IMMUNE RESPONSIVENESS TO EXOERYTHROCYTIC STAGES

A. Exoerythrocytic Stages in Avian Hosts

1. Acquired Resistance in Experimental Infections

The work of several investigators allows a general presentation of characteristics of infection with *P. gallinaceum* in chickens (Huff and Coulston, 1944, 1946; Haas *et al.*, 1948; Coulston and Huff, 1948). Three patterns may be characterized according to the parasite stage used to initiate infection. First, sporozoite-induced infections follow a predictable pattern in which cryptozoite and metacryptozoite generations of EE stages precede erythrocyte invasion. A fulminating parasitemia may follow and result in death of the host, but some chickens may develop a parasitemia crisis, i.e., a precipitous decrease in the percentage of parasitized erythrocytes. Later some birds may die with many EE stages (phanerozoites) in organs but with few parasitized red cells. Second, birds inoculated with parasitized erythrocytes exhibit increasing parasitemia and often die before EE stages can be detected in organs. Some birds may exhibit a parasitemia crisis but later die (at 3–4 weeks postinfection) with numerous EE forms in organs but with few parasites within red cells. A third pattern is seen in chickens inoculated with infected tissue containing EE forms. An early increase in the number of EE stages in various organs occurs, and birds often die within 2 weeks with many EE stages in organs but with low parasitemia. However, some birds survive infections initiated by any of the three methods, suggesting immunological responsiveness or age-related acquisition of resistance. Huff (1952) saw apparently degenerate *P. gallinaceum* EE forms in several organs of a chicken injected with sporozoites and suggested that antibody might play a role in EE stage degeneration. The bird was sacrificed just 3 days after sporozoite inoculation, however, and acquired immunity was unlikely to have been present at that early a stage of infection.

Corradetti (1955) injected chickens with infected RBCs and found *P. gallinaceum* EE stages in the brain 11 days later, but by day 34 EE forms were no longer seen. In birds inoculated with tissue containing EE stages these forms were detected between days 8 and 25 postinfection, but no EE stages were found thereafter. These results suggested immunological responsiveness against EE stages. While splenectomy of recovered chickens resulted in renewed multiplication of blood stages, no effect on EE forms was detected. Two convalescent birds seemed to exhibit acquired resistance to EE forms. Sixteen days after challenge with tissue containing EE forms no EE stage was seen in brain smears from the recovered birds, but these forms were present in two previously uninfected control chickens infected at the same time. In another experiment splenectomy of recovered birds did not lessen resistance to a later challenge with EE stages.

Graham *et al.* (1973a) studied the course of *P. fallax* infection in turkeys initiated with parasitized red cells and with EE forms from cell cultures. Following the injection of parasitized RBCs, turkey poults exhibited an early increase in parasitemia and some birds died. Others exhibited a parasitemia crisis but died 1–2 weeks later, and numerous EE stages were seen in brain smears. Birds injected with EE stages in fibroblasts from cell cultures exhibited an early increase in the number of EE stages in brain smears, but these forms were found in fewer numbers in birds sacrificed later. In birds injected with EE stages the parasitemia increased as the number of EE stages appeared to decrease, suggesting immune responsiveness against EE forms.

Despite these implications that birds acquire resistance to EE stages appearing subsequent to infection initiated with blood forms or infected tissue, it is clear that cryptozoites resulting from sporozoite inoculation are unaffected by demonstrated immunity in recovered birds. Huff and Coulston (1946) observed normal development of cryptozoites after the injection of sporozoites into the wing skin of chickens which had been initially infected with sporozoites and had subsequently resisted several challenge infections.

2. Passive Transfer of Immunity

Several investigators using immunofluorescence methods demonstrated antibodies which reacted with EE stages in serum from chickens which had recovered from *P. gallinaceum* infection (Ingram and Carver, 1963; Voller and Taffs, 1963; El-Nahal, 1967). Since chickens harbor both EE forms and RBC stages during *P. gallinaceum* infection, the use of convalescent serum does not differentiate between antibodies which may be stage-specific and those which react with antigens shared by EE and RBC forms.

Graham *et al.* (1973b) produced antisera specific for EE stages of *P. fallax* in the following manner. One-month-old turkeys received an initial intravenous injection of 10^8 EE stages in fibroblast cells from culture. Two challenge infections containing, respectively, 2.5×10^8 and about 1.7×10^8 EE stages were given 17 and 27 days later, and poults received chloroquine throughout the experiment in order to suppress erythrocytic stages. Two of 18 poults treated in this manner died. A control group was injected with uninfected fibroblasts from culture and treated with chloroquine, while another group of poults received EE forms in fibroblasts but without the drug regimen (3 of 18 birds in this group died). A final group was injected with uninfected fibroblasts, and no chloroquine was given. Sera were harvested 7 days after the second injection of infected or uninfected fibroblasts for use in passive transfer experiments. Normal serum was collected from previously untreated birds of the same age.

Passive transfer of immunity was tested in 30-day-old poults injected with 2×10^8 EE-infected cells from culture. Groups of birds were injected intravenously with hyperimmune or control serum (6 ml/kg body weight) on days 0 (day of infection), 1, 2, and 3. Infections were monitored by recording daily body weight changes of birds (Graham *et al.*, 1973a). From day 7 to day 8 after infection a weight gain of at least 2% was exhibited by 7 of 8 poult which had received hyperimmune serum, while only 4 of 20 recipients of control serum displayed this degree of weight gain. By day 9 all poults had lost weight. This 1-day delay in the onset of weight loss in birds receiving hyperimmune serum equates with a 90% reduction in parasite number in the infecting inoculum (Graham *et al.*, 1973a).

A similar effect on body weight change was seen in younger poults (17 days old) receiving anti-EE stage serum, and Graham *et al.* (1973b) also estimated the number of EE stages in brain smears of birds sacrificed 7 days after infection. Infected turkeys injected with anti-EE stage serum gained weight 1 day longer and had fewer EE forms in brain smears than birds receiving control serum (Table II).

An important point in these experiments is the stage specificity of passive transfer against EE forms. Successful passive transfer against EE forms was with serum from turkeys which had resisted two challenges with EE stages while

TABLE II

Effect of Passive Transfer of Serum on the Course of the Exoerythrocytic Form Infection in 17-Day-Old Poults as Determined by Body Weight and Degree of Exoerythrocytic Form Parasitization of Cerebral Cells[a]

Treatment	Infected or uninfected	Percentage of poults gaining weight daily as of day			EE stages per 50 fields from two poults killed on day 7
		6	7	8	
Anti-EE form serum	Infected	100	100	25	6, 5
Anti-tissue culture					
Cell tissue	Infected	100	25		30, 78
Normal turkey serum	Infected	100	0		22, 14
Saline	Infected	100	25		11, 52
None	Infected	100	0		30, 78
None	Uninfected	100	100	100	

[a] All groups contained four birds except the untreated, infected group and the anti-EE form serum-treated, infected group (six birds each). All infected birds were inoculated intravenously on day 0 with 6000 parasitized tissue culture cells per kilogram body weight.

receiving chloroquine, but the serum donors were fully susceptible to a subsequent challenge with RBC stages of *P. fallax*.

3. Immunoglobulins Involved in Immunity against Exoerythrocytic Stages

Marion *et al.* (1974) confirmed that hyperimmune anti-EE stage serum from turkeys conferred immunity against EE forms and extended these results by testing immunoglobulin components of serum in passive transfer experiments. IgG and IgM components of hyperimmune turkey serum were harvested by ammonium sulfate precipitation and chromatography on Sephadex G-200. With the use of passive transfer methods similar to those of Graham *et al.* (1973b), most protective activity was found in the IgG fraction, although IgM from the same sera also slightly delayed body weight loss in turkeys infected with EE forms.

These results demonstrated that the resistance of turkeys to EE stages was mediated, at least in part, by antibody. Antibodies seem to be specific for EE stages, since serum from birds immune to EE stages, but susceptible to RBC-stage challenge, conferred resistance to EE forms by passive transfer (Graham *et al.*, 1973b).

Whether antibodies against erythrocytic stages provide protection against EE forms is not clear. Manwell and Goldstein (1938) protected birds against RBC forms of *P. circumflexum* by passive transfer of immune serum and noted that

EE stages were present in various organs of serum recipients, but no effect of serum transfer on these forms was mentioned. Manresa (1953) noted that passive transfer of serum from turkeys and chickens which had recovered from *P. lophurae* infection had no effect on the appearance of EE forms (i.e., phanerozoites) in serum recipients following the injection of RBC forms. The last of six serum injections was on day 5 after infection, but the greatest phanerozoite density occurred from day 18 to day 21 in the brain of turkeys receiving immune serum. It would be of interest to determine whether the injection of anti-RBC stage serum has an effect during the time EE stages appear to be developing in demonstrable numbers. Manresa (1953) also noted that neither the intensity of the initial parasitemia nor the sex of the serum recipients had an apparent effect on the appearance of phanerozoites.

B. Immunization against Avian Exoerythrocytic Stages

1. Plasmodium fallax

Holbrook *et al.* (1974) conducted a series of experiments testing the immunogenicity of merozoites from EE stages of *P. fallax* in turkeys. Merozoites were harvested by centrifugation of medium overlay from fibroblast cultures initiated from infected turkey embryo brain. Parasites were killed by suspension in 0.1% Formalin for 30 minutes at room temperature and kept at 4°C overnight. The immunization schedule for the initial experiment in their study is presented in Table III. Groups 1 and 2 consisted of 4-week-old poults which received Formalin-killed merozoites (FKMs). Control birds received equivalent injections of Formalin-treated centrifugate of overlay from cultures of uninfected fibroblasts (groups 3 and 4) or no treatment prior to challenge (group 5). In this experiment poults were challenged intravenously with merozoites from cell cultures and received a single chloroquine treatment (6.0 mg/kg) 6 days later to

TABLE III

Schedule for the Immunization of Turkeys with Formalin-Killed Merozoites from Cell Cultures[a]

Group	Day −21	Day −14	Day −7
1	1.5×10^6 FKMs with FCA im	2.3×10^6 FKMs in EBSS iv	1.2×10^6 FKMs in EBSS iv
2	NT	2.3×10^6 FKMs in EBSS iv	1.2×10^6 FKMs in EBSS iv
3	NO with FCA im	NO in EBSS iv	NO in EBSS iv
4	NT	NO in EBSS iv	NO in EBSS iv
5	NT	NT	NT

[a] On day 0 all birds were challenged with 5.0×10^4 merozoites from cell culture. NO, centrifugate of normal uninfected culture medium overlay; NT, no treatment; EBSS, Earle's alanced salt solution; im, intramuscularly; iv, intravenously.

TABLE IV

Number of Turkeys Surviving after Challenge on Day 0 with 5.0 $\times$ 10^4 Merozoites from Cell Culture

Group[a] no.	Number of survivors on day					
	10	11	12	13	14	15
1	10	10	10	10	10	10
2	10	10	10	10	9	8
3	10	9	8	4	3	3
4	10	10	9	8	5	4
5	10	10	6	3	2	2

[a] Groups 1 and 2 were immunized with FKMs prior to challenge; groups 3 and 4 received formalin-treated centrifugate to challenge; and group 5 was untreated before challenge.

suppress RBC stages which might kill the birds before an effect of FKM immunization would be apparent. Eighteen of 20 FKM-immunized turkeys survived the challenge infection, while 21 of 30 control birds died, most with numerous EE stages in brain smears (Table IV). Neither of the two FKM-immunized poults which died had detectable EE stages in brain smears, but each had parasitemia greater than 70% at death.

In a second experiment in this study FKM-immunized and previously untreated poults were challenged with EE merozoites from culture, but chloroquine was not given. Five of the 6 FKM-immunized birds survived. One bird in this group died with high parasitemia (81.1%), but no EE stage was seen in brain smears. Five of 7 control birds died, and 3 had numerous EE forms in the brain. In another experiment FKM-immunized and control turkeys were challenged with RBC stages. No effect of FKM immunization on the course of parasitemia was seen (Table V), but 4 of 14 FKM-immunized poults survived while all 28 control turkeys died, either during the initial increase in parasitemia or as a consequence of developing EE forms. One FKM-immunized bird exhibited high parasitemia (ranging from 38.9 to 77.7%) for 13 consecutive days and died on the seventeenth day after challenge.

Immunization with FKMs appears to have a specific protective effect against the development of EE stages after a challenge with merozoites from cell culture or with RBC stages. A total of 40 birds was immunized with FKMs of *P. fallax* in the study, and only 1 died with detectable EE stages after challenge. These forms were numerous in brain smears from most control birds which died (Holbrook et al., 1974). The mechanism of this protective effect is not known.

TABLE V

Result of Infection of Immunized and Control Turkeys Injected iv with 17.6 $\times$ 10^6 Parasitized Turkey Erythrocytes

Group[a]	No. of turkeys	Mean peak parasitemia (%)	No. surviving parasitemia	No. dying later with EE stages	No. survivors
FKM + S	7	73.3	3	1	2
FKM − S	7	77.2	2	0	2
NO + S	7	65.5	2	2	0
NO − S	7	72.1	2	2	0
NT + S	7	72.3	0	0	0
NT − S	7	69.0	0	0	0

[a] FKM, turkeys immunized with FKMs; NO and NT, controls. Birds in some groups received 2.0 ml normal turkey serum on day of challenge (+S); others received no serum (−S).

Immunization with FKMs may prevent the entry of merozoites into cells which could support EE development or inhibit maturation of EE forms after cell invasion. The possible effect of FKM immunization on the development of preerythrocytic stages (i.e., cryptozoites and metacryptozoites) developing after sporozoite inoculation has not been tested in the *P. fallax*–turkey system.

2. *Plasmodium gallinaceum*

Richards and Latter (1977) immunized chickens with Formalin-treated EE forms of *P. gallinaceum*. Birds injected twice with Formalin-treated brain or infected cells from culture (with saponin as an adjuvant) survived longer than control chicks after a challenge with EE forms in infected brain or from cell culture. Immunization with emulsions of infected kidney provided no protection, perhaps because of inadequate numbers of EE stages in the preparation. Immunization with EE stages had no apparent effect on a challenge with sporozoites or blood stages.

C. Exoerythrocytic Stages in Mammals

A striking observation in histological studies on EE forms in mammalian hosts is the absence of a discernible host reaction to the developing parasite in the liver. The maturing EE trophozoite seems to be ignored by the infected animal and causes only distortion of the host cells and eventual displacement of adjacent tissue. Following rupture of the mature EE schizont with the release of merozoites, cellular infiltration is seen in the area formerly occupied by the parasite (Shortt and Garnham, 1948b; 1956; Garnham *et al.*, 1957; Yoeli and Most, 1965), but the reparative process seems to be remarkably efficient. Little evidence of the previous presence of EE stages is detected even in animals which had earlier harbored large numbers of EE forms in the liver (Garnham and Bray, 1956). Most evidence suggests that the developing intracellular EE schizont is sufficiently "hidden" to render it insusceptible to immunological recognition in mammals.

Demonstrable protective immunity against erythrocytic stages appears to have no effect on the development of EE stages following sporozoite challenge in mammals. The initial demonstration of EE forms of *P. vivax* was in a human subject who had recovered from a previous infection with blood stages of this parasite. Shortt and Garnham (1948b) found EE stages in the liver 7 days after sporozoite injection, but no RBC forms were seen subsequently in blood films although the subject experienced a transitory fever 15 days after sporozoite injection.

Hawking and Thurston (1952) demonstrated that immunity against RBC stages of *P. cynomolgi* did not influence the development of EE stages following sporozoite inoculation. Monkeys initially infected with RBC stages or sporozoites were later splenectomized and resisted two challenges with RBC stages of this parasite. When these animals were injected with *P. cynomolgi* sporozoites, EE stages were detected in liver sections of each monkey 9 days later, and each animal exhibited low-grade parasitemia on day 14. Microscopic examination of EE forms revealed no altered morphology of the EE stages, despite the demonstrable immunity of the host animals against RBC stages.

Garnham and Bray (1956) studied EE stages of *P. cynomolgi* in monkeys which had resisted repeated challenges with RBC stages or sporozoites. After the injection of *P. cynomolgi* sporozoites the density of EE stages in the liver of immune and control animals varied considerably, but these stages were morphologically similar. An unexpected finding in this study was the presence of numerous EE stages in the liver of two immune monkeys 35 days after sporozoite inoculation, when no EE forms were seen in a control animal.

Although demonstrable immunity of mammals against RBC stages of malaria parasites seems to have no deleterious effect on EE forms, several investigators have shown that antiserum from mammals which have recovered from a RBC stage infection reacts with EE stages *in vitro* (Ingram and Carver, 1963; El-Nahal, 1967; Ward and Conran, 1968;). Using indirect immunofluorescence, El-Nahal (1967) demonstrated that anti-RBC stage serum from animals, including humans, reacted with EE stages in liver sections. Cross-reactions between EE stages of species of rodent malaria parasites were seen, but antisera from primates reacted only with EE forms of the homologous parasite species. However, using a similar method, Krotoski *et al.* (1973) described serological cross-reactivity between EE forms of *P. cynomolgi* and *P. knowlesi*.

A recent study on *P. berghei* in rats showed that antigens were shared by sporozoites, EE stages, and RBC forms of this parasite (Golenser *et al.*, 1977).

Antiserum from rats which had recovered from an infection initiated with RBC stages reacted in indirect fluorescent antibody tests with RBC forms, EE stages in liver sections, and sporozoites. Rats exposed at least twice to mosquito-transmitted *P. berghei* sporozoites produced antibodies which reacted against EE and RBC forms, but titers were highest against sporozoites.

Nardin and Nussenzweig (1978) also found that RBC forms and sporozoites possessed cross-reacting antigens, demonstrable only when sporozoites were air-dried and frozen before reacting with antiserum against RBC stages, suggesting that cross-reacting antigens on sporozoites were exposed by membrane disruption.

Danforth *et al.* (1978) confirmed the reaction of anti-RBC stage serum with EE stages of *P. berghei*. They also found that antiserum from mice immunized with irradiated sporozoites reacted strongly with EE stages in liver taken 14–24 hours after infection but the reaction was much weaker at 36 and 42 hours postinfection. Conversely, anti-RBC serum reacted more strongly with late than with early EE forms.

It seem clear that EE stages of mammalian plasmodia are not adversely affected by demonstrable immunity against erythrocytic stages. That these parasite stages share antigens has been shown by *in vitro* reactions of EE stages with antiserum from animals which have recovered from blood stage infection. Positive *in vitro* serological reactions with EE stages in the absence of a detectable *in vivo* protective response suggest (1) that antibody demonstrated by immunofluorescence reacts with antigen that plays no role in the induction of acquired immunity, (2) that the developing EE form is not susceptible to the action of antibody *in vivo,* or (3) that potentially protective antibody simply does not reach the EE stage within the liver parenchyma cell.

D. Immunization of Mammals against Exoerythrocytic Stages

Technical problems imposed by the biological characteristics of mammalian malaria parasites have prevented direct tests of immunogenicity of EE stages. The EE forms of mammalian Plasmodia develop only as a consequence of sporozoite inoculation and mature *in vivo* only within parenchymal cells in the liver. No culture system has been available to support complete development of EE forms of mammalian malaria parasites, and these forms are not presently available for immunogenic tests. Strome *et al.* (1979) recently initiated EE stage development by *P. berghei* sporozoite inoculation of cells cultured from embryonic rat and turkey organs and Foley *et al.* (1978a) found that EE forms of *P. berghei* retained infectivity for up to 44 hours in cultures of liver cells from infected rats. These important studies suggest that a test of the immunogenicity of mammalian EE stages will be feasible.

Most notable success in attempts to immunize mammals against malaria parasites has been achieved using sporozoites or merozoites derived from RBC stages as immunogens. These approaches are discussed in detail elsewhere in this volume (Chapters 4 and 6, but a brief review of the effects of immunization with these stages on EE forms is presented here.

Merozoites from RBC forms of *P. knowlesi*, combined with Freund's complete adjuvant (FCA), have been used to elicit strong stage-specific and parasite species-specific immunity in monkeys. Some immunized monkeys exhibit brief low-grade parasitemia after a challenge with RBC stages, but other animals appear to be completely immune to a challenge with this form (Mitchell *et al.*, 1975; Cohen *et al.*, 1977a,b; Mitchell, 1977). A delay in the appearance of parasitized red cells was seen in merozoite-immunized monkeys following a challenge with *P. knowlesi* sporozoites (Richards *et al.*, 1977) but may have been due to the inhibition or destruction of merozoites produced by early generations of erythrocytic forms following normal preerythrocytic development in the liver rather than specific inhibition of developing EE forms.

Golenser *et al.* (1977) immunized rats against sporozoites of *P. berghei* by exposing the animals to infected mosquitoes while treating with chloroquine to suppress development of emerging RBC stages. After a later sporozoite challenge the immunized rats harbored fewer EE stages in the liver than control animals. These investigators also found fewer EE stages in the liver of rats injected with sporozoites while the animals were experiencing a parasitemia, than in previously uninfected controls. The lower density of EE forms was particularly notable in rats challenged while experiencing rising parasitemia. Golenser *et al.* (1977) suggested as possible mechanisms that antibodies against RBC forms reacted with inoculated sporozoites, that nonspecific immunological stimulation participated, or that the capability of the liver parenchymal cell to support EE development was impaired during the period RBC forms were multiplying.

Mice receiving multiple intravenous injections of irradiated *P. berghei* sporozoites completely resist subsequent challenge with normal sporozoites (Nussenzweig *et al.*, 1969). Injections of heat-killed or frozen and thawed sporozoites provide less effective protection (Spitalny and Nussenzweig, 1972), suggesting that some degree of preerythrocytic development following inoculation of irradiated sporozoites may be needed to elicit immunity. Vanderberg *et al.* (1968) examined liver sections taken 45 hours after intravenous inoculation of irradiated *P. berghei* sporozoites into young rats and found that the EE forms were smaller and fewer in number than in animals inoculated with untreated sporozoites. Small parasities easily recognized as EE stages and other forms which may have been retarded EE stages were seen in the liver of two rats 16 days after the injection of irradiated sporozoites. This indicated that EE stages could play a role in protective immunity elicited by injections of irradiated sporozoites (Vanderberg *et al.*, 1968). Mackaness (1977) recently suggested that cell-mediated responsiveness against EE stages may be a mechanism in sporozoite-induced immunity. While sporozoite-induced immunity appears to depend in part on cell-mediated responsiveness (Verhave *et al.*, 1978), whether the response acts against the EE form or solely against inoculated sporozoites is not known. Although the mechanisms of acquired immunity elicited by immunization with irradiated sporozoites are not completely known, it appears that a humoral component is involved. A precipitate forms on normal sporozoites incubated in serum from sporozoite-immunized animals, and infectivity of sporozoites for previously uninfected mice is decreased by *in vitro* incubation in antisporozoite serum (Vanderberg *et al.*, 1969). Also, following intravenous injection normal sporozoites can be demonstrated by blood subinoculation for a longer time in the circulating blood of normal mice than in sporozoite-immunized mice (Nussenzweig *et al.*, 1972).

Efforts to detect specific responsiveness against EE forms in sporozoite-immune animals have been few. Vanderberg (1973) attempted to determine whether antiserum from mice immunized with irradiated *P. berghei* sporozoites reacted with the EE stages of this parasite. Mice were injected with normal sporozoites and received 0.5 ml antiserum from sporozoite-immunized mice 3 and 27 hours later. No effect of antiserum transfer was seen on the number, morphology, or size of the EE forms in liver sections from serum recipients. In a similar experiment injections of antisporozoite serum had no effect on the length of the prepatent period following the injection of sporozoites into serum recipients. The EE stages dissociated from infected rat liver by enzymatic methods apparently were not affected by *in vitro* exposure to antisporozoite serum. These results demonstrated that antisporozoite serum had no effect on EE forms after the infection was established in the liver but did not disprove a possible participation of EE stages in the induction of protective immunity by irradiated sporozoites. After intravenous inoculation normal sporozoites disappear from the circulating blood of nonimmune animals within 1 hour (Nussenzweig *et al.*, 1972), and the parasite presumably occupied an intracellular position before the first injection of antiserum was made by Vanderberg (1973) (i.e., 3 hours after sporozoite injection). If the developing EE stages within the liver parenchyma cell are inaccessible to antibody, no effect of antisporozoite serum on the morphology of EE stages or on the length of the prepatent period would be expected. Also, EE stages freed from infected liver could have been enclosed in the parenchyma cell membrane and not accessible to antibody. A possible participation of cell-mediated responsiveness in sporozoite-induced immunity would not be expected to be demonstrable by passive serum transfer.

Foley and Vanderberg (1977) demonstrated that mice immunized with irradiated *P. berghei* sporozoites (which were resistant to a challenge with infective sporozoites) were susceptible to a challenge with EE stages. These forms were obtained from the liver of rats which had been injected with sporozoites 2.5 or 21–28 hours earlier. The demonstrated infectivity of the EE stages in liver from sporozoite-infected rats is an important finding and may allow a more direct approach for studies on these forms. However, merozoites produced by the inoculated EE forms presumably were infective only for red cells, and the study further demonstrates the stage specificity of sporozoite-induced immunity, relative to RBC stages, without disproving participation of EE forms in the induction of sporozoite-induced immunity.

No direct test of the immunogenicity of mammalian EE stages has been made, but Holbrook *et al.* (1976) studied the effect of injections of avian EE stages on subsequent challenge of mice with *P. berghei* sporozoites. In the initial experiment in the study merozoites of *P. fallax* EE forms were harvested from a medium overlay of turkey fibroblast cultures which had been initiated as explants of infected embryo brain 2–3 months earlier. The EE merozoites were killed by suspension in 0.1% Formalin. One group of mice received an intramuscular inoculation of FKMs combined with FCA, followed by two intravenous injections of FKMs in Earle's balanced salt solution at weekly intervals. Another group of mice received equivalent FKM inoculations, but FCA was not included. Control mice in the experiment received a Formalin-treated centrifugate of medium overlay from uninfected fibroblast cultures or no treatment. The result of intravenous challenge with 10^4 *P. berghei* sporozoites is presented in Table VI. A small proportion of FKM-immunized mice, (i.e., 25% overall) exhibited no parasites in blood cells after sporozoite challenge, while all control animals became infected. Mice immunized with FKMs which were not completely pro-

TABLE VI

Result of Intravenous Challenge of Formalin-Killed Merozoite-Immunized and Control Mice with 10^4 *Plasmodium berghei* Sporozoites

Group no. and no. of mice	Mean prepatent period (days)	Percentage protected
1 (8)	6.0	12.5
2 (8)	4.8	37.5
3 (6)	4.5	0
4 (8)	4.3	0
5 (7)	4.3	0

[a] Group-1 mice received 6.3×10^5 FKMs with FCA intramuscularly on day −29 and 1.0×10^5 FKMs in Earle's balanced salt solution intravenously on days −22 and −15. Group 2 received the same injections, but FCA was not included. Groups 3 and 4 were corresponding control groups which received a Formalin-treated centrifugate of medium overlay from uninfected cell cultures. Group 5 was not treated prior to challenge. Calculation excludes mice which did not exhibit parasitized erythrocytes after challenge.

tected against sporozoite challenge exhibited an increased prepatent period as compared with control animals.

In a subsequent experiment groups of mice received FKMs from 3- to 5–week-old cell cultures in three injections at weekly intervals. All eight mice injected with FKMs via an initial intramuscular inoculation (without adjuvant) and two weekly intravenous injections completely resisted *P. berghei* sporozoite challenge. Six of eight animals receiving three intravenous injections of FKMs also resisted sporozoite challenge, but animals receiving FKMs from the same cultures via three intramuscular or intraperitoneal injections were not protected.

When this experiment was repeated, using the same number of FKMs injected via an initial intramuscular and two subsequent intravenous inoculations, a slightly increased prepatent period was observed, but no mice were completely protected. The FKMs used in this experiment were harvested from fibroblast cultures which had been maintained for longer than 3 months, suggesting a possible loss of merozoite immunogenicity with increased time in culture. In an additional experiment an attempt was made to compensate for possible decreased immungenicity by increasing the number of FKMs injected and the number of weekly FKM inoculations from three to seven. Two of the five FKM-immunized mice completely resisted a *P. berghei* sporozoite challenge after receiving the extended FKM regimen, and the three susceptible animals in this group exhibited a 1-day increase in the prepatent period as compared with appropriate control animals.

In each of these experiments FKM-immunized mice not completely protected against sporozoite challenge were as susceptible as control animals to the multiplication of erythrocytic stages appearing subsequent to sporozoite inoculation. However, the appearance of parasitized red cells in microscopically detectable numbers in FKM recipients was delayed approximately 1 day. Mice immunized with FKM which were completely protected from sporozoite challenge were fully susceptible to infection initiated with RBC stages of *P. berghei*. Thus, resistance elicited by FKM injections was directed against the sporozoite before entrance into the liver parenchyma cell or against the developing EE stage. The mechanism of resistance to *P. berghei* sporozoite challenge in FKM-immunized mice is not known. Sera harvested from mice completely protected against subsequent sporozoite challenge did not react with *P. berghei* sporozoites *in vitro*. No reaction resembling circumsporozoite precipitation activity was detected nor was infectivity of *P. berghei* sporozoites altered by *in vitro* incubation in sera from FKM-immunized mice (Holbrook *et al.*, 1976). El-Nahal (1967) noted that the EE forms of avian and mammalian malaria parasites did not cross-react in immunofluorescent antibody tests, and it seems unlikely that EE stages of *P. fallax* and *P. berghei* share antigens which stimulate specific acquired immunity. Resistance conferred by FKM injections likely represents a form of nonspecific stimulation previously demonstrated in other studies on rodent malaria (Nussenzweig, 1967; Jahiel et al., 1969; Clark et al., 1976).

Two experiments were subsequently conducted in an attempt to confirm that EE merozoites of avian plasmodia can stimulate resistance against P. berghei sporozoite challenge (T. W. Holbrook, unpublished). The first attempt was made to determine whether EE forms of another avian parasite, P. gallinaceum, could alter the response of mice to a P. berghei sporozoite challenge. The avian parasite was provided by R. B. McGhee. Cell cultures were initiated as explants of chick embryo brain heavily infected with EE stages, but the number of P. gallinaceum EE forms in cultured cells decreased soon after cultures were established. Thus, parasites with relatively large amounts of tissue debris were harvested 7 days after culture initiation and killed by suspension in 0.1% Formalin. The preparations were sent to the laboratory of R. S. Nussenzweig, and mice received five intravenous injections at weekly intervals. No protection was evident when these animals were challenged by an intravenous injection of P. berghei sporozoites.

In the second study mice received five intravenous injections of P. fallax FKMs (a total of about 4×10^6 per mouse) at weekly intervals from turkey fibroblast cultures initiated 4–8 weeks earlier. Animals immunized with FKMs and appropriate control groups were sent to R. L. Beaudoin for a P. berghei sporozoite challenge 1 week after the final inoculation. These animals exhibited a delay of about 1 day in the appearance of parasitized red cells in peripheral blood films compared with controls, but no mice were completely resistant to sporozoite challenge.

The results of these preliminary trials using P. fallax EE stages are highly variable with respect to the number of FKM-immunized animals completely resistant to a P. berghei sporozoite challenge. One consistent feature in experiments using P. fallax FKMs is an increased prepatent period in stimulated mice following a challenge with P. berghei sporozoites.

III. DISCUSSION

A. Comparison of Avian and Mammalian Responsiveness to Exoerythrocytic Stages

An effort to immunize against any developmental stage of malaria parasites must presume that the animal can be stimulated to mount an effective immunological response against this stage. It is clear that birds respond immunologically to sporozoites (Mulligan et al., 1941; Richards, 1966), EE stages (Graham et al., 1973b; Marion et al., 1974), and both asexual and sexual erythrocytic forms (Manwell and Goldstein, 1938; Richards, 1966; Gwadz, 1976). Immunization of mammals against sporozoites (Nussenzweig *et al.*, 1969), merozoites from RBC stages (Mitchell *et al.*, 1975) and sexual stages (Gwadz and Green, 1978) has been demonstrated, but as yet no definitive evidence of a specific acquired protective response against EE stages of mammalian malaria parasites has been shown.

The apparent nonresponsiveness of mammals to EE forms is probably a consequence of the events which occur after sporozoite inoculation rather than a lack of immunogenicity of EE stages. Sporozoites introduced by intravascular injection disappear from the circulation relatively quickly (Nussenzweig *et al.*, 1972), and blood is not infective for subinoculated animals until the preerythrocytic phase is completed. In mammals EE forms have only been demonstrated within parenchyma cells of the liver and elicit little discernible host reaction at this site until the mature EE forms burst and release merozoites. In the liver the parasite seems to be effectively sequestered at an intracellular site which does not allow the immunological system of the mammalian host to recognize the parasite as "foreign." If one assumes (perhaps incorrectly) that only one preerythrocytic phase occurs in mammalian malaria, the infected animal is exposed to the sporozoite before invasion of the host cell and to merozoites liberated after maturation of the EE stage. In this view the host is never exposed to potential antigens of the developing EE stage.

Merozoites produced by preerythrocytic schizogony in mammalian malaria preseumably are destined to invade erythrocytes and apparently are no different in this physiological characteristic from merozoites produced by erythrocytic schizogony. Whether merozoites produced by EE schizogony differ antigenically from RBC stage merozoites is pertinent to their possible use in immunization studies. Monkeys immunized with merozoites from RBC stages of *P. knowlesi* exhibit an increased prepatent period after sporozoite challenge (Richards *et al.*, 1977), but whether this response affects merozoites emerging from EE stages or is directed exclusively at merozoites produced by early generations of erythrocytic stages is not known.

A system for *in vitro* cultivation of mammalian EE stages is needed to determine whether these forms can be used to stimulate protective immune responsiveness, and technical problems which must be resolved in developing such a system have been discussed (Beaudoin, 1977). If an immunogenic preparation from mammalian EE stages becomes available, the process of immunization will require not only the induction of an effective protective response but must also render the EE form accessible to the response. If sporozoite entrance into the liver paraenchyma cell is direct, the EE stage may avoid immunological recognition within the cell despite the mammal's ability to respond. However, infection of the parenchyma cell may be secondary to a brief period within another cell type, possibly phagocytic in function. The mechanism by which the sporozoite gains entrance into the parenchyma cell is not known, and clarification of this aspect of the vertebrate cycle is significant in attempts to establish EE stages in cell culture and the possible use of EE forms in immunization trials. The recent advances in cultivation of EE stages of *P. berghei* (Foley *et al.*, 1978a, Strome *et al.*, 1979) should allow detailed study of EE stage development and provide parasites for immunogenic trials.

Avian hosts can be shown to respond immunologically against EE stages. This is in part a consequence of the cyclic nature of these forms in birds. The injection of sporozoites into a susceptible bird results in the development of two preerythrocytic phases (i.e., cryptozoites and metacryptozoites) and the subsequent appearance of successive generations of EE forms (i.e., phanerozoites) in various organs. Birds that survive have been exposed to relatively large numbers of EE stages and respond immunologically to these forms. The relative ease with which the EE forms of avian plasmodia can be cultivated and used for immunization or infection has allowed studies which cannot presently be made with mammalian malaria systems.

B. Areas for Research in Avian Systems

Several aspects of the immune responsiveness of birds against EE stages need further study. The mechanism by which birds recover from infection and resist subsequent challenge with EE stages appears to be mediated in part by antibodies (Graham *et al.*, 1973b), especially those of the IgG class (Marion *et al.*, 1974), but the humoral response seems to be incomplete. Thus, passive transfer of large volumes of antiserum prolongs the life of turkey recipients about 24 hours, but the birds usually die. Further study of humoral mechanisms and of the possible participation of cell-mediated resistance can provide a better understanding of the response of birds to EE stages and may have broader application to the responses of avian hosts to other intracellular parasites.

Immunization of turkeys with merozoites from EE stages of *P. fallax* elicits protection in a proportion of birds, which is sufficient to prevent death if erythrocytic stages are specifically drug-suppressed (Holbrook *et al.*, 1974). The response appears to be stage-specific, since protection is not afforded against RBC stages, suggesting an antigenic difference between merozoites which are destined for intraerythrocytic development and those which can invade and mature within endothelial cells. The question of whether invasion of erythrocyte or endothelial cells is opportunistic or a predetermined characteristic of an individual merozoite is of interest. The former possibility seems more likely, since the inoculation of a single parasitized erythrocyte can eventually produce EE stages in a susceptible bird (Manwell and Goldstein, 1938). Inoculation of *P. fallax* EE merozoites from culture into adult chickens, hosts normally refractory to EE stages of this parasite (Huff, 1957), produces parasitemia in the apparent absence of EE stages in organs.

Several aspects of the immunization of birds against EE stages need to be explored. The effect of the immunization route, mechanism of resistance to challenge, duration of protective resistance, and stage of development of the EE form against which resistance is expressed are factors which need study. Richards and Latter (1977) reported that immunization of chickens with Formalin-treated EE forms of *P. gallinaceum* did not affect sporozoite-induced infection. This suggests that preerythrocytic EE forms and phanerozoites are antigenically different or that the preerythrocytic stages of *P. gallinaceum* are sequestered within cells and immunological responsiveness that could affect these stages is inactive because of the inaccessibility of the developing parasite.

C. Application of Studies of Avian Exoerythrocytic Forms to Mammalian Malaria

Differences in biological characteristics of avian and mammalian EE stages (Table I) raise the question of whether studies on EE forms of birds have relevance to mammalian malaria. Despite these differences the parasites of birds and mammals share a characteristic relevant to the use of EE stages in immunization studies. In sporozoite-induced malaria of birds or mammals, preerythrocytic development is obligatory before merozoites infective for erythrocytes are produced. The sequence of events occurring between sporozoite inoculation and erythrocyte invasion is better known for avian than mammalian malaria parasites. The mechanism by which sporozoites of mammalian malaria parasites gain entrance into hepatic parenchyma cells is not known, but an understanding of this process is important from the aspect of *in vitro* cultivation of EE stages and the potential use of these forms in immunization studies. Immunization with EE forms from culture system may have little protective effect if sporozoites in a challenge inoculum directly invade hepatic parenchyma cells. Despite the theoretical capability of the immunized mammal to respond against EE forms, these intracellular stages might be inaccessible to immune mechanisms. If the sporozoite is first engulfed by phagocytic cells within the liver and undergoes some developmental change before entering the parenchyma cell, specific immunization against the EE stage may be more effective. Parenthetically, the latter sequence of events parallels the cryptozoite-to-metacryptozoite developmental process in avian malaria.

With the limited data available it is not possible to assess the significance of stimulation with EE merozoites of the avian parasite *P. fallax* against sporozoite-induced *P. berghei* malaria in mice (Holbrook *et al.*, 1976). Only a small proportion of mice were completely protected against sporozoite challenge in this study, but a consistent feature in mice stimulated with FKMs was a delay in the appearance of microsopically detectable parasitized red cells after sporozoite injection. The infective sporozoite inoculum was, in effect, decreased. Resistance elicited by this method almost certainly represents nonspecific stimulation but a test of specific immunization using mammalian EE forms appears to be a realistic goal (Foley *et al.*, 1978a,b; Strome *et al.*, 1979).

Development of a practical vaccine which will prevent or modify malaria in human subjects seems to be possible. Immunization with irradiated sporozoites or with merozoites from RBC stages elicits strong stage-specific resistance, but problems attend the use of either method on a practical scale. A source of suitable numbers of merozoites of human plasmodia and an acceptable adjuvant for use in humans are major problems associated with the use of RBC stage merozoites. These problems appear to be more amenable to resolution than the production of sporozoites in necessary numbers for use on a practical scale. Immunization with gamete-enriched preparations not only blocks vector transmission but elicits resistance against asexual erythrocytic stage in mammals (Mendis and Targett, 1979; Gwadz and Green, 1978).

A direct test of immunogenicity of mammalian EE forms is dependent on the development of a culture system which will allow production of these stages in adequate numbers and free of tissue. We need a culture system for EE stages of mammalian malaria parasites before we can evaluate the use of EE stages in vaccination studies. Cultivation of these forms might permit the investigation of biological interactions of the parasite and host cell. The system might allow important studies on the physiology of EE forms and contribute to a rational chemotherapeutic approach. Answers to questions concerning basic phenomena such as the mechanism of sporozoite entrance and transformation to the EE form within the hepatic parenchyma cell are not known. The system might permit studies on relapse mechanisms.

The recent advances in methods for the cultivation of hepatocytes, particularly those of rodents (Jeejebhoy and Phillips, 1976), seem to be appliable in attempts to cultivate mammalian EE forms (Foley *et al.*, 1978). Initiation of EE stage development in cells cultivated from organs of embryonic rats and turkeys by inoculation of *P. berghei* sporozoites (Strome *et al.*, 1979) is an important advance and should allow a better understanding of mammalian EE stages and their interaction with the host.

ACKNOWLEDGMENTS

The writer is grateful to Dr. W. B. Lushbaugh for helpful discussion and comments during preparation of the manuscript, and to Ms. Patricia Platts for typing and editorial assistance. Parts of the work in which the writer participated were supported by the World Health Organization and the South Carolina Appropriation for Biomedical Research. Table II has been reproduced with permission of Academic Press, and Tables III, IV, V, and VI with permission of the American Society of Parasitologists.

REFERENCES

Beaudoin, R. L. (1977). Should cultivated exoerythrocytic parasites be considered as a source of antigen for a malaria vaccine? *Bull. W.H.O.* **55**, 373-376.

Beaudoin, R. L., Strome, C. P. A., and Clutter, W. G. (1974). Cultivation of avian malaria parasites in mammalian liver cells. *Exp. Parasitol.* **36**, 355-359.

Boyd, M. F., and Stratman-Thomas, W. K. (1934). Studies on benign tertian malaria. 7. Some observations on inoculation and onset. *Am. J. Hyg.* **20**, 488-495.

Bray, R. S. (1957a). Studies on malaria in chimpanzees. II. *Plasmodium vivax. Am. J. Trop. Med. Hyg.* **6**, 514-520.

Bray, R. S. (1957b). Additional notes on the tissue stages of *Plasmodium cynomolgi. Trans. R. Soc. Trop. Med. Hyg.* **51**, 248-252.

Bray, R. S. (1960). Studies on malaria in chimpanzees. III. The experimental transmission and pre-erythrocytic phase of *Plasmodium malariae,* with a note on the host range of the parasite. *Am. J. Trop. Med. Hyg.* **9**, 455-465.

Clark, I. A., Allison, A. C., and Cox, F. E. (1976). Protection of mice against *Babesia* and *Plasmodium* with BCG. *Nature (London)* **259**, 309-311.

Clyde, D. F., Most, H., McCarthy, V. C., and Vanderberg, J. P. (1973). Immunization of man against sporozoite-induced falciparum malaria. *Am. J. Med. Sci.* **266**, 169-177.

Clyde, D. F., McCarthy, V. C., Miller, R. M., and Woodward, W. E. (1975). Immunization of man against falciparum and vivax malaria by use of attenuated sporozoites. *Am. J. Trop. Med. Hyg.* **24**, 397-401.

Cohen, S., Butcher, G. A., Mitchell, G. H., Deas, J. A., and Langhorne, J. (1977a). Acquired immunity and vaccination in malaria. *Am. J. Trop. Med. Hyg.* **26**, Suppl., 223-229.

Cohen, S., Butcher, G. A., and Mitchell, G. H. (1977b). Immunization against erythrocytic forms of malaria parasites. *In* "Immunity to Blood Parasites of Animals and Man" (L. H. Miller, J. A. Pino, and J. J. McKelvey, Jr., eds.), pp. 89-112. Plenum, New York.

Corradetti, A. (1955). Studies on comparative pathology and immunity in *Plasmodium* infections of mammals and birds. *Trans. R. Soc. Trop. Med. Hyg.* **49**, 311-333.

Coulston, F., and Huff, C. G. (1948). Symposium on exoerythrocytic forms of malarial parasites. IV. The chemotherapy and immunology of preerythrocytic stages in avian malaria. *J. Parasitol.* **34**, 290-299.

Coulston, F., and Manwell, R. (1941). Single-parasite infections and exoerythrocytic schizogony in *Plasmodium circumflexum. Am. J. Hyg.* **34**, Sect. C, 119-125.

Danforth, H. D., Onjih, A. U., and Nussenzweig, R. S. (1978). Immunofluorescent staining of exoerythrocytic schizonts of *Plasmodium berghei* in fixed liver tissue with stage-specific immune serum. *J. Parasitol.* **64**, 1123-1125.

Davey, D. G. (1946). Concerning exoerythrocytic forms and the evidence for their existence in human malaria. *Trans. R. Soc. Trop. Med. Hyg.* **40**, 171-182.

Davis, A. G., Huff, C. G., and Palmer, T. T. (1966). Procedures for maximum production of exoerythrocytic stages of *Plasmodium fallax* in tissue culture. *Exp. Parasitol.* **19**, 1-8.

Doby, J. M., and Barker, R. (1976). Essais d'obtention *in vitro* des formes pre-erythrocytaires de *Plasmodium vivax* en cultures de cellules hepatiques humaines inoculees par sporozoites. *C. R. Seances Soc. Biol. Ses Fil.* **170**, 661-665.

Dubin, I. N., Laird, R. L., and Drinnon, V. P. (1949). The development of sporozoites of *Plasmodium gallinaceum* into cryptozoites in tissue culture. *J. Nat. Malar. Soc.* **8**, 175-180.

Dubin, I. N., Laird, R. L., and Drinnon, V. P. (1950). Further observations on the development of sporozoites of *Plasmodium gallinaceum* into cryptozoites in tissue culture. *J. Nat. Malar. Soc.* **9,** 119–127.

El-Nahal, H. M. S. (1967). Study of serological cross-reactions of exoerythrocytic schizonts of avian, rodent and primate malaria parasites by the fluorescent antibody technique. *Bull. W.H.O.* **37,** 154–158.

Fairley, N. H. (1947). Sidelights on malaria in man obtained by subinoculation experiments. *Trans. R. Soc. Trop. Med. Hyg.* **40,** 621–676.

Foley, D. A., and Vanderberg, J. P. (1977). *Plasmodium berghei:* Transmission by intraperitoneal inoculation of immature exoerythrocytic schizonts from rats into rats, mice, and hamsters. *Exp. Parasitol.* **43,** 69–81.

Foley, D. A., Kennard, J., and Vanderberg, J. P. (1978a). *Plasmodium berghei:* Infective exoerythrocytic schizonts in primary monolayer cultures of rat liver cells. *Exp. Parasitol.* **46,** 166–178.

Foley, D. A., Kennard, J., and Vanderberg, J. P. (1978b). *Plasmodium berghei:* Preparation of rat hepatic cell suspension that include infective exoerythrocytic shizonts. *Exp. Parasitol.* **46,** 179–188.

Garnham, P. C. C., and Bray, R. S. (1956). The influence of immunity upon the stages (including late exo-erythrocytic schizonts) of mammalian malaria parasites. *Rev. Bras. Malariol. Doencas Trop.* **8,** 151–160.

Garnham, P. C. C., Bray, R. S., Cooper, W., Lainson, R., Awad, F. I., and Williamson, J. (1955). The pre-erythrocytic stage of *Plasmodium ovale. Trans. R. Soc. Trop. Med. Hyg.* **49,** 158–167.

Garnham, P. C. C., Lainson, R., and Cooper, W. (1957). The tissue stages and sporogony of *Plasmodium knowlesi. Trans. R. Soc. Trop. Med. Hyg.* **51,** 384–396.

Golenser, J., Heeren, J., Verhave, J. P., Kaay, H. J. V. D., and Meuwissen, J. H. E. (1977). Crossreactivity with sporozoites, exoerythrocytic forms and blood-schizonts of *Plasmodium berghei* in indirect fluorescent antibody tests with sera of rats immunized with sporozoites or infected blood. *Clin. Exp. Immunol.* **29,** 43–51.

Graham, H. A., Stauber, L. A., Palczuk, N. C., and Barnes, W. D. (1973a). Immunity to exoerythrocytic forms of malaria. I. Course of infection of *Plasmodium fallax* in turkeys. *Exp. Parasitol.* **34,** 364–371.

Graham, H. A., Palczuk, N. C., and Stauber, L. A. (1973b). Immunity to exoerythrocytic forms of malaria. II. Passive transfer of immunity to exoerythrocytic forms. *Exp. Parasitol.* **34,** 372–381.

Gwadz, R. W. (1976). Malaria: Successful immunization against the sexual stages of *Plasmodium gallinaceum. Science* **193,** 1150–1151.

Gwadz, R. W., and Green, I. (1978). Malaria immunization in rhesus monkeys. A vaccine effective against both the sexual and asexual stages of *Plasmodium knowlesi. J. Exp. Med.* **148,** 1311–1323.

Haas, V. H., Wilcox, A., Laird, R. L., Ewing, F. M., and Coleman, N. (1948). Symposium on exoerythrocytic forms of malarial parasites. VI. Response of exoerythrocytic forms to alterations in the life cycle of *Plasmodium gallinaceum. J. Parasitol.* **34,** 306–320.

Hawking, F. (1948). Growth of protozoa in tissue culture. I. *Plasmodium gallinaceum,* exoerythrocytic forms. *Trans. R. Soc. Trop. Med. Hyg.* **39,** 245–263.

Hawking, F., and Thurston, J. P. (1952). Chemotherapeutic and other studies on the pre-erythrocytic forms of simian malaria (*Plasmodium cynomolgi*). *Trans. R. Soc. Trop. Med. Hyg.* **46,** 293–300.

Hawking, F., Perry, W. L. M., and Thurston, J. P. (1948). Tissue forms of a malaria parasite, *Plasmodium cynomolgi. Lancet* **1,** ccliv, 783–788.

Hegner, R., and Wolfson, F. (1939). Tissue-culture studies of parasites in reticulo-endothelial cells of birds infected with *Plasmodium*. *Am. J. Hyg.* **29**, 83–85.

Holbrook, T. W., Palczuk, N. C., and Stauber, L. A. (1974). Immunity to exoerythrocytic forms of malaria. III. Stage-specific immunization of turkeys against exoerythrocytic forms of *Plasmodium fallax*. *J. Parasitol.* **60**, 348–354.

Holbrook, T. W., Spitalny, G. L., and Palczuk, N. C. (1976). Stimulation of resistance in mice to sporozoite-induced *Plasmodium berghei* malaria by injections of avian exoerythrocytic forms. *J. Parasitol.* **62**, 670–675.

Huff, C. G. (1952). Studies on the exoerythrocytic stages of *Plasmodium gallinaceum* during the "transitional phase." *Exp. Parasitol.* **1**, 392–405.

Huff, C. G. (1957). Organ and tissue distribution of the exoerythrocytic stages of various avian malarial parasites. *Exp. Parasitol.* **6**, 143–162.

Huff, C. G. (1969). Exoerythrocytic stages of avian and reptilian malarial parasites. *Exp. Parasitol.* **24**, 383–421.

Huff, C. G., and Bloom, W. (1935). A malarial parasite infecting all blood and blood-forming cells of birds. *J. Infect. Dis.* **57**, 315–336.

Huff, C. G., and Coulston, F. (1944). The development of *Plasmodium gallinaceum* from sporozoite to erythrocytic trophozoite. *J. Infect. Dis.* **75**, 231–249.

Huff, C. G., and Coulston, F. (1946). The relation of natural and acquired immunity of various avian hosts to the cryptozoites and metacryptozoites of *Plasmodium gallinaceum* and *P. relictum*. *J. Infect. Dis.* **78**, 99–117.

Huff, C. G., and Coulston, F. (1947). A search for the pre-erythrocytic stages of *Plasmodium vivax* and of *P. cynomolgi*. *J. Parasitol.* **33**, II, 27.

Huff, C. G., Pipkin, A. C., Weathersby, A. B., and Jensen, D. V. (1960). The morphology and behavior of living exoerythrocytic stages of *Plasmodium gallinaceum* and *P. fallax* and their host cells. *J. Biophys. Biochem. Cytol.* **7**, 93–102.

Ingram, R. L., and Carver, R. K. (1963). Malaria parasites: Fluorescent antibody technique for tissue stage study. *Science* **139**, 405–406.

Jahiel, R. I., Nussenzweig, R. S., Vilcek, J., and Vanderberg, J. (1969). Protective effect of interferon inducers on *Plasmodium berghei* malaria. *Am. J. Trop. Med. Hyg.* **18**, 823–835.

James, S. P., and Tate, P. (1937). New knowledge of the life cycle of malaria parasites. *Nature (London)* **139**, 545.

Jeejebhoy, K. N., and Phillips, M. J. (1976). Isolated mammalian hepatocytes in culture. *Gastroenterology* **71**, 1086–1096.

Krotoski, W. A., Jumper, J. R., and Collins, W. E. (1973). Immunofluorescent staining of exoerythrocytic schizonts of simian plasmodia in fixed tissue. *Am. J. Trop. Med. Hyg.* **22**, 159–162.

McCarthy, V. C., and Clyde, D. F. (1977). *Plasmodium vivax:* Correlation of circumsporozoite precipitation (CSP) reaction with sporozoite-induced protective immunity in man. *Exp. Parasitol.* **41**, 167–171.

Mackaness, G. B. (1977). Cellular immunity and the parasite. *In* "Immunity to Blood Parasites of Animals and Man" (L. H. Miller, J. A. Pino, and J. J. McKelvey, Jr., eds.), pp. 65–73. Plenum, New York.

Manresa, M., Jr. (1953). The occurrence of phanerozoites of *Plasmodium lophurae* in blood-inoculated turkeys. *J. Parasitol.* **39**, 452–455.

Manwell, R., and Goldstein, F. (1938). Life history and immunity studies of the avian malaria parasite, *Plasmodium circumflexum*. *Proc. Soc. Exp. Biol. Med.* **39**, 426–428.

Marion, G. R., Palczuk, N. C., and Holbrook, T. W. (1974). Immunoglobulin fraction conveying passive immunity against infection with exoerythrocytic merozoites of *Plasmodium fallax* in turkeys. *Bull., N. J. Acad. Sci.* **19**, 27.

Mendis, K. N., and Targett, G. A. T. (1979). Immunization against gametes and asexual erythrocytic stages of a rodent malaria parasite. *Nature (London)* **277**, 389–391.

Meyer, H. (1947), Cultivation of the erythrocytic form of *Plasmodium gallinaceum* in tissue cultures of embryonic chicken brain. *Nature (London)* **160**, 155–156.

Miller, L. H. (1977a). Current prospects and problems for a malaria vaccine. *J. Infect. Dis.* **135**, 855–864.

Miller, L. H. (1977b). A critique of merozoite and sporozoite vaccines in malaria. *In* "Immunity to Blood Parasites of Animals and Man" (L. H. Miller, J. A. Pino, and J. J. McKelvey, Jr., eds.), pp. 113–120. Plenum, New York.

Mitchell, G. H. (1977). A review of merozoite vaccination against *Plasmodium knowlesi* malaria. *Trans. R. Soc. Trop. Med. Hyg.* **71**, 281–282.

Mitchell, G. H., Butcher, G. A., and Cohen, S. (1975). Merozoite vaccination against *Plasmodium knowlesi* malaria. *Immunology* **29**, 397–407.

Mulligan, H. W., Russell, P. F., and Mohan, B. N. (1941). Active immunization of fowls against *Plasmodium gallinceum* by injections of killed homologous sporozoites. *J. Malar. Inst. India* **4**, 25–34.

Nardin, E. H., and Nussenzweig, R. S. (1978). Stage-specific antigens on the surface membrane of sporozoites of malaria parasites. *Nature (London)* **274**, 55–57.

Nussenzweig, R. S. (1967). Increased non-specific resistance to malaria produced by administration of killed *Corynebacterium parvum*. *Exp. Parasitol.* **21**, 224–231.

Nussenzweig, R. S., Vanderberg, J., and Most, H. (1969). Protective immunity produced by the injection of X-irradiated sporozoites of *Plasmodium berghei*. IV. Dose response, specificity and humoral immunity. *Mil. Med.* **134**, 1176–1182.

Nussenzweig, R. S., Vanderberg, J. P., Sanabria, Y., and Most, H. (1972). *Plasmodium berghei:* Accelerated clearance of sporozoites from blood as part of immune-mechanism in mice. *Exp. Parasitol.* **31**, 88–97.

Porter, R. J., and Huff, C. G. (1940). Review of the literature on exoerythrocytic schizogony in certain malarial parasites and its relation to the schizogonic cycle in *Plasmodium elongatum*. *Am. J. Trop. Med.* **20**, 869–888.

Raffaele, G. (1934). Un ceppo italiano di *Plasmodium elongatum*. *Riv. Malariol.* **13**, 332–337.

Raffaele, G. (1936). Presumibili forme iniziale di evoluzione di *P. relictum*. *Riv. Malariol.* **15**, 318–324.

Richards, W. H. G. (1966). Active immunization of chicks against *Plasmodium gallinaceum* by inactivated homologous sporozoites and erythrocytic parasites. *Nature (London)* **212**, 1492–1494.

Richards, W. H. G., and Latter, V. S. (1977). Malarial immunity in *Plasmodium gallinaceum*. *Parasitology* **75**, xxix.

Richards, W. H. G., Mitchell, G. H., Butcher, G. A., and Cohen, S. (1977). Merozoite vaccination of rhesus monkeys against *Plasmodium knowlesi* malaria: Immunity to sporozoite (mosquito-transmitted) challenge. *Parasitology* **74**, 191–198.

Rieckmann, K. H., Carson, P. E., Beaudoin, R. L., Cassells, J. S., and Sell, K. M. (1974). Sporozoite-induced immunity in man against an Ethiopian strain of *Plasmodium falciparum*. *Trans. R. Soc. Trop. Med. Hyg.* **68**, 258–259.

Rodhain, J., Gavrilov, W., and Cowez, S. (1940). Essais d'infection de culture de tissus d'embryon de poulet par les sporozoites de *Plasmodium gallinaceum*. *C. R. Seances Soc. Biol. Ses Fil.* **134**, 261.

Schaudinn, F. (1903). Studien uber krankheitserregende Protozoen. *Arb. Kais. Gesund.* **19**, 169–250.

Shortt, H. E., and Garnham, P. C. C. (1948a). Pre-erythrocytic stage in mammalian malaria. *Nature (London)* **161**, 126.

Shortt, H. E., and Garnham, P. C. C. (1948b). The pre-erythrocytic development of *Plasmodium cynomolgi* and *Plasmodium vivax*. *Trans. R. Soc. Trop. Med. Hyg.* **41,** 785–795.

Shortt, H. E., Garnham, P. C. C., and Malamos, B. (1948a). The pre-erythrocytic stage of mammalian malaria. *Br. Med. J.* **1,** 192–194.

Shortt, H. E., Garnham, P. C. C., Covell, G., and Shute, P. G. (1948b). The preerythrocytic stage of human malaria, *Plasmodium vivax*. *Br. Med. J.* **1,** 547.

Shortt, H. E., Fairly, N. H., Covell, G., Shute, P. G., and Garnham, P. C. C. (1949). The prererythrocytic stage of *Plasmodium falciparum—A preliminary note*. *Br. Med. J.* **2,** 1006–1008.

Shortt, H. E., Fairley, N. H., Covell, G., Shute, P. G., and Garnham, P. C. C. (1951). The pre-erythrocytic stage of *Plasmodium falciparium*. *Trans. R. Soc. Trop. Med. Hyg.* **44,** 405–419.

Sodeman, T., Schnitzer, B., Durkee, T., and Contacos, P. (1970). The fine structure of the exoerythrocytic stage of *Plasmodium cynomolgi*. *Science* **170,** 340–341.

Spitalny, G. L., and Nussenzweig, R. S. (1972). Effect of various routes of immunization and methods of parasite attentuation on the development of protection against sporozoite-induced rodent malaria. *Proc. Helminthol. Soc. Wash.* **39,** Spec. Issue, 506–514.

Strome, C. P. A., De Santos, P. L., and Beaudoin, R. L. (1979). The cultivation of the exoerythrocytic stage of *Plasmodium berghei* from sporozoites. *In Vitro* **15,** 531–536.

Vanderberg, J. P. (1973). Inactivity of rodent malaria anti-sporozoite antibodies against exoerythrocytic forms. *Am. J. Trop. Med. Hyg.* **22,** 573–577.

Vanderberg, J. P., Nussenzweig, R. S., Most, H., and Orton, C. G. (1968). Protective immunity produced by the injection of X-irradiated sporozoites of *Plasmodium berghei*. II. Effects of radiation on sporozoites. *J. Parasitol.* **54,** 1175–1180.

Vanderberg, J. P., Nussenzweig, R. S., and Most, H. (1969). Protective immunity produced by the injection of X-irradiated sporozoites of *Plasmodium berghei*. V. *In vitro* effects of immune serum on sporozoites. *Mil. Med.* **134,** 1183–1190.

Verhave, J. P., Meuwissen, J. H. E., and Golenser, J. (1978). Cell-mediated reactions and protection after immunization with sporozoites. *Isr. J. Med. Sci.* **14,** 611–613.

Voller, A., and Taffs, L. F. (1963). Fluorescent-antibody staining of exoerythrocytic stages of *Plasmodium gallinaceum*. *Trans. R. Soc. Trop. Med. Hyg.* **57,** 32–33.

Ward, P. A., and Conran, P. B. (1968). Application of fluorescent antibody to exoerythrocytic stages of simian malaria. *J. Parasitol.* **54,** 171–172.

Warren, A. J., and Coggeshall, L. T. (1937). Infectivity of blood and organs in canaries after inoculation with sporozoites. *Am. J. Hyg.* **26,** 1–10.

Yoeli, M., and Most, H. (1965). Studies on sporozoite-induced infection of rodent malaria. I. The pre-erythrocytic tissue stage of *Plasmodium berghei*. *Am. J. Trop. Med. Hyg.* **14,** 700–714.

Yorke, W., and Macfie, J. W. S. (1924). Observations on malaria made during treatment of general paralysis. *Trans. R. Soc. Trop. Med. Hyg.* **18,** 1–3.

Immunization against Asexual
Blood-Inhabiting Stages of Plasmodia

Wasim A. Siddiqui

I. INTRODUCTION

Attempts to develop a vaccine against malaria were initiated half a century ago but gave way to searches for new drugs during World War II and to the anti-mosquito programs that followed. During the late 1930s, recognition of the insecticidal effect of dichlorodiphenyltrichloroethane (DDT) turned the eyes of the world toward the possibility of eradicating the disease. From 1956 to 1962, a large-scale malaria eradication program was initiated by the World Health Organization in many of the countries of Asia, North Africa, Central and South America, and Europe, resulting in a reduced prevalence of malaria from an estimated 300 million cases in 1940 to 90 million cases in 1975. The overwhelming success and impact of the control program was so impressive that by 1961 a rapid decline in scientific research and in the training of malaria workers had resulted. The initial success and momentum, however, have since been replaced by a gradual, unrelenting battle with the disease that has now undergone a sudden resurgence in many areas of the world. Continuation of the malaria eradication program has been hampered by operational, administrative, and financial problems in many malarious countries. In addition, such underlying technical diffi-

Malaria, Vol. 3

231

culties as the resistance of *Plasmodium falciparum* to 4-aminoquinolines and of certain anopheline species to insecticides have aided the resurgence of malaria. Thus "at the end of 1976, the population of originally malarious areas of the world was 2.05 billion, of whom 436 million (21%) were living in areas where malaria is reported to have been eradicated, and 1.26 billion (62%) were living in areas where antimalaria activities were implemented. The remaining 352 million (17%) were living in places where no antimalaria measures were undertaken" (Noguer *et al.*, 1978).

In view of the precarious situation of malaria control, it seems obvious that neither insecticides nor antimalarial drugs are sufficient to control the vectors and parasites, hence the disease. Consequently, there has been renewed interest in the search for an alternate or supplemental means aimed toward solution of the malaria problem. Research activities for developing an immunological solution have accelerated in recent years. A marked change in view about the possibility of developing a vaccine against malaria has developed. Formerly, much of the pessimism concerning the use of such a vaccine was founded on the belief that, since natural infections did not induce complete immunity, vaccination was unlikely to succeed. Fortunately, however, recent advances made in knowledge of the immune response and demonstration of the immunization of various animals against malaria have brought about considerable revision of this viewpoint. With the availability of *Aotus trivirgatus griseimembra* (the owl monkey) for direct experimentation with human malaria (Young *et al.*, 1966; Geiman and Meagher, 1967; Geiman and Siddiqui, 1969) has also come the availability of techniques for producing large quantities of *P. falciparum* antigen through continuous or short-term *in vitro* cultivation (Trager and Jensen, 1976; Siddiqui *et al.*, 1974). These developments, together with the more recent demonstration of effective immunization of owl monkeys against *P. falciparum* (Siddiqui, 1977; Mitchell *et al.*, 1977b), have given real hope of producing a vaccine against at least one species of human malaria parasite, *P. falciparum*.

At present, there are five different kinds of malaria vaccine under investigation: exoerythrocytic merozoites from tissue culture, irradiated sporozoites from the mosquito, extracts from blood schizonts, emulsified erythrocytic merozoites, and extracellular gametes. The objective of this chapter is to review vaccination studies conducted against avian, rodent, simian, and human malaria parasites using blood stage vaccines. The discussion is confined to studies on active immunization using attenuated or killed parasite antigen. No attempt has been made to review the literature on serology or the mechanism of acquired immunity in malaria, as these topics form independent chapters of this book. For obvious reasons, special attention has been given to studies on vaccination against *P. falciparum*, with the results critically reviewed for their applicability to immunization of humans.

II. IMMUNIZATION AGAINST BIRD MALARIA PARASITES

The protection of canaries against *P. cathemerium* was demonstrated by Redmond (1939) and Gingrich (1941) by immunization with large numbers of asexual blood parasites killed by Formalin or heat treatment. Birds with no previous experience of malaria were administered 12 intravenous injections of 1 ml of a 50% suspension of 40–60% parasitized red blood cells. The effectiveness of the immunity produced in the birds was demonstrated by the unusually low-grade parasitemia of short duration which developed after challenge. Jacobs (1943), on the other hand, showed that ducks vaccinated subcutaneously with killed, free *P. lophurae* parasites acquired only a small degree of resistance and that such protection was elicited only by the water-insoluble residues of the parasite material. It was found that the degree of protection could be heightened by adding small quantities of *Staphylococcus* toxoid to the vaccine.

Freund *et al.* (1945a) showed for the first time the effectiveness of Formalin-killed *P. lophurae* incorporated with Freund's complete adjuvant (FCA). Ducks were vaccinated three times 1 month apart with multiple subcutaneous and intramuscular injections. When challenged a month after the last injection with 10^9 *P. lophurae* parasites, seven of the eight vaccinated birds survived with parasitemias well below those found in control birds, and of much shorter duration. Ducks similarly vaccinated against *P. cathemerium* (Thomson *et al.*, 1947) developed a more significant protection when the vaccine was incorporated into FCA than when it was not, and the resistance acquired lasted for at least 6 months. Coffin (1951) confirmed that ducks could be immunized against *P. lophurae* using Freund's technique, but he was unable to immunize chickens against *P. gallinaceum* effectively. A particularly interesting point drawn from Coffin's work was that two chickens immunized with killed *P. lophurae* and FCA, and subsequently twice infected with *P. lophurae,* acquired a high level of resistance to *P. gallinaceum*. Richards (1966), using saponin as an adjuvant and killed, free *P. gallinaceum* parasites, immunized 80 chickens by giving three intravenous injections of vaccine. Fourteen days after the last injection, only 23 of the 80 chickens developed partial resistance to a challenge of 2.5×10^4 *P. gallinaceum* parasitized cells.

Immunization against malaria with a purified protein was done for the first time by Kilejian (1978). Ducklings immunized with a histidine-rich protein (HRP) isolated from *P. lophurae*-infected red blood cells survived an otherwise fatal *P. lophurae* challenge. Most significant in this work by Kilejian was that adjuvant was not required for this protective effect and immunity could be passively transferred with serum. HRP was found to have an unusual composition of approximately 70% histidine and 30% of four other amino acids: alanine, aspartic acid, glutamic acid, and proline (Kilejian, 1974). The testing of this protein as a vaccine was undertaken because of indirect evidence that it could have a role in the penetration of merozoites into erythrocytes (Kilejian, 1976). On day 0, 4½-week-old ducklings were injected intramuscularly with an emulsion of 1 mg of HRP in 0.5 ml of phosphate-buffered saline, 0.25 ml of FCA, and 0.25 ml of Freund's incomplete adjuvant (FIA). On days 4 and 7, the ducklings to be immunized were intravenously administered 0.7 mg and 1 mg of antigen, respectively. When challenged on day 14, only one of five immunized ducklings survived. In the next experiment, however, when the purified HRP dosage was increased to a total of 4 mg, seven of eight immunized ducklings survived the lethal challenging dose. Indication that HRP could induce protective immunity without the aid of adjuvant was demonstrated when three out of four ducks receiving HRP only survived challenge. It was found that commercially available synthentic polyhistidine was completely ineffective when substituted for *P. lophurae*-derived HRP antigen. Kilejian (1978) went on to demonstrate that three young 8-day-old ducklings given the globulin fraction obtained from 5–6 ml of serum of a surviving immunized challenged duckling survived a challenge with 9×10^6 parasitized erythrocytes. Globulin fractions collected from sera of immunized ducklings which had not been challenged also yielded protection of young ducks, but these sera have given less consistent results. It may be of interest to point out that, although ducklings become immunologically mature at about 6 weeks of age, immunization in the above experiments had of necessity to be initiated in birds 4–4½ weeks old. Since some ducklings developed a natural resistance to the infection when 8–9 weeks of age, a massive challenge dose was required within 15 days.

III. IMMUNIZATION AGAINST RODENT MALARIA PARASITES

A degree of acquired immunity was demonstrated in rats by Zuckerman *et al.* (1967) who administered a cell-free extract of *P. berghei*, both with and without adjuvant. The cell-free extract was obtained from saponin-lysed parasitized cells which were subsequently disintegrated in a Hughes press. Each rat received one to five vaccinating doses subcutaneously, with partial immunity occurring after the third dose of antigenic material. A single dosage of extract also in adjuvant produced an equivalent effect. The criteria of immunity were changes in the degree of parasitemia, mortality rate, duration of patency, and incubation period, as compared to control rats. The parasitemia peaks and mortality rates which occurred in the vaccinated rats were one-third those in the control rats. The duration of patency was only slightly longer among the vaccinated than among the control rats. Prepatency in the vaccinated rats was 4 days longer than in the control rats. Employing a similar technique, Desowitz (1967) was able to improve the immunogenicity of soluble homogenates of *P. berghei* by binding the antigens to carboxymethyl cellulose. This study also showed that injection of immune globulin before challenge did not reduce the parasitemia below that which occurred in immunized rats not given globulin. The median prepatent period in the rats given globulin was extended from 4 to 7 days beyond that which occurred in immunized rats not given globulin, however.

With the use of vaccines of roentgen-irradiated blood infected with *P. berghei*, Corradetti *et al.* (1966) and Wellde and Sadun (1967) were able to induce relatively effective immunity against *P. berghei* in rodents. Jerusalem and Eling (1969) effectively immunized mice with freed *P. berghei* (K 173 strain) parasites. No significant differences were observed in the antigenicity of plasmodial preparations obtained from parasites freed from host cells by the use of saponin or antierythrocyte serum. Surprisingly, it was the route of inoculation of the vaccinating material that proved to be of importance in immunization. The best survival rates and the greatest degree of antiparasitic immunity occurred in rodents immunized by the intravenous route.

In 1966, D'Antonio *et al.* (1966b) described a new method utilizing a French pressure cell (FPC) for releasing *P. berghei* from host erythrocytes and for disrupting them, and a column procedure for the isolation of a partially purified plasmodial fraction (PPF). This fraction was found to fix complement in the presence of specific plasmodial antibody and to be free of host material which could be detected serologically (D'Antonio *et al.*, 1966a,b). The fraction was subsequently found to be able to induce immunity in mice against *P. berghei* infection (D'Antonio *et al.*, 1969, 1970). In 1972, using the FPC technique, D'Antonio (1972a) described in detail a method of preparation of four *P. berghei* fractions: A, the FPC-isolated free parasites and associated large parasite fragments; E, the large parasite fragments remaining after high-pressure disintegration of isolated parasites; G, the Sephadex G-200 void volume eluate of the disintegrated parasite fraction A; C, the Sephadex G-200 void volume eluate of the mixture containing disintegrated erythrocytes and parasites. The immunogencity of the various parasite fractions was tested in A/J mice. The mice were injected once intraperitoneally with the parasite fractions, and 8 weeks later they were challenged intraperitoneally with 10^7 virulent *P. berghei* (NK 65 D strain). Of the mice given the above preparations, 31 of 34 administered either A or E were protected, 16 of 20 receiving G were protected, and 11 of 15 receiving C were protected. Thus, a 70–80% survival rate after a normally 100% lethal challenge occurred in mice vaccinated with the free parasites (A), the parasite fragments (E), and the Sephadex void volume eluates (G and C). Based on these results, D'Antonio suggested that the antigen may be of membrane origin and, moreover, that the parasite antigen (G) appearing in the void volume eluate of Sephadex G-200 columns was the most highly purified *P. berghei* antigen obtained up to that time. D'Antonio (1972b) achieved significant protection in mice by immunization with heat-inactivated parasitized blood of *P. berghei* (NK 65 strain)-infected mice. The type and degree of protection against *P. berghei* in mice of DDS and CFI mouse strains were essentially the same as those reported for A/J mice vaccinated with the various fractions of *P. berghei* (D'Antonio *et al.*, 1969, 1970). Desowitz (1975) reported the results of a series of experiments for screening adjuvants. The adjuvants were tested for their ability to enhance immunogenicity of a soluble *P. berghei* antigen in weanling white rats. Mortality rate, parasitemia, and course of infection, were the parameters used to evaluate the vaccination procedures. Protective immunity was induced by antigen in combination with the following adjuvants: saponin, hexylamine, *Bordetella pertussis* vaccine, levamisole, and polyinosinic-polycytidylic acid [poly (I:C)]. Neither the antigen alone or combined with FCA, bacterial endotoxin, vitamin A, and/or polyinosinic-polyuridlic acid [poly (A:U)] induced significant protective immunity. Injection into the footpad of *P. berghei* parasites isolated by a freezing and thawing method, in combination with FCA, did not induce immunity in mice against a lethal challenge with *P. berghei* (Reisen and Hillis, 1975).

Clark *et al.* (1976a) protected four out of four female CBA mice against challenge with *P. berghei yoelii* (strain 17X) by intravenous injection of 2×10^7 live Bacillus Calmette-Guérin (BCG). Challenge was 1 month after vaccination. In another experiment only two out of four CBA mice were protected. With the same procedure, an appreciable degree of protection was conferred on eight mice against *P. vinckei*. Normally lethal in mice, this parasite killed four control mice on day 8, while all the mice in the BCG-treated group survived. To explain the intraerythrocytic death of parasites observed in these experiments, these investigators suggested that the likely mechanism of immunity was the release of nonantibody mediators. The previous infection with BCG caused an enhanced output of nonantibody mediators of immunity, thus augmenting protection. Clark *et al.* (1976b) also investigated the use of another nonspecific immunostimulant, *Corynebacterium parvum*, to protect mice against rodent babesial, *P. vinckei*, and *P. chabaudi* infections. Mice were injected intravenously, intraperitoneally, or subcutaneously with killed *C. parvum* and later challenged by known numbers of babesia, *P. vinckei*, or *P. chabaudi*. Injection of *C. parvum* did not protect mice against *P. vinckei* or *P. chabaudi* challenge as absolutely as against challenge with *Babesia*. The malaria parasitemias in immunized mice always reached levels at least half those in control mice, while the mice were completely immune to the *Babesia*. These authors contended that *P. vinckei* and *P. chabaudi* were less susceptible to the effects of the nonantibody mediators than rodent babesia. In studies on *P. berghei*, no evidence was obtained that BCG induced immunity or intracellular death, thus, the mediators may have had little or no effect on this parasite. Because of the duration of patent parasitemias in the *P. vinckei*- and *P. chabaudi*-infected mice pretreated with *C. parvum* these authors did not attribute the intracellular death observed solely to a nonspecific action of *C. parvum*, as there was adequate time for generation of a specific immune response. Nonetheless, *C. parvum* pretreatment made the difference between recovery and death. Pretreatment with *C. parvum* did not prevent the generation of specific immunity in the challenged mice since, when the recovered mice were rechallenged 60 days later, no parasitemia developed.

A highly effective immunity in CB57BI × BALB/c F^1 mice was demonstrated by Playfair *et al.* (1977) when these mice were vaccinated with 10^8 saponin-lysed, Formalin-fixed *P. yoelii* parasitized cells mixed with 10^8 *B. pertussis* organisms. Vaccinated mice showed normal or slightly enhanced parasitemia over a 4-day period, after which their parasitemia suddenly cleared. Ten days later, subinoculation into fresh recipients revealed that there were no living parasites in the blood, spleen, liver, or bone marrow. Protection could also be transferred to normal recipients by the transfer of serum and peripheral blood cells from the vaccinated and challenged mice after they had recovered from the challenge infection. These researchers assert that, with the *P. yoelii* system, the vital requirements for obtaining highly effective sterilizing immunity in mice are (1) a sizable vaccine dosage (10^8 parasites), (2) inoculation via the intravenous route, and (3) the use of *B. pertussis* as an adjuvant. With a similar technique, a lesser degree of protective effect was obtained against *P. berghei*. Since the protection was species-specific, it was therefore unlikely to be related to the nonspecific immunopotentiation induced by such agents as BCG (Clark *et al.*, 1976a) and stilbestrol (Cottrell *et al.*, 1977).

Sonic oscillation carried out in a continuous-flow sonication system releases intraerythrocytic *P. berghei*. When subjected to differential centrifugation, the sonicated preparation yields populations of *P. berghei* rich in merozoites (Prior and Kreier, 1972; Prior *et al.*, 1973; Kreier *et al.*, 1976). The parasites obtained by these procedures were used as immunogens in vaccination studies by Saul and Kreier (1977) and Grothaus and Kreier (1980). Single-dose vaccination with this antigen of 40 to 50-g rats resulted in enhanced infection. On adding adjuvant, however, infections in vaccinated rats were milder than in controls, with reduced parasitemia peaks and patent periods, although complete protection was not attained. Comparing the efficiency of saponin and FCA as adjuvants, Saul and Kreier (1977) found that rats receiving *P. berghei* antigen combined with saponin had immunity as good as or better than that of rats receiving antigen incorporated with FCA. These authors also demonstrated that, when a frozen and thawed parasite preparation was separated into soluble and insoluble components by centrifugation, protective ability resided in both components. Freezing and thawing may dislodge some but not all of the antigen from the membrane. If, in fact, this occurs, the authors suggest that antigen capable of stimulating a protective response may be membrane-associated, as suggested by Spear *et al.* (1976), though still appearing in the soluble component of the frozen and thawed parasites. Saul and Kreier (1977) and Grothaus and Kreier (1980) also obtained an immunogen by washing free parasites in physiological saline. This soluble material, which contained a small subset of the antigens which could be released by freezing and thawing the free parasites, was as potent an immunogen as the intact parasites form which it was obtained.

IV. IMMUNIZATION AGAINST SIMIAN MALARIA PARASITES

The earliest attempts to immunize rhesus monkeys (*Macaca mulatta*) against *P. knowlesi* were unsuccessful (Eaton and Coggeshall, 1939; Short and Menon, 1940), however, these attempts did induce the monkeys to produce malarial antibody detectable by serological means (Eaton and Coggshall, 1939; Ray *et al.*, 1941). In later studies, monkeys immunized subcutaneously with two doses of Formalin-treated *P. knowlesi*—parasitized blood (optimally about 15 × 10⁹ schizonts) emulsified with FCA—became extremely resistant to otherwise lethal challenges of *P. knowlesi* (Freund *et al.*, 1945b, 1948). The course of infection in control monkeys was highly variable. In one experiment (Freund *et al.*, 1945b), out of 14 control monkeys challenged, 1 survived infection, 3 died with low parasitemias (1.5–8%), and the remaining 10 had parasitemias ranging from 8 to 53%. Immunized monkeys, if they became infected, often developed a low-grade parasitemia of short duration only. These monkeys did not subsequently relapse during an observation period of at least 6 months. This was the first successful vaccination with a nonhuman primate malaria. The key to success was the use of paraffin oil containing killed tubercle bacilli as an adjuvant, which today bears the name of Freund.

The components most vital to this adjuvant's composition are the killed tubercle bacilli for which no satisfactory substitute could be found. Cerotic acid was tried but yielded inconsistent results; lipid extracts of mycobacteria, cholesterol, and lecithin were all found ineffective (Freund *et al.*, 1948). When peanut oil was substituted for paraffin oil, and Arlacel for Falba, no protection whatsoever resulted. The comparative immunogenicity of various antigenic preparations of schizont stage *P. knowlesi,* both with and without FCA, was studied by Targett and Fulton (1965). These workers also studied the effects of different routes of administration on immunogenicity. Freund's technique of subcutaneous injection did not produce as strong protection as intramuscular injection of killed parasites in FCA. The injection of free parasites in FCA also proved highly protective. These investigators attributed the superior protection afforded by intramuscular injection to the route of administration. It should be pointed out, however, that, while the interval between the first and second intramuscular injections was 76 days, the interval between the subcutaneous injections was 46 days. The two studies, therefore, are rot strictly comparable, as the difference in time could well be of critical importance. In studies by Targett and Voller (1965) correlating the serological response with the degree of protective immunity, it was concluded that "there was no correlation between gamma-globulin and the level of protective immunity. The increase was as great in monkeys which showed little or no resistance to the challenge as in those which were successfully immunized. The fluorescent antibody titers were mostly high and, again, the levels were as high in animals which remained susceptible to challenge as in those which were protected. Targett & Voller (1965)"

In spite of antigenic variation in *P. knowlesi* (Brown and Brown, 1965), the results of both Freund *et al.* (1948) and Targett and Fulton (1965) indicate that effective vaccination is possible. In related studies by Brown *et al.* (1968), it was shown that monkeys immunized with killed *P. knowlesi* schizont-infected cells in FIA responded with only a variant-specific immunity. When challenged with the same variant as that used for immunization, such monkeys suffered fatal infections from an antigenic variant which appeared after challenge. In contrast, monkeys immunized with parasites in FCA experienced prolonged latent periods after challenge, and they eliminated their infections after a brief parasitemic breakthrough. Still, the survival rate in the vaccinated monkeys was not 100%. Elimination of infection was confirmed by subinoculation of blood from vaccinated into normal monkeys. No infection developed in the test monkeys. Splenectomy of the vaccinated monkeys produced no recrudescence of parasitemia. Later, Brown *et al.* (1970) compared the degree of protection against *P. knowlesi* induced in rhesus monkeys by drug-suppressed infections to that induced by the injection of killed parasites in FCA. Rhesus monkeys immunized by drug-treated H. Nuri strain *P. knowlesi* infections developed only partial immunity and had long-lasting chronic infections. Their immunity was largely ineffective against other strains of *P. knowlesi*. By comparison, monkeys immunized with killed schizont-infected cells in FCA (provided they had survived the initial infection after primary challenge) soon lost their infection but were able to maintain an immunity effective against other strains of *P. knowlesi*. Immunization with killed parasitized cells in FIA proved to have no protective effect at all.

In extending these studies, Brown and Tanaka (1975) compared the immunogenic aspects of various adjuvant combinations. They found that monkeys vaccinated with *P. knowlesi* schizont-infected cell antigen emulsified in FIA plus *Mycobacterium butyricum,* BCG, AD5 (a subfraction of wax D from *Mycobacterium tuberculosis*), or poly (A:U) had on challenge a significant degree of protection in 50% of the monkeys immunized. Of the remaining half, some monkeys developed chronic infections on challenge and others died of acute parasitemia. Immunization with antigen in FIA containing ADG (another fraction of wax D), poly (I:C), and reduced doses of poly (A:U) did not produce any protection at all.

D'Antonio *et al.* (1971) used the FPC technique for separating plasmodia from erythrocyte stromata, and a column technique for the isolation of a complement-fixing PPF of *P. knowlesi*, D'Antonio *et al.* (1971) then sought to protect rhesus monkeys against *P. knowlesi* with this PPF. The resulting protection was only partial. Subsequently, following the D'Antonio technique and using the PPF antigen, Schenkel *et al.* (1973) explored the effectiveness of several adjuvants. Of five monkeys vaccinated with PPF and FCA, three survived challenge infection. Both BCG and poly (A:U) proved ineffective as adjuvants. D'Antonio (1974) later showed that one monkey vaccinated with PPF and BCG survived challenge.

Simpson *et al.* (1974) reported studies on the vaccination of rhesus monkeys against *P. knowlesi* with fractions of *P. knowlesi* schizont antigen prepared on sucrose density gradients. Thirteen juvenile rhesus monkeys were inoculated with a variety of nonviable products derived from *P. knowlesi*-parasitized cells in the schizont stage by these gradient techniques. Samples were prepared from parasitized erythrocytes by FPC disintegration followed by differential centrifugation, by BioGel column chromatographic separation, and by linear sucrose density gradient fractionation. Two injections of the antigen preparation emulsified in Freund's adjuvant (the first dose containing FCA and the second dosage FIA) were given at 4-week intervals followed 4 weeks later by blood stage challenge with the homologous *P. knowlesi* strain. Six out of nine vaccinated monkeys survived; all the control monkeys died. Unlike most of the studies employing the *P. knowlesi*-rhesus monkey model system, in this particular experiment 1.5-kg juvenile rhesus monkeys rather than adult monkeys (6–7 kg) were used; thus the immune status of children was closely simulated.

In extending these studies, Schenkel *et al.* (1975) used lyophilized antigen to compare the immunopotentiation of adjuvant 65, BCG, and FCA. No protective effect was observed using adjuvant 65 alone as an adjuvant. Vaccination with adjuvant 65 and BCG emulsified with antigen gave the same degree of protection (75% survival) as vaccination with antigen emulsified with FCA. Thus, apart from suggesting a new adjuvant for use in malaria vaccination, this study was the first to demonstrate the success of vaccination against primate malaria using lyophilized antigen. Studies extended by Cabrera *et al.* (1976) confirmed that *P. knowlesi* antigen could be lyophilized and still retain its immunogenicity. An experiment showed that it was possible to reduce the concentration of antigen from 1 mg to 250 μg protein antigen per injection. With the smaller dose of antigen 11 of 18 vaccinated monkeys survived challenge. In another experiment, it was found that 16 of 18 vaccinated monkeys developed a positive delayed hypersensitivity response when skin-tested with the immunizing antigen. However, only 10 of the 16 positive reactors survived *P. knowlesi* challenge, demonstrating that there was no correlation between the delayed hypersensitivity response and protection. Ultrastructural evidence presented by Spear *et al.* (1976) supported the view that the active protection-inducing antigen used in these vaccination experiments (Schenkel *et al.*, 1973, 1975; D'Antonio, 1974;

Simpson *et al.*, 1974; Schenkel *et al.*, 1975; Cabrera *et al.*, 1976) was in large part material of parasite membrane origin. These data, however, did not exclude the possibility that other soluble materials may also have been present in the antigen preparations and could possibly be important components of the vaccine. Cabrera *et al.* (1977) noted that over 60% of the specific anti-*P. knowlesi* immunoglobulin G found in monkeys immunized with an antigenic preparation from the H strain challenged with the H strain of *P. knowlesi* reacted with a similar antigenic preparation prepared from the W strain of *P. knowlesi*, suggesting that antigens made from these two strains by the FPC procedure have many antigenic sites in common. Further investigations of this antigen indicate that both ultrastructurally (Spear *et al.*, 1976) and biochemically (Beckwith *et al.*, 1975; Cabrera *et al.*, 1976) most of it is parasite-derived membrane.

Collins *et al.* (1977) attempted to immunize rhesus monkeys against *P. knowlesi* with heat-stable, serum-soluble antigens. The serum-soluble S antigens were prepared by the technique of Wilson *et al.* (1969). The serum from which the antigen was prepared was collected at the time of or shortly after schizont rupture when 25% of the erythrocytes were parasitized. The first dose of antigen was mixed with FCA and injected subcutaneously; booster immunization doses mixed with FIA were administered intramuscularly. All the monkeys were then challenged with sporozoites of the homologous strain of *P. knowlesi*, either by the bites of four or five infected *Anopheles balabacensis* mosquitoes or by intravenous inoculation of at least 12,000 sporozoites from dissected salivary glands of infected mosquitoes. The death rate among the control animals was 57% (8 of 14), well below that anticipated following sporozoite inoculation, making it difficult to evaluate the effect of vaccine. The death rate among the immunized monkeys was 53% (19 of 36). These results suggest that S antigens cannot be used to protect animals from parasitemia or from death by this parasite following challenge by sporozoites. Had a few of the monkeys used in this experiment been challenged with blood stage parasites, comparisons of this study's results with those of other investigators who used the rhesus monkey– *P. knowlesi* host–parasite system might well have made broader evaluation possible.

A team led by S. Cohen at Guy's Hospital in London initiated a series of relatively unique vaccination studies in which extracellular merozoites were used as the immunizing agent. These studies were undertaken to test the hypothesis that extracellular merozoites might provide an excellent malaria vaccine. The hypothesis that merozoites are important in immunity to malaria developed from studies on the mechanism of acquired malarial immunity *in vivo* (Cohen *et al.*, 1961) and *in vitro* (Cohen *et al.*, 1969). These studies suggested that protective antibodies did not affect intracellular parasites but interrupted the development of malarial parasites when the merozoites were released into the plasma. Butcher and Cohen (1970) and Butcher *et al.* (1973) determined that immune serum agglutinated free merozoites and thus prevented their attachment to the red cells of susceptible host species. The results of all these studies added an important dimension to the role of merozoite antigens in specific malarial immunity. Consequently, an *in vitro* technique was developed for isolating extracellular blood stage merozoites (Mitchell *et al.*, 1973) for use in subsequent vaccination studies in the rhesus monkey–*P. knowlesi* host–parasite system (Mitchell *et al.*, 1974, 1975). The merozoite isolation method devised by this group (Mitchell *et al.*, 1973) involved obtaining parasitized blood with high parasitemia (ranging from 20 to 70%) and when the parasites were multinucleated schizonts. After gentle centrifugation of the parasitized blood, a brownish layer of concentrated schizonts was obtained which, when incubated at 37°C in a suitable flask containing medium 199, matured, ruptured, and released the parasites. By adding phytohemagglutinin (PHA), agglutination of the unruptured schizont-infected cells was induced. After centrifugation a supernatant rich in merozoites was obtained. Freshly isolated merozoites suspended in 1 ml of medium 199 were emulsified in 1-ml volumes of FCA or FIA. Two rhesus monkeys were immunized with three doses of mature schizonts given intramuscularly at approximately 2- to 4-week intervals; 12 others were immunized with two to four doses of merozoites in FIA or FCA. In addition to the 14 vaccinated monkeys, 12 control monkeys were challenged with *P. knowlesi* of known strain and variant specificity. In 7–11 days following challenge, 9 of the unvaccinated monkeys died, and the remaining 3 had parasitemias of 1.3–5.0%. These 2 monkeys were cured by treatment with antimalarial drugs. Of the 2 schizont-vaccinated monkeys, 1 died, with the single survivor sustaining an 11-day parasitemia peaking at 1.3%. About 2–5 weeks later, 6 (of the original 12 merozoite-immunized) monkeys were challenged with the same immunizing variant (W_1). Not only did all these monkeys survive challenge, but only 3 developed parasitemia. The parasitemias in these 3 ranged from 0.04 to 1.5% and persisted for 6–8 days. The remaining 6 merozoite-immunized animals were challenged with a *P. knowlesi* variant (W_3) different from that used for vaccination. The 4 monkeys receiving two or more inoculations of merozoites in FCA survived the challenge. They developed peak parasitemias of only 0.1 to 1.5%, and their infections lasted from 1 to 12 days. The 2 remaining monkeys were inoculated with merozoites in either FIA or were only given the initial dose in FCA, followed by booster doses in FIA; both these monkeys developed progressive parasitemia and died within a few days' time. These results were the first demonstration of a vaccine that gave 100% survival against *P. knowlesi* among immunized monkeys. Moreover, these results reinforced the concept that merozoites emulsified in FCA were able to induce immunity against challenge with a heterologous variant of *P. knowlesi* and that FCA was essential for achieving resistance to an initial homologous variant challenge.

In subsequent work extending these studies, Mitchell *et al.* (1977a) explored the effectiveness of a freeze-dried merozoite vaccine for protection of rhesus monkeys against both homologous and heterologous variants of *P. knowlesi*. A total of 11 monkeys were used to evaluate freeze-dried vaccines. Three were not vaccinated and served as control animals, and 8 were vaccinated. The 8 vaccinated monkeys each received W_1 strain merozoites isolated from *in vitro* cultures by differential agglutination with PHA (Mitchell *et al.*, 1975). Within 3 hours of isolation, these organisms were suspended in phosphate-buffered saline, frozen by inversion in liquid nitrogen, and stored at $-80°C$; alternatively, merozoites were freeze-dried after suspension in 10% normal rhesus serum in water. Both the frozen and freeze-dried vaccines were stored for up to 12 weeks before use. The merozoite antigens were emulsified in FCA, and two intramuscular injections of the preparations were given between 3 and 4 weeks apart. Of the 8 vaccinated monkeys, 2 received injections containing merozoites which had been stored frozen, and the remaining 6 were given the freeze-dried merozoite preparation. All the animals were challenged about 3–4 weeks later with either W_1 or W_3 *P. knowlesi* variants. The nonvaccinated monkeys developed rapidly rising parasitemias and expired on days 6 and 8 after inoculation by either variant. In contrast, each of the 8 vaccinated monkeys survived challenge, with 3 experiencing no parasitemia; the remaining 5 developed parasitemias which peaked between 0.5 and 5.9%. These results clearly indicate that merozoites stored after freeze-drying or in a frozen state are as effective immunogenically as freshly isolated merozoites (Mitchell *et al.*, 1975).

Adjuvants other than FCA, e.g., FIA, adjuvant 65-4, Alhydrogel, and BCG, were all found to be completely ineffective in inducing immunity with the merozoite antigen. Pretreatment of merozoites with formol also reduced the efficacy of vaccination (Butcher *et al.*, 1978).

Richards *et al.* (1977) investigated the effectiveness of merozoite vaccination against sporozoite challenge, the natural form of transmission. Rhesus monkeys were injected with W_1 strain merozoites isolated from *in vitro* cultures following the removal of red cell material by agglutination with PHA (Mitchell *et al.*, 1975). Merozoites were also prepared for these studies by the cell-sieving technique of Dennis *et al.* (1975). In the latter method, schizont-infected cells derived from infected monkeys were incubated in a cell sieve, a specially designed culture chamber incorporating a polycarbonate membrane of 2 μm pore size through which culture medium can be pumped continuously. As merozoites are released from rupturing schizonts, they are swept from the chamber in the medium passing through the membrane, while the unruptured schizonts are retained. Some of the merozoites thus collected were then emulsified in FCA within 3 hours of isolation, and others after treatment with a formol–saline solution (1:1000) for 16 hours at 4°C and freeze-drying in 10% (v/v) normal rhesus serum in water. The freeze-dried preparations were stored at 4°C for up to 4 weeks before use. Of 5 normal monkeys challenged by the bites of 10 infected

A. balabacensis or by intravenous injection of 10^3 sporozoites, only 2 died of acute malaria; the remaining 3 developed peak parasitemias of 4–7% and were subsequently drug-cured. Of 6 merozoite-vaccinated monkeys challenged with sporozoites, 1 died with a peak parasitemia of only 7.0%. The other 5 monkeys in the group survived but had peak parasitemias ranging from 0.4 to 6.0%. Vaccination with formol-treated, freeze-dried merozoites in FCA proved to be less effective than vaccination with untreated freeze-dried merozoites.

In another study in which resistance to sporozoite challenge was evaluated 4 monkeys were vaccinated with W_1 strain merozoites, challenged repeatedly by the injection of blood stage parasites, and then challenged by the bites of 10 infected *A. balabacensis* mosquitoes. All these monkeys developed transient infections with a peak parasitemia of 0.24%, which resolved within 1–5 days after the sporozoite challenge administered by the mosquito bites. Had a more virulent sporozoite inoculum been utilized, which would have caused higher parasitemia in the control monkeys, it would have been easier to interpret these results. Drug treatment of the surviving control animals also complicated interpretation. In any case, these results demonstrate that merozoite vaccination did not completely inhibit preerythrocytic parasite development, since all monkeys developed some blood infection after sporozoite challenge. The blood stage infections which developed in the vaccinated monkeys after sporozoite challenge were short and mild, however.

Recently, Mitchell *et al.* (1978) evaluated Nor-muramyl dipeptide (MDP) (a synthetic derivative of *N*-acetylmuramyl-L-alanyl-D-isoglutamine), *Mycobacterium butyricum,* and *B. pertussis* organisms as immunological adjuvants. He compared their activity as adjuvants to the activity of FCA in vaccination studies on rhesus monkeys infected by *P. knowlesi*. Merozoite antigens were prepared following the technique of Mitchell *et al.* (1975). Of 6 monkeys immunized using FCA as adjuvant, only 1 died after challenge, whereas of 6 monkeys vaccinated using Nor-MDP and FIA as adjuvant, 4 died after challenge. In another group of 3 monkeys, vaccinated using adjuvant 65 and Nor-MDP combined, all the monkeys died after challenge. Neither of 2 monkeys immunized using *B. pertussis* as an adjuvant survived challenge. Only one monkey in a group of 3 monkeys vaccinated with merozoites and *M. butyricum* in adjuvant 65 survived challenge. These results confirm the ineffectiveness of most of the adjuvants tested but show that Nor-MDP in FIA emulsion has some useful adjuvant activity. Adjuvant 65 was not an adequate substitute for the oil phase normally used in FCA.

An exhaustive study was recently conducted to compare the relative immunigenicity of viable blood stage antigens (schizont, FPC, and merozoite) of *P. knowlesi* emulsified in FCA (Rieckman *et al.,* 1978). The frozen and thawed schizont stage *P. knowlesi* antigen was made according to the procedure outlined by Brown *et al.* (1970); lyophilized fractions of *P. knowlesi* (schizont stage) antigen that had been disintegrated in a FPC were prepared according to the method described by *Schenkel et al.* (1973); the merozoite antigen was made by the technique of Mitchell *et al.* (1975), except that merozoites were collected with the use of Bacto PHA instead of filtration through polycarbonate membranes (Nucleopore). The PHA technique was used because it gave better yields of merozoites than the filtration technique. A total of 32 rhesus monkeys were used in this study—8 as controls and 8 each for testing the 3 antigenic materials. Following two immunizations with frozen or lyophilized schizont antigens or merozoites emulsified in FCA administered intramuscularly at 6-week intervals, all the monkeys were challenged with blood stage *P. knowlesi* of a variant different from that used for immunization. All 8 control monkeys developed severe parasitemia and died of infection within 12 days after challenge. Six of the 8 monkeys died in the group receiving the schizont antigen. The 2 surviving monkeys had parasitmeia peaks at 0.7 and 3.2%, and their infections lasted for 10–13 days. Similarly, 6 of the 8 monkeys which received merozoite antigens died. The 2 surviving monkeys developed infections which lasted for 10–14 days, with peak parasitemias of 0.01 and 2.7%. Only 4 of the 8 monkeys which received the FPC antigen died. The remaining 4 survived with infections that persisted over a 9- to 15-day period with parasitemia peaks of 0.07, 0.4, 0.9 and 1.2%. These results in monkeys given the schizont antigen were similar to those reported earlier (Brown *et al.*, 1970). However, the results in monkeys given FPC antigen were different from the results obtained in a similar study (Schenkel *et al.*, 1975). Schenkel *et al.* (1975) reported that 75% of immunized monkeys survived blood-induced infection, while in this study only 50% survived. The difference in these two studies may not have statistical significance, however, since the number of monkeys used by Schenkel *et al.* (1975) was 4, and 8 monkeys were used by Rieckmann *et al.* (1978). It was most surprising, however, that only 2 monkeys out of the 8 receiving merozoite antigen survived. Other investigators obtained 100% protection with merozoite antigen in similar studies (Mitchell *et al.*, 1975, 1977a). Some variations in experimental detail in the two laboratories may account for the difference in the degree of protection observed. Nevertheless, the results of these studies (Rieckmann *et al.*, 1978) do not provide evidence for the superiority of any one of the three antigenic preparations in protection of rhesus monkeys against *P. knowlesi*.

V. IMMUNIZATION AGAINST HUMAN MALARIA PARASITES

The earliest attempts to immunize against *P. vivax* were those of Boyd and Kitchen (1936, 1943) and Heidelberger *et al.* (1946a–d). Despite continuing efforts there have been no successes in vaccinating human subjects using blood stage vaccines. Boyd and Kitchen (1943) succeeded in reducing the severity of

P. vivax infection by prior inducement of infection with living parasites in two susceptible, uninfected human volunteers. The immunizing infections were controlled by quinacrine. Heidelberger, *et al.* (1946b) inoculated 200 volunteers who had *P. vivax* infections with 2–4 × 10⁹ killed *P. vivax* (some volunteers received two and three injections of killed parasites). The injections had no effect on the relapse rate in the volunteers.

Only now, about three decades after those pioneering experiments, has direct experimentation with human malaria parasites become really feasible. This is because of the discovery that owl monkeys (*A. trivirgatus griseimembra*) are susceptible to the three species of human malaria parasites—*P. vivax* (Young *et al.*, 1966; Porter and Young, 1966), *P. falciparum* (Geiman and Meagher, 1967; Siddiqui *et al.*, 1967; Geiman *et al.*, 1969b), and *P. malariae* (Geiman and Siddiqui, 1969a). The demonstration that human plasmodia would grow in a small primate made possible for the first time studies on the biological, chemotherapeutic, and immunological aspects of human malaria parasites in an experimental animal and greatly facilitated *in vitro* cultivation. Many strains of *P. falciparum* are now regularly maintained in owl monkeys (Geiman *et al.*, 1969b; Hickman, 1969; Richards and Voller, 1969; Siddiqui *et al.*, 1972; Schmidt, 1973). The use of a commercially available medium for short-term *in vitro* cultivation of *P. falciparum* in *Aotus* red blood cells provides high yields of various intraerythrocytic stages of these parasites (Siddiqui *et al.*, 1970, 1974). The recent landmark discovery that continuous *in vitro* cultivation of *P. falciparum* in human erythrocytes is possible (Trager and Jensen, 1976) has opened new vistas for biological and immunological studies. It has now become possible to conduct vaccination studies against *P. falciparum*. In the past few years many significant studies have been made on human malaria parasites using the newly developed culture techniques and newly discovered experimental hosts. These studies are reviewed in the following section.

The first, though unsuccessful, immunization study against *P. falciparum* in owl monkeys using killed antigen was reported by Voller and Richards (1968). The antigen was obtained from a splenectomized owl monkey infected with the Camp strain of *P. falciparum* which was bled out when the parasitemia reached 60% and when a significant percentage of the parasites were schizonts. The vaccine was prepared by the technique of Targett and Fulton (1965). The infected red blood cells were washed free of plasma, treated with 0.1% neutral Formalin, and then emulsified in FCA. Into two owl monkeys 5 × 10⁹ parasites were injected intramuscularly. A second, similar dosage was given 5 weeks later. The parasites for challenge were obtained from an owl monkey in which an infection was initiated with the original stabilate of the Camp strain of *P. falciparum*. For this challenge a sample of blood containing 2000 parasites was given intraperitoneally to each of the two vaccinated and two control monkeys. All the monkeys subsequently expired with fulminating parasitemia. The parasitemia reached peaks ranging from 48.7 to 64.0%. The only beneficial effect of the vaccination was a prolongation of the prepatent period by 4 days. The time between vaccination and challenge was considered by these reseachers to be one of the prime causes for the negative results obtained in this study. In addition, however, the adverse effect of Formalin (Richards *et al.*, 1977) and the antigenic nature of the vaccine could also have played an important role in causing the failure of the vaccination to provide protection in these monkeys. Contrary to what is claimed in this report, short-term *in vitro* cultivation of parasitized blood derived from heavily infected owl monkeys is required if high schizont yields are to be obtained (Siddiqui *et al.*, 1974).

Because of the encouraging results obtained from the use of a vaccine comprised of roentgen-irradiated blood infected with *P. berghei* (Wellde and Sadun, 1967), an exhaustive study was undertaken to determine whether protective immunity in owl monkeys could be induced by inoculation of irradiated *P. falciparum*-infected erythrocytes (Sadun *et al.*, 1969). The inoculation of owl monkeys with four doses of irradiated (25,000 rads) parasitized *Aotus* red cells (Camp strain) derived from owl monkeys with ongoing infections conferred significant protection against challenge. The vaccinated monkeys had lower parasite levels after challenge than the control monkeys. Four of the seven vaccinated monkeys died within 5 weeks, but 100% of the control monkeys died within 8 days. Less striking protection was obtained by giving only three rather than four immunizing inoculations at weekly intervals. In this group only two of four immunized monkeys survived. No protection was obtained by the administration of a single immunizing dose. Using the experimental protocol reported earlier (Sadun *et al.* (1969), Wellde *et al.* (1978) in the same laboratory confirmed the aforementioned findings (Sadun *et al.*, 1969). Two owl monkeys given a single immunizing dose of gamma-irradiated parasitized blood (*P. falciparum*, Camp strain) died with fulminating parasitemia following challenge. However, only one of three monkeys receiving four immunizing doses died after challenge; the two surviving vaccinated monkeys developed only low-level parasitemias. The protection obtained in this group of immunized monkeys (75% survival) was greater than that found in the previous study (Sadun *et al.*, 1969), where only 43% of the animals survived challenge. These are the only two studies reported in the literature in which irradiated blood stage *P. falciparum* was used to induce immunity in owl monkeys against *P. falciparum*. The significant aspects of these results are the degree of protection obtained without the use of adjuvant and the requirement for four immunizing doses to produce a significant degree of immunity. Further evaluation of this technique must await further research.

Siddiqui (1977) reported the first successful immunization of owl monkeys against *P. falciparum* employing *P. falciparum* blood stage antigen derived from an ongoing owl monkey infection. The Uganda–Palo Alto (FUP) strain of *P.*

falciparum was used in this study. Through short-term *In vitro* cultivation of parasitized blood from donor monkeys, mature segmenters were produced (Siddiqui *et al.*, 1974). These mature segmenters were harvested and concentrated. Merozoites relatively free of other cellular elements were then harvested from the mature segmenters (Siddiqui *et al.*, 1978a). The final preparation of antigenic material consisted of 60–70% merozoites, with the remainder trophozoites and immature schizonts. Two owl monkeys were used as controls, and three other owl monkeys were immunized with *P. falciparum* (FUP strain) segmenters containing fully developed merozoites emulsified with equal volumes of FCA. Two doses of the vaccine were administered intramuscularly at 3-week intervals. Each vaccine dose contained 2.73 mg of protein. No vaccinated monkey developed a detectable infection as a result of vaccination. Three weeks following the second vaccination, all five animals were challenged by intravenous injection of 6.2×10^5 parasites of the FUP strain of *P. falciparum*. Each of the control monkeys developed fatal fulminating infections. The parasitemias in these monkeys ranged from 64 to 81%. Death occurred within 2 weeks after challenge. The three vaccinated monkeys, in contrast, survived; one was completely protected, and the second became patent on day 18 postchallenge with a mild infection. The maximum parasitemia was 0.1%, and the blood became negative in 2 weeks' time. In the third immunized monkey, however, parasites were first detected on day 11. This monkey had a peak parasitemia of 7.0% on day 17; by day 30, the parasitemia had dropped to below 0.1%. The blood of this monkey became negative on day 34. It can be concluded from these results that it is possible to immunize owl monkeys successfully against lethal challenges with a homologous strain of *P. falciparum* by the use of *P. falciparum* blood stage antigen. The antigen must consist of mature segmenters prepared via short-term *in vitro* cultivation of the parasitized blood of owl monkeys and must be given in FCA.

An independent study conducted in another laboratory (Mitchell *et al.*, 1977b) confirmed the above findings. Short-term *in vitro* cultivation of *P. falciparum*-parasitized blood derived from Gambian children with parasitemias ranging from 2 to 32% was used to obtain mature stages (schizonts) of the parasites. One wonders about the clinical status of these children in whom the parasitemia had reached such high levels. From these cultures, merozoites were isolated using CF11 cellulose-powder columns. One owl monkey was used as a control, and three were vaccinated three times at 2- to 3-week intervals. The *P. falciparum* merozoites were emulsified in FCA before administration. Three to 6 weeks following the second vaccination, all the monkeys were challenged with a West African (Lagos) isolate of *P. falciparum* obtained from a donor owl monkey. All four monkeys, including the control, survived the challenge. The prepatent period, however, was prolonged from 4 days in the controls to 16–20 days in the vaccinated monkeys. The parasitemias (0.5–10.0%) were much lower in the vaccinated monkeys than in the control monkey (22.0%). Apart from one vaccinated monkey that died by accident, the remaining monkeys survived but had intermittent low-grade parasitemia for up to 11 weeks after challenge. These monkeys later showed good resistance when challenged with an East African *P. falciparum* (FUP) strain.

In another study (Siddiqui *et al.*, 1978b), similar cross-resistance was observed in owl monkeys vaccinated with an East African–*P. falciparum* (FUP) strain. When these monkeys, after recovery from the homologous challenge, underwent challenge with a Vietnam–Oak Knoll (FVO) strain of *P. falciparum*, they were resistant. The vaccinating FUP strain was chloroquine-sensitive, and the challenge FVO strain was chloroquine-resistant. Despite the fact that resistance was demonstrated in these vaccinated monkeys after an initial homologous challenge, the role of merozoite vaccination in resistance to heterologous challenge is evident (Mitchell *et al.*, 1977b). An unvaccinated monkey which had recovered from an infection with a homologous strain developed a parasitemia of 9% when challenged with a heterologous strain, while the parasitemias in two vaccinated monkeys were only 0.4–1.0%. However, we do not yet know whether vaccination alone will protect owl monkeys against a primary challenge with a heterologous strain.

Very recently, another study on the vaccination of owl monkeys against *P. falciparum* was reported (Reese *et al.*, 1978a). The unique feature of this study was the use of antigen obtained from *in vitro* cultivated *P. falciparum* maintained in continuous culture for over a year. The FCR-3/FMG strain of *P. falciparum* was used throughout, and flow vial, petri dish (Trager and Jensen, 1976), and mechanized tipper flask (Trager, 1978) techniques were used for culture. When the parasitemia exceeded 10%, parasitized red blood cells containing mature trophozoites and schizonts were selectively concentrated and isolated using Physiogel (Reese *et al.*, 1978b); merozoites harvested by saponin lysis of schizonts were used as the antigen. The first experiment employed six monkeys; three of the animals received 5×10^8 merozoites emulsified with FCA; a booster vaccination dose was given 3 weeks later consisting of the same number of merozoites but emulsified in FIA. The remaining 3 monkeys, used as controls, received adjuvant only. All injections were intramuscular. Three weeks after the second vaccination, all six animals were challenged by intravenous injection of 1 $\times 10^6$ fresh parasitized red blood cells (FCR-3/FMG strain of *P. falciparum*) derived from an infected splenectomized owl monkey. Within 2–3 weeks after challenge, all six monkeys died with peak parasitemias ranging from 10 to 55%. However, some amelioration of the course of infection during the first 2 weeks of infection in at least two of the immunized monkeys was evident. In a later experiment, the following alterations were introduced in the experimental protocol (1) Three vaccination doses 3 weeks apart were administered; (2) the first two vaccine preparations consisted of merozoite antigen emulsified with MDP and mineral oil (FIA), with the third comprised solely of antigen mixed with mineral oil (FIA); (3) the total number of merozoites given to each monkey was approximately 1.7×10^9 in contrast to the 1.0×10^9 of the first experiment; and (4) the challenge inoculum given was reduced to 5×10^5, or about half that used in experiment 1. Of the six monkeys used in this experiment, five died on challenge—three controls and two immunized. A comparable result was reported from another laboratory (Siddiqui et al., 1978c) when MDP in peanut oil was substituted for FCA. However, on evaluation of both studies one can conclude that the course of infection in immunized monkeys was definitely ameliorated as judged by (1) the lower level of parasitemia, and (2) the 7- to 12-day delay in time to death in the two immunized monkeys, as compared with that in the controls. The immunity induced in the third immunized monkey was indeed impressive, the parasitemia never exceeding 0.4%. The latter experiment was based on the hypothesis that the amount of antigen injected may be of more importance than the manner in which it is administered (Reese et al., 1978a). The role of adjuvant, however, may be of even more importance. Mitchell et al. (1977b) used approximately 2.0×10^9 merozoites; Siddiqui (1977) used 2.8 mg of parasite protein per monkey. In each study, when the antigen was given with FCA, 100% of the vaccinated monkeys survived challenge. Reese et al. (1978a), who used 1.7×10^9 merozoites (approximately the dosage used by Mitchell et al., 1977b) but used FIC, in some cases with MDP added to the vaccine, protected only 33% of the vaccinated monkeys from death following challenge.

All the aforementioned studies point to FCA as an essential requisite for effective immunization of owl monkeys against P. falciparum infection. The use of this adjuvant in human subjects is considered unsafe because of the extensively documented data that it produces problems including potentiation of plasma cell tumors in mice, induction of autoimmune reactions, formation of disseminated focal granulomata, and long-term persistence of mineral oil in animals (Freund, 1956; Lieberman et al, 1961; Stebly, 1963; Heymann et al., 1959; Cutler et al., 1962).

The ultimate objective of all malaria vaccine studies is to develop a vaccine which can be used to immunize and protect man, not monkeys or rodents. Therefore the development of an immunologically satisfactory and pharmacologically acceptable adjuvant is imperative in the development of a malaria vaccine acceptable for use in man.

The synthesis of MDP—which could replace the whole tubercle bacilli in FCA and which has been shown to enhance the immunological response of an animal against an antigen when injected with mineral oil (FIA)—was recently achieved in two laboratories (Ellouz et al, 1974; Kotani et al., 1975). In the two most recent studies, however, MDP in mineral or peanut oil was not completely successful for vaccinating owl monkeys against P. falciparum (Reese et al., 1978a; Siddiqui et al., 1978c). Furthermore, MDP or its derivatives could only be used for human immunization without mineral oil, which is partially responsible for creating undesirable side effects from vaccination.

A study by Kotani *et al.* (1977) has demonstrated that replacement of the primary hydroxyl group at the C-6 position of *N*-acetylmuramyl-L-alanyl-D-isoglutamine (MDP) by a lauroyl, steroyl, or docosanoyl group yields an MDP derivative with adjuvant properties. Siddiqui *et al.* (1978d) recently demonstrated that stearoyl-MDP (6-0-stearoyl-*N*-acetylmuramyl-L-alanyl-D-isoglutamine) could replace FCA in effective immunization of owl monkeys against infection with *P. falciparum*. The immunizing agent [*P. falciparum* (FUP strain) and merozoite-enriched segmenters] was prepared following the technique of Siddiqui (1977) and Siddiqui *et al.* (1978a). The bulk of the antigenic material consisted of 50–60% segmenters with individual merozoites; the remainder consisted of parasites in other developmental stages. Antigen was stored at $-20°C$ for several weeks. The stearoyl-MDP adjuvant was used with carrier liposomes (cholesterol plus lecithin). The adjuvant-incorporated liposomes were prepared by the method of Inoue (1974). The preparation of the vaccine involved thoroughly mixing the antigen and the liposomes incorporated with adjuvant by passing them between two syringes connected by a double-hubbed needle. Seven owl monkeys (*A. trivirgatus griseimembra,* karyotype II and phenotype B) were used in this study. Three of the seven were used as controls, and the remaining four were immunized with the vaccine. Each of the monkeys was given two intramuscular injections of vaccine containing about 2.86 mg parasite protein at intervals 4 weeks apart. Vaccination never produced a detectable infection. About 17 days following the second dose of vaccine, all seven monkeys were challenged by intravenous injection of 7.5×10^5 parasites of the homologous strain (FUP) of *P. falciparum* derived from an ongoing infection in an owl monkey. Two of the control animals died within 2 weeks after challenge; the third, though it eventually survived, had more than 25% of its erythrocytes infected at the peak of its parasitemia. In contrast, all four of the immunized monkeys survived. Two of them developed only a low-grade infection that lasted for 1 week. The remaining two developed parasitemias that ranged from between 5 and 15.0% and which lasted 1 week. By the fourth week after challenge, all the vaccinated monkeys became negative for parasites on blood examination. The most important finding from this study was that the administration of *P. falciparum* antigen with stearoyl-MDP adjuvant and liposomes did not produce any reaction at the injection site. This is in sharp contrast to the mild-to-severe ulceration which occurs upon injection of *P. falciparum* in FCA or FIA. The only adjuvant-related side effect seen was anorexia for a few days immediately following vaccination, which resulted in some loss of weight. All the vaccinated and adjuvant control monkeys, however, regained the weight lost within 2 weeks after immunization. Loss of weight was minimal in one of the monkeys that had received only one-third the concentration of the adjuvant given to the other monkeys—an indication of some correlation between the concentration of adjuvant and the degree of side effects produced. The results of this study are significant, as they indicate that there may be a safe adjuvant for effective immunization of experimental monkeys against *P. falciparum* and suggests that an effective, safe human malaria vaccine may be possible.

There are about seven reports to date on the vaccination of owl monkeys with *P. falciparum* antigens. Three of these studies utilized relatively unselected peripheral blood stages of *P. falciparum* as antigen but failed to obtain complete protection of vaccinated monkeys (Voller and Richards, 1968; Sadun *et al.*, 1969; Wellde *et al.*, 1978). The techniques employed in the other two studies (Siddiqui, 1977; Mitchell *et al.*, 1978) using, in contrast, *P. falciparum* merozoites emulsified with FCA as a vaccine induced complete protection of vaccinated monkeys. The substitution of MDP for FCA did not produce 100% protection in two other studies (Siddiqui *et al.*, 1978e; Reese *et al.*, 1978a). However, the most recent report of Siddiqui *et al.* (1978d) describes the first successful replacement of FCA by another adjuvant. This adjuvant, stearoyl-MDP, permitted effective immunization of owl monkeys against infection with *P. falciparum* in the absence of FCA.

VI. SUMMARY AND CONCLUSION

Based on our present knowledge, we may conclude that immunization using blood stage antigens derived from avian, rodent, simian, and human malaria parasites gives impressive protection to appropriate host animals. The degree of protection has varied, of course, depending largely upon the nature of antigen used and the form in which it is administered to the host.

Irradiated parasitized erythrocytes have been used extensively as experimental immunogens. Because of some success achieved with rodent malaria (Corradetti *et al.*, 1966; Wellde and Sadun, 1967), irradiated erythrocytes infected with *P. falciparum* were used to vaccinate owl monkeys (Sadun *et al.*, 1969; Wellde *et al.*, 1978). The significant aspects of the results obtained in these studies were the degree of protection (43–75% survival) obtained without the use of adjuvant and the requirement for four immunizing doses to achieve any significant degree of immunity. Subsequent investigations of irradiated antigens should evaluate irradiated schizonts and merozoites.

Parasitized blood containing schizonts, the mature, intraerythrocytic stages of the parasite, has been used in vaccine trials (Freund *et al.*, 1945b, 1948; Targett and Fulton, 1965; Brown *et al.*, 1970). Brown *et al.* (1970), showed that injection of frozen and thawed schizonts of *P. knowlesi* in FCA protected approximately 50% of monkeys against homologous challenge, although no protection was provided against a heterologous variant. However, monkeys immunized in this manner which had recovered from challenge with the homologous variant subsequently exhibited immunity to a heterologous variant.

Significant protection has also been achieved in experimental animals with the use of fractions derived from parasites or parasitized erythrocytes. Utilizing the FPC to release *P. berghei* from host erythrocytes, D'Antonio *et al.* (1966b, D'Antonio, 1972b) isolated a PPF which, when used as vaccine, was able to protect a proportion of mice from challenge. In a study using a similar technique, *P. knowlesi* fractions were isolated and used as antigen to immunize rhesus monkeys (Schenkel *et al.,* 1973; Simpson *et al.,* 1974). The immunizing material effectively suppressed parasite development in most of the immunized monkeys, although not all those immunized survived challenge. In rats given a cell-free extract of *P. berghei* as antigen limited success was achieved in producing effective protection.

Merozoites were shown to be the most effective immunogen by Mitchell *et al.* (1974, 1975). These studies demonstrated for the first time a 100% survival rate in rhesus monkeys immunized with *P. knowlesi* merozoites. In contrast to schizont or plasmodial fraction immunization, merozoite immunization induced an immunity far greater in degree that was also broader in specificity. Comparable protection was obtained in ducklings immunized with *P. gallinaceum* merozoite-enriched antigen emulsified in FCA (Kilejian, as referenced in a review by Cohen *et al.,* 1977). In contrast, vaccination with *P. yoelli* merozoites has failed to protect mice of several inbred strains (Butcher *et al.,* as referenced in a review by Cohen *et al.,* 1977). Using *P. berghei* merozoites as antigen in rats, however, Saul and Kreier (1977) found it possible to procure some degree of protection. These workers also demonstrated that a soluble material obtained by washing sonically released merozoites stimulated the rats' protective response to plasmodial infection.

Our confidence in the immunizing effectiveness of merozoites as antigenic material was strengthened by the protection demonstrated by *P. knowlesi* merozoite-vaccinated rhesus monkeys against sporozoite-induced infection with *P. knowlesi* (Richards *et al.,* 1977).

Rieckmann *et al.* (1978) compared the efficacy of three nonviable blood stage antigens (schizonts, a schizont fraction obtained by FPC disruption of parasitized erythrocytes, and merozoites) of *P. knowlesi* in inducing protective immunity in rhesus monkeys. No clear evidence of the superiority of any of the three specific antigenic preparations was found. The survival of only two monkeys of eight receiving merozoite antigen was most surprising, as other investigators had reported 100% protection with this material (Mitchell *et al.,* 1975, 1977a). However, some variation in experimental detail within the two respective laboratories may account for the difference in the degree of protection realized.

Utilizing *P. falciparum* merozoite-containing schizonts, however, or extracellular merozoites as antigenic material, Siddiqui (1977) and Mitchell *et al.*

(1977b) obtained 100% survival of immunized owl monkeys challenged with a homologous strain of *P. falciparum*. These studies were the first to demonstrate effective immunization of an experimental animal against *P. falciparum*, the most dreaded of the human malaria species. It may be well to point out that extracellular merozoites are not required to produce effective immunity (Siddiqui, 1977; Siddiqui *et al.*, 1978d). Moreover, these studies show that saponin-lysed schizonts rich in merozoites can be maintained at −20°C for several weeks and that the frozen and thawed preparations of this material retain their immunogenic potency. While further research on the relative immunogenic efficacy of trophozoites, schizonts, and merozoites is desirable, this line of investigation may have to await the development of techniques for obtaining synchrony in continuous *P. falciparum* cultures.

Freund *et al.* (1948) was the first to demonstrate the importance of using FCA in conjunction with parasite antigenic material for achieving protective immunity against plasmodia. Subsequent vaccination studies reviewed in Sections II–IV confirmed this finding. It has generally been established that FCA is essential for immunizing owl monkeys against *P. falciparum*. Each of the following adjuvant materials has been tried as a substitute for FCA, only to prove ineffective in producing the degree of protection elicited by FCA: FIA, adjuvant 65/4, BCG, aluminum hydrogel, saponin, hexylamine, *B. pertussis*, levamisole, poly (I:C), poly (A:U), MDP, and Nor-MDP.

The recent work of Siddiqui *et al.* (1978d), has shown for the first time that there may be a possible safe, effective adjuvant for immunization against plasmodia—stearoyl-MDP. Until clinical trials are carried out the safety of stearoyl-MDP for humans remains to be demonstrated.

Methods for obtaining purified parasite antigen free of red cell debris, pigment, etc., may hopefully become available in the not too distant future. There are indications that lectins may prove useful in the selective removal of red cell membranes. The ability of concanavalin A to bind red cell membrane (Nicolson, 1974) but not malaria parasites (Seed and Kreier, 1976) was recently exploited in isolating *P. chabaudi* and *P. knowlesi* merozoites naturally released from contaminating debris (David *et al.*, 1978). The ability of membrane glycoproteins to bind concanavalin A is shared by the erythrocytes of many species, including man.

The duration of the protective immunity produced by immunization with plasmodial merozoites has yet to be established. In studies on the time span of vaccination-induced immunity, a major consideration is the use of adequate controls. It is not proper to use vaccinated animals challenged shortly after vaccination to establish the long-term effect of vaccination, since these vaccinated animals receive not only the antigenic material in the vaccine but also the challenging dose of parasites. However, Cabrera *et al.* (1977) used a vaccinated and then challenged rhesus monkey that had overcome a *P. knowlesi* challenge infection to demonstrate that protective immunity persisted in immunized monkeys for over a 4-year period. What cannot be ruled out in such experiments is the possibility that there was a synergistic effect between the vaccination and the infection produced by the challenge.

We do not know if the protective immunity acquired through vaccination in the experimental animal is strain-specific, or whether it also affords protection against heterologous strains. Based on the results of two studies involving only a few owl monkeys vaccinated with *P. falciparum* merozoites, it has been suggested that vaccination confers cross-immunity between geographically remote strains of *P. falciparum* (Mitchell *et al.*, 1977b; Siddiqui *et al.*, 1978b). What cannot be ruled out, however, is the possibility that the immunity demonstrated in these tests is the result of a synergistic effect between the vaccination and the exposure of the monkeys to homologous challenge. To determine if there is cross-immunity, the truest test would be to challenge vaccinated monkeys with a heterologous strain without previous exposure of the vaccinated monkeys to a homologous challenge. Monkeys that have undergone spontaneous or drug-induced recovery from a homologous infection should ideally be used as one of the sets of controls.

Complete immunity to malaria develops under natural conditions; this is especially true in holoendemic areas. For complete immunity to be acquired through natural infection, repeated infections are required, and immunity takes years to develop. Even after years of exposure, immunity may still not be absolute in naturally infected individuals, as parasitemia often continues in the absence of clinical symptoms. Similarly, repeated infection with *P. knowlesi* and *P. falciparum* and drug cure lead to an acquired immunity associated with chronic relapsing parasitemia in rhesus and owl monkeys, respectively. Challenged rhesus monkeys (Mitchell *et al.*, 1975) and owl monkeys (Siddiqui, 1977; Mitchell *et al.*, 1977b) previously vaccinated with merozoites emulsified in FCA, on the other hand, may develop a low-grade infection and completely eliminate their parasites after approximately 2–4 weeks. Commenting on the prospects of developing human malaria vaccines, Neva (1977) has noted that "if vaccines are to be used, they will have to be an improvement upon nature." The results of most of the vaccination studies reviewed here indeed suggest that this may be possible.

In proposing guidelines for the development of human malaria vaccines, the Scientific Working Group on the Immunology of Malaria of the World Health Organization recently stated (WHO, 1976): "Vaccines should be developed having regard to ease of use under field conditions, i.e., they should be cheap, stable under various conditions of temperature and humidity and preferably in a freeze-dried form, require few booster doses, and induce protection of long duration." When considering the initiation of clinical trials, the group felt that "trials with vaccines in man should not be started until clear evidence from extensive investigations is available that the vaccine provides an effective immunity and is free of side-effects in animal models including primates.''

Vaccines incorporating merozoites and merozoite-enriched schizonts have been demonstated to be effective immunogens. Many of the data on vaccination studies reviewed here indicate that most of the technical difficulties which preclude the initiation of clinical trials have been overcome. In this connection, the success in achieving continuous propagation of *P. falciparum* in human erythrocytes (Trager and Jensen, 1976), the development of techniques for large-scale production of *P. falciparum* antigen (Trager, 1978; Siddiqui *et al.*, 1978e), the demonstration of effective immunization of owl monkeys against *P. falciparum* (Siddiqui, 1977; Mitchell *et al.*, 1977b), the demonstration that *in vitro* cultured *P. falciparum* parasites are immunogenic (Reese *et al.*, 1978a) and that freeze-dried merozoites and lyophilized schizonts of *P. knowlesi* are immunogenic (Mitchell *et al.*, 1977a), and, lastly but significantly, the replacement of FCA with a possible safe agent that leads to effective immunization of owl monkeys against *P. falciparum* (Siddiqui *et al.*, 1978d) are noteworthy. Together, these developments provide the most significant reasons for us to hope that we will soon realize our ultimate goal of development of a safe, effective vaccine for human malaria.

In a highly significant study, it was recently demonstrated that ducklings could be effectively immunized with HRP isolated from *P. lophurae*-infected erythrocytes. This was done without the use of an adjuvant. The immunity produced was effective against a normally fatal *P. lophurae* infection (Kilejian, 1978). This is the first instance where it has been possible to immunize against malaria with a purified protein. If the same results can be obtained against *P. falciparum* in owl monkeys, then this purified protein will prove a good candidate for a vaccine.

Some questions have been raised about the applicability of *P. falciparum* vaccination studies in *Aotus* (Siddiqui, 1977; Mitchell *et al.*, 1977b; Siddiqui *et al.*, 1978d) to human trials, owing to the failure of the monkeys to develop sterile immunity after the primary challenge.

The objective of vaccination against microbial infections is to prevent disease and mortality. The fact that populations immunized against polio continue to excrete virulent viruses, or that clostridial spores can be isolated from symptom-free hosts, is accepted by microbiologists as indicative of successful vaccination. Reduction in morbidity and mortality are the main criteria for assessing the potency of vaccines against tetanus, cholera, smallpox, poliomyelitis, rabies, pertussis, and diphtheria. It is unnecessary to demonstrate that the protected host is completely free of the infecting agent, i.e., that sterile immunity exists. The aim of human malaria vaccination at present is not to obtain sterile immunity but to lower the parasitemia and to modify the clinical course of the disease. The time has come to deliberate and debate this subject. Commenting on this, Zuckerman (1969) has stated

Finally, it would seem highly appropriate that the following proposition dealing with any future global program of vaccination against malaria be widely debated, namely, whether it is desirable to aim at eradicating the malarial parasite from the body of an inhabitant of an endemic area, or rather to aim at curbing his infection within clinically tolerable limits. . . . This procedure might permit the vaccinated patient in an endemic area to survive the most dangerous period of the disease, primary infection, while establishing acquired immunity associated with progressively increasing resistance to superinfection with the local strains of plasmodia to which he is constantly being exposed.

REFERENCES

Beckwith, R., Schenkel, R. H., and Silverman, P. H. (1975). Qualitative analysis of phospholipids isolated from nonviable plasmodium antigens. *Exp. Parasitol.* **37**, 164–172.

Boyd, M. F., and Kitchen, S. F. (1936). Is the acquired homologous immunity to *Plasmodium vivax* equally effective against sporozoites and trophozoites? *Am. J. Trop. Med.* **16**, 317–322.

Boyd, M. F., and Kitchen, S. F. (1943). On attempts to hyperimmunize convalescents from vivax malaria. *Am. J. Trop. Med.* **23**, 209–225.

Brown, K. N., and Brown, I. N. (1965). Immunity to malaria: Antigenic variation in chronic infections of *Plasmodium knowlesi*. *Nature (London)* **208**, 1286–1288.

Brown, K. N., and Tanaka, A. (1975). Vaccination against *Plasmodium knowlesi* malaria. *Trans. R. Soc. Trop. Med. Hyg.* **69**, 350–353.

Brown, K. N., Brown, I. N., and Trigg, P. I. (1968). Immunization against *Plasmodium knowlesi:* Studies on the mode of action of Freund's adjuvant in stimulating protection. Proceedings of the British Society for Parasitology. *Parasitology* **58**, 18P (abstr.).

Brown, K. N., Brown, I. N., and Hills, W. A. (1970). Immunity to malaria. I. Protection against *Plasmodium knowlesi* shown by monkeys sensitized with drug-suppressed infections or by dead parasites in Freund's adjuvant. *Exp. Parasitol.* **28**, 304–317.

Butcher, G. A., and Cohen, S. (1970). Schizogony of *Plasmodium knowlesi* in the presence of normal and immune sera. *Trans. R. Soc. Trop. Med. Hyg.* **64**, 470.

Butcher, G. A., Mitchell, G. H., and Cohen, S. (1973). Mechanism of host specificity in malarial infection. *Nature (London)* **244**, 40–42.

Butcher, G. A., Mitchell, G. H., and Cohen, S. (1978). Antibody mediated mechanisms of immunity to malaria induced by vaccination with *Plasmodium knowlesi* merozoites. *Immunology* **34**, 77–86.

Cabrera, E. J., Speer, C. A., Schenkel, R. H., Barr, M. L., and Silverman, P. H. (1976). Delayed dermal hypersensitivity in rhesus monkeys (*Macaca mulatta*) immunized against *Plasmodium knowlesi*. *Z. Parasitenk.* **50**, 31–42.

Cabrera, E. J., Barr, M. L., and Silverman, P. H. (1977). Long term studies on rhesus monkeys (*Macaca mulatta*) immunized against *Plasmodium knowlesi*. *Infec. Immun.* **15**, 461–465.

Clark, I. A., Allison, A. C., and Cox, F. E. G. (1976a). Protection of mice against *Babesia* and *Plasmodia* with BCG. *Lancet* **1**, 309–311.

Clark, I. A., Cox, F. E. G., and Allison, A. C. (1976b). Protection: *Corynebacterium: Babesia; Plasmodium:* mice (To, CNA, *mi/nu*). *Science* **194**, 204–206.

Coffin, G. S. (1951). Active immunization of birds against malaria. *J. Infect. Dis.* **89**, 1–7.

Cohen, S., McGregor, I. A., and Carrington, S. C. (1961). Gamma globulin and acquired immunity to human malaria. *Nature (London)* **192**, 733–737.

Cohen, S., Butcher, G. A., and Crandall, R. B. (1969). Action of malarial antibody *in-vitro*. *Nature (London)* **223**, 368–371.

Cohen, S., Butcher, G. A., Mitchell, G. H., Deans, J. A., and Langhorne, J. (1977). Acquired immunity and vaccination in malaria. *Am. J. Trop. Med. Hyg.* **26**, 223–229.

Collins, W. E., Contacos, P. G., Harrison, A. J., Stanfill, P. S., and Skinner, J. C. (1977). Attempts to immunize monkeys against *Plasmodium knowlesi* by using heat-stable, serum-soluble antigens. *Am. J. Trop. Med. Hyg.* **26**, 373–376.

Corradetti, A., Verolini, F., and Bucei, A. (1966). Resistenza a *Plasmodium berghei* da parte di ratti albini precedentemente immunizatti con *P. berghei* irradiato. *Parassitologia* **8**, 133–145.

Cottrell, B. J., Playfair, J. H. L., and de Souza, J. B. (1977). *Plasmodium yoelii* and *Plasmodium vinckei:* The effects of non-specific immunostimulation on murine malaria. *Exp. Parasitol.* **43**, 45–53.

Cutler, J. C., Lesesne, L., and Vaughn, I. (1962). Use of poliomyelitis virus vaccine in light mineral oil adjuvant: A community immunization program and report of reactions encountered. *J. Allergy* **33**, 193–209.

D'Antonio, L. E. (1972a). *Plasmodium:* A resume of the isolation of a vaccine fraction by the French pressure cell technique. *Exp. Parasitol.* **31**, 75–81.

D'Antonio, L. E. (1972b). *Plasmodium berghei:* Vaccination of mice against malaria with heat inactivated parasitized blood. *Exp. Parasitol.* **31**, 82–87.

D'Antonio, L. E. (1974). Vaccination against malaria: Evaluation of a plasmodial vaccine fraction and a preliminary study of some immunologic adjuvants in a primate model system: A brief report. *J. Am. Osteopath. Assoc.* **73**, 649–652.

D'Antonio, L. E., and Silverman, P. H. (1970). Malaria resistance induced by a plasmodial particulate fraction. *Fed. Proc., Fed. Am. Soc. Exp. Biol.* **29**, 638.

D'Antonio, L. E., von Doenhoff, A. E., Jr., and Fife, E. H., Jr. (1966a). A new method for isolation and fractionation of complement fixing antigens from *Plasmodium knowlesi*. *Proc. Soc. Exp. Biol. Med.* **123**, 30–34.

D'Antonio, L. E., von Doenhoff, A. E., Jr., and Fife, E. H., Jr. (1966b). Serological evaluation of the specificity and sensitivity of purified malaria antigens prepared by a new method. *Mil. Med.* **131**, 1152–1156.

D'Antonio, L. E., Dagnillo, D. M., and Silverman, P. H. (1971) Vaccination of rhesus monkeys against *Plasmodium knowlesi* malaria with a partially purified plasmodial fraction. Federation Proceedings, **30**, 303 (Abstr.).

D'Antonio, L. E., Dagnillo, D. M., and Silverman, P. H. (1969). Induction of resistance to malaria with a partially isolated plasmodial fraction. *J. Protozool.* **16**, 17 (abstr.).

David, P. H., Hommel, M., Benichou, J.-C., Eisen, H. A., and Da Silva, L. H. P. (1978). Isolation of merozoites: Release of *Plasmodium chabaudi* merozoites from schizonts bound to immobilized concanavalin A. *Proc. Natl. Acad. Sci. U.S.A.* **75**, 5081–5084.

Dennis E. D., Mitchell, G. H., Butcher, G. A., and Cohen, S. (1975). *In-vitro* isolation of *Plasmodium knowlesi* merozoites using polycarbonate sieves. *Parasitology* **71**, 475–481.

Desowitz, R. S. (1967). Immunization of rats against *Plasmodium berghei* with plasmodial homogenate, carboxymethyl cellulose (CMC) bound homogenate and CMC-homogenate followed by administration of "immune" gamma globulin. *Protozoology* **2**, 105–111.

Desowitz, R. S. (1975). *Plasmodium berghei:* Immunogenic enhancement of antigen by adjuvant addition. *Exp. Parasitol.* **38**, 6–13.

Eaton, M. D., and Coggshall, L. T. (1939). Production in monkeys of complement-fixing antibodies without active immunity by injection of killed *Plasmodium knowlesi*. *J. Exp. Med.* **70**, 141–146.

Ellouz, F., Adam, A., Ciorbaru, R., and Lederer, E. (1974). Minimal structural requirements for adjuvant activity of bacterial peptidoglycan derivatives. *Biochem. Biophys. Res. Commun.* **59**, 1317–1325.

Freund, J. (1956). The mode of action of immunologic adjuvants. *Adv. Tuberc. Res.* **7,** 130–148.

Freund, J., Sommer, H. E., and Walter, A. W. (1945a). Immunization against malaria vaccination of ducks with killed parasites, incorporated with adjuvants. *Science* **102,** 200–204.

Freund, J., Thompson, K. J., Sommer, H. E., Walter, A. W., and Schenkein, E. L. (1945b). Immunization of rhesus monkeys against malarial infection (*P. knowlesi*) with killed parasites and adjuvants. *Science* **102,** 202–204.

Freund, J., Thompson, K. J., Sommer, H. E., Walter, A. W., and Pisani, T. M. (1948). Immunization of monkeys against malaria by means of killed parasites with adjuvants. *Am. J. Trop. Med.* **28,** 1–22.

Geiman, Q. M., and Meagher, M. J. (1967). Susceptibility of a New World monkey to *Plasmodium falciparum* from man. *Nature (London)* **215,** 437–439.

Geiman, Q. M., and Siddiqui, W. A. (1969a). Susceptibility of a New World monkey to *Plasmodium malariae* from man. *Am. J. Trop. Med. Hyg.* **18,** 351–354.

Geiman, Q. M., Siddiqui, W. A., and Schnell, J. V. (1969b). Biological basis for susceptibility of *Aotus trivirgatus* to species of plasmodia from man. *Mil. Med.* **134,** 780–786.

Gingrich, W. D. (1941). Immunization of birds to *Plasmodium cathemerium. J. Infect. Dis.* **68,** 46–52.

Grothaus, G. D., and Kreier, J. P. (1980). Isolation of a soluble component of *P. berghei* which induces immunity in rats. *Infect. Immunol.* **28,** 245–253.

Heidelberger, M., Mayer, M. M., and Demarest, C. R. (1946a). Studies in human malaria. I. The preparation of vaccines and suspensions containing plasmodia. *J. Immunol.* **52,** 325–330.

Heidelberger, M., Coates, W. A., and Mayer, M. M. (1946b). Studies in human malaria. II. Attempts to influence relapsing vivax malaria by treatment of patients with vaccine. *J. Immunol.* **53,** 101–107.

Heidelberger, M., Prout, C., Hindle, J. A., and Rose, A. S. (1946c). Studies in human malaria. III. An attempt at vaccination of paretics against blood-borne infections with *Plasmodium vivax. J. Immunol.* **53,** 109–112.

Heidelberger, M., Mayer, M. M., Alving, A. S., Craige, B., Jones, R., Pullman, T. N., and Wharton, M. (1946d). Studies in human malaria. IV. An attempt at vaccination of volunteers against mosquito-borne infection with *Plasmodium vivax. J. Immunol.* **53,** 113–118.

Heymann, W., Hackel, D., Harwood, S., Wilson, S., and Hunter, J. (1959). Production of nephrotic syndrome in rats by Freund's adjuvants and rat kidney suspension. *Proc. Soc. Exp. Biol. Med.* **100,** 660–664.

Hickman, R. L. (1969). The use of subhuman primates for experimental studies of human malaria. *Mil. Med.* **134,** 741–756.

Inoue, K. (1974). Permeability properties of liposomes prepared from dipalmitoyllecithin, dimyristoyllecithin, egg lecithin, rat liver lecithin and beef brain sphingomyelin. *Biochim. Biophys. Acta* **339,** 390–402.

Jacobs, H. R. (1943). Immunization against malaria: Increased protection by vaccination of ducklings with saline-insoluble residues of *Plasmodium lophurae* mixed with bacterial toxins. *Am. J. Trop. Med. Hyg.* **23,** 597–606.

Jerusalem, C., and Eling, W. (1969). Active immunization against *Plasmodium berghei* malaria in mice, using different preparations of plasmodial antigen and different pathways of administration. *Bull. W.H.O.* **40,** 807–818.

Kilejian, A. (1974). A unique histidine-rich polypeptide from malaria parasite, *Plasmodium lophurae. J. Biol. Chem.* **249,** 4650–4655.

Kilejian, A. (1976). Does a histidine-rich protein from *Plasmodium lophurae* have a function in merozoite penetration? *J. Protozool.* **23,** 272–277.

Kilejian, A. (1978). Histidine-rich protein as a model malaria vaccine. *Science* **201,** 922–924.

Kotani, S., Watanabe, J., Kinoshita, F., Shimono, T., Morisaki, I., Shiba, T., Kusumoto, S., Tarumi, Y., and Ikenaka, K. (1975). Immunoadjuvant activities of synthentic N-acetylmuramyl-peptides or amino acids. *Biken J.* **18**, 105–111.

Kotani, S., Kinoshita, F., Morisaki, I., Shimono, T., Okunaga, T., Takada, H., Tsujimoto, M., Watanabe, Y., and Kato, K. (1977). Immunoadjuvant activities of synthetic 6-O-acyl-N-acetylmuramyl-ʟ-alanyl-ᴅ-isoglutamine with reference to the effect of its administration with liposomes. *Biken J.* **20**, 95–103.

Kreier, J. P., Hamburger, J., Seed, T. M., Saul, K., and Green, T. (1976). *Plasmodium berghei:* Characteristics of a selected population of small free blood stage parasites. *Tropenmed. Parasitol.* **27**, 82–88.

Lieberman, R., Mantel, N., and Humphrey, W., Jr. (1961). Ascites production in 17 mouse strains. *Proc. Soc. Exp. Biol. Med.* **107**, 163–165.

Mitchell, G. H., Butcher, G. A., and Cohen, S. (1973). Isolation of blood-stage merozoites from *Plasmodium knowlesi* malaria. *Int. J. Parasitol.* **3**, 443–445.

Mitchell, G. H., Butcher, G. A., and Cohen, S. (1974). A merozoite vaccine against *Plasmodium knowlesi* malaria. *Nature (London)* **252**, 311–313.

Mitchell, G. H., Butcher, G. A., and Cohen, S. (1975). Merozoite vaccination against *Plasmodium knowlesi* malaria. *Immunology* **29**, 397–407.

Mitchell, G. H., Butcher, G. A., Langhorne, J., and Cohen, S. (1977a). A freeze-dried merozoite vaccine effective against *Plasmodium knowlesi* malaria. *Clin. Exp. Immunol.* **28**, 276–279.

Mitchell, G. H., Butcher, G. A., Richards, W. H. G., and Cohen, S. (1977b). Merozoite vaccination of douroucouli monkeys against falciparum malaria. *Lancet* **1**, 1335–1338.

Mitchell, G. H., Richards, W. H. G., Voller, A., Dietrich, F. R. M., and Dukor, P. (1979). An investigation of Nor-MDP, saponin, corynebacteria and pertussis organisms as immunological adjuvants in experimental malaria vaccination of macaques. *Bull. W.H.O.* **57**, 189–197.

Neva, F. A. (1977). Looking back for a view of the future: Observations on immunity to induced malaria. *Am. J. Trop. Med. Hyg.* **26**, 211–214.

Nicolson, G. L. (1974). The interactions of lectins with animal cell surfaces. *Int. Rev. Cytol.* **39**, 89–188.

Noguer, A., Wernsdorfer, W., Kouznetsow, R., and Hempel, J. (1978). The malaria situation in 1976. *WHO Chron.* **32**, 9–17.

Playfair, J. H. L., de Souza, J. B., and Cottrell, B. J. (1977). Protection of mice against malaria by a killed vaccine: Difference in effectiveness against *P. yoelii* and *P. berghei. Immunology* **33**, 507–515.

Porter, J. A., Jr., and Young, M. D. (1966). Susceptibility of Panamanian primates to *Plasmodium vivax. Mil. Med.* **131**, 952–958.

Prior, R., and Kreier, J. P. (1972). *Plasmodium berghei* freed from host erythrocytes by a continuous flow ultrasonic system. *Exp. Parasitol.* **32**, 239–243.

Prior R., Smucker, R. A., Kreier, J. P., and Pfister, R. M. (1973). A comparison by electron microscopy of *Plasmodium berghei* freed by ammonium chloride lysis to *P. berghei* freed by ultrasound in a continuous flow system. *J. Parasitol.* **59**, 200–201.

Ray, J. C., Muckerjee, S., and Roy, A. N. (1941). Agglutination reaction in experimental animals in response to *Plasmodium knowlesi* antigen. *Ann. Biochem. Exp. Med.* **1**, 207–218.

Redmond, W. B. (1939). Immunization of birds to malaria by vaccination. *J. Parasitol.* **25**, 28 (abstr.).

Reese, R. T., Trager, W., Jensen, J. B., Miller, D. R., and Tantravati, R. (1978a). Immunization against malaria with antigen from *in-vitro* cultivated *Plasmodium falciparum. Proc. Natl. Acad. Sci. U.S.A.* **75**, 5665.

Reese, R. T., Langreth, S. G., and Trager, W. (1979). Isolation of stages of the human parasite, *Plasmodium falciparum,* from culture and from animal blood. *Bull. W.H.O.* **57**, 53–61.

Reisen, W. K., and Hillis, T. C. (1975). Failure to protect *Mus musculus* against *Plasmodium berghei* with footpad injections of killed parasites incorporated in complete Freund's adjuvant. *J. Parasitol.* **61,** 937–940.

Richards, W. H. G. (1966). Active immunization of chicks against *Plasmodium gallinaceum* by inactivated homologous sporozoites and erythrocytic parasites. *Nature (London)* **212,** 1492–1494.

Richards, W. H. G., and Voller, A. (1969). The normal course of infection of *Plasmodium falciparum* in owl monkeys. *Trans. R. Soc. Trop. Med. Hyg.* **63,** 2.

Richards, W. H. G., Mitchell, G. H., Butcher, G. A., and Cohen, S. (1977). Merozoite vaccination of rhesus monkeys against *Plasmodium knowlesi* malaria: Immunity to sporozoite (mosquito-transmitted) challenge. *Parasitology* **74,** 191–198.

Rieckmann, K. H., Cabrera, H. J., Campbell, G. H., Jost, R. C., Miranda, R., and O'Leary, T. R. (1979). Immunization of rhesus monkeys with blood stage antigens of *Plasmodium knowlesi*. *Bull. W.H.O.* **57,** 139–151.

Sadun, E. H., Wellde, B. T., and Hickman, R. L. (1969). Resistance produced in owl monkeys (*Aotus trivirgatus*) by inoculation with irradiated *Plasmodium falciparum*. *Mil. Med.* **134,** 1165–1175.

Saul, K. W., and Kreier, J. P. (1977). *Plasmodium berghei:* Immunization of rats with antigens from a population of free parasites rich in merozoites. *Tropenmed. Parasitol.* **28,** 302–318.

Schenkel, R. H., Simpson, G. L., and Silverman, P. H. (1973). Vaccination of rhesus monkeys (*Macaca mulatta*) against *Plasmodium knowlesi* by the use of non-viable antigen. *Bull. W.H.O.* **48,** 597–604.

Schenkel, R. H., Cabrera, E. J., Barr, M. L., and Silverman, P. (1975). A new adjuvant for use in vaccination against malaria. *J. Parasitol.* **63,** 549–550.

Schmidt, L. H. (1973). Infection with *Plasmodium falciparum* and *Plasmodium vivax* in the owl monkey—Model systems for basic biological and chemotherapeutic studies. *Trans. R. Soc. Trop. Med. Hyg.* **67,** 446–474.

Seed, T. M., and Kreier, J. P. (1976). Surface properties of extracellular malaria parasites: Electrophoretic and lectin-binding characteristics. *Infect. Immun.* **14,** 1339–1347.

Short, H. E., and Menon, K. P. (1940). Attempt to produce active immunity to malaria in monkeys by vaccination with parasitic substance. *J. Malar. Inst. India* **3,** 191–193.

Siddiqui, W. A. (1977). An effective immunization of experimental monkeys against a human malaria parasite, *Plasmodium falciparum*. *Science* **197,** 388–389.

Siddiqui, W. A., Geiman, Q. M., and Meagher, M. (1967). The course of infection and gametocyte development of *Plasmodium falciparum* in *Aotus trivirgatus*. *Proc. Annu. Meet. Soc. Parasitol.* Abstract.

Siddiqui, W. A., Schnell, J. V., and Geiman, Q. M. (1970). Use of a commercially available culture medium to test the susceptibility of human malarial parasites to antimalarial drugs. *J. Parasitol.* **56,** 188–189.

Siddiqui, W. A., Schnell, J. V., and Geiman, Q. M. (1972). A model *in-vitro* system to test the susceptibility of human malarial parasites to antimalarial drugs. *Am. J. Trop. Med. Hyg.* **21,** 392–399.

Siddiqui, W. A., Schnell, J. V., and Richmond-Crum, S. (1974). *In-vitro* cultivation of *Plasmodium falciparum* at high parasitemia. *Am. J. Trop. Med. Hyg.* **23,** 1015–1018.

Siddiqui, W. A., Kramer, K., and Richmond-Crum, S. (1978a). *In-vitro* cultivation of partial purification of *Plasmodium falciparum* antigen suitable for vaccination studies in *Aotus* monkeys. *J. Parasitol.* **64,** 168–169.

Siddiqui, W. A., Taylor, D. W., Kan, S. C., Kramer, K., and Richmond-Crum, S. (1978b). Partial protection of *Plasmodium falciparum*-vaccinated *Aotus trivirgatus* against a challenge of a heterologous strain. *Am. J. Trop. Med. Hyg.* **27,** 1277–1278.

Siddiqui, W. A., Taylor, D. W., Kan, S. C., Kramer, K., Richmond-Crum, S. M., Kotani, S., Shiba, T., and Kusumoto, S. (1979). Vaccination of experimental monkeys against a human malaria parasite, *Plasmodium falciparum:* Use of synthetic adjuvants. *Bull. W.H.O.* **57**, 199–203.

Siddiqui, W. A., Taylor, D. W., Kan, S. C., Kramer, K., Richmond-Crum, S. M., Kotani, S., Shiba, T., and Kusumoto, S. (1978d). Vaccination of experimental monkeys against *Plasmodium falciparum:* A possible safe adjuvant. *Science* **201**, 1237–1239.

Siddiqui, W. A., Kan, S. C., Kramer, K., and Richmond-Crum, S. M. (1979). *In-vitro* production and partial purification of *Plasmodium falciparum* antigen. *Bull. W.H.O.* **57**, 75–82.

Simpson, G. L., Schenkel, R. H., and Silverman, P. H. (1974). Vaccination of rhesus monkeys against malaria by use of sucrose density gradient fractions of *P. knowlesi* antigens. *Nature (London)* **247**, 304–305.

Spear, C. A., Silverman, P. H., and Barr, M. L. (1976). Ultrastructural study of *Plasmodium knowlesi* antigen used in vaccination of rhesus monkeys. *J. Protozool.* **23**, 437–442.

Stebly, R. W. (1963). Glomerulonephritis induced in monkeys by injection of heterologous glomerular basement membrane and Freund's adjuvant. *Nature (London)* **197**, 1173–1176.

Targett, G. A. T., and Fulton, J. D. (1965). Immunization of rhesus monkeys against *Plasmodium knowlesi* malaria. *Exp. Parasitol.* **17**, 180–193.

Targett, G. A. T., and Voller, A. (1965). Studies on antibody levels during vaccination of rhesus monkeys against *Plasmodium knowlesi*. *Br. Med. J.* **2**, 1104–1106.

Thomson, K. J., Freund, J., Sommer, H. E., and Walter, A. W. (1947). Immunization of ducks against malaria by means of killed parasites with or without adjuvant. *Am. J. Trop. Med.* **27**, 79–105.

Trager, W. (1979). Recent developments in enlarging the scale of production of *Plasmodium falciparum in-vitro*. *Bull. W.H.O.* **57**, 85–86.

Targer, W., and Jensen, J. B. (1976). Human malaria parasites in continuous culture. *Science* **193**, 673–675.

Voller, A., and Richards, W. H. G. (1968). An attempt to vaccinate owl monkeys (*Aotus trivirgatus*) against falciparum malaria. *Lancet* ii, 1172–1174.

Wellde, B. T., and Sadun, E. H. (1967). Resistance produced in rats and mice by exposure to irradiated *Plasmodium berghei*. *Exp. Parasitol.* **21**, 310–324.

Wellde, B. T., Diggs, C. L., and Anderson, S. (1979). Immunization of *Aotus trivirgatus* against *Plasmodium falciparum* with irradiated blood forms. *Bull. W.H.O.* **57**, 153–157.

Wilson, R. J. M., McGregor, I. A., Hall, P., Williams, K., and Bartholomew, R. (1969). Antigens associated with *Plasmodium falciparum* infections in man. *Lancet* **2**, 201–205.

World Health Organization (1976). "Report of the Scientific Working Group on the Immunology of Malaria," TDR/IM/76.3. WHO, Geneva.

Young, M. D., Porter, J. A., Jr., and Johnson, C. M. (1966). *Plasmodium vivax* transmitted from man to monkey to man. *Science* **153**, 1006–1007.

Zuckerman, A. (1969). Vaccination against Plasmodia. *Isr. J. Med. Sci.* **5**, 429–434.

Zuckerman, A., Hamburger, J., and Spira, D. (1967). Active immunization of rats with a cell-free extract of the erythrocytic parasites of *Plasmodium berghei*. *Exp. Parasitol.* **21**, 84–97.

7

Infectiousness and Gamete Immunization in Malaria

Richard Carter and Robert W. Gwadz

I. INTRODUCTION

The sources of infectiousness of a malarious individual are the gametocytes of the malaria parasite. These are the sexual stages produced under obscure circumstances during multiplication of the asexual parasites in the bloodstream. On

Malaria, Vol. 3

263

completing their maturation, the gametocytes [male (microgametocytes) and female (macrogametocytes)] undergo no further development in the blood. Their destiny, should they survive, is to establish the parasite in the tissues of the mosquito vector following their ingestion by the insect during a blood meal.

Following ingestion by a mosquito, the gametocytes are immediately stimulated to undergo gametogenesis. The factors involved in initiating gametogenesis in the mosquito appear to be manifold. The existence of a mosquito factor responsible for this transformation was implied by the results of Micks *et al.* (1948) and recently demonstrated conclusively by Nijhout (1979). Spontaneous gametogenesis also occurs on exposùre of gametocyte-carrying blood to air. In *Plasmodium gallinaceum* this has been shown to depend upon the presence of bicarbonate ion (but no further constituents of blood other than sodium chloride) and a rise in pH from that of circulating blood, about pH 7.4, to between pH 7.8 and 8.3 (Bishop and McConnachie, 1960; Nijhout and Carter, 1978). A fall in temperature below 37°C is also essential for gametogenesis whether stimulated by the pH–bicarbonate-dependent process or by the mosquito factor (Sinden and Croll, 1975; Sinden and Smalley, 1976; R. Carter, unpublished observations).

Within 2–5 minutes of initiation of gametogenesis at 24°C, the gametocytes, which in *P. gallinaceum* are elongated, oval forms in their quiescent state, become perfectly spherical within the host red blood cell (RBC). Shortly thereafter the membranes of the host cell begin to disintegrate, and the gametocytes become extracellular. The extracellular macrogametocyte is now in effect a macrogamete and undergoes no further obvious changes prior to fertilization. The extracellular microgametocyte, on the other hand, completes its development with the release of eight highly motile spermlike microgametes. This process, known as exflagellation, occurs at 24°C mainly between 8 and 12 minutes after initiation. Fertilization proceeds rapidly, the peak of fertilization being almost coincident with the peak of exflagellation (Carter *et al.,* 1979b). Both processes are largely complete within 20 minutes following the initiation of gametogenesis.

The fertilized zygote transforms during the next 18–24 hours into the motile vermiform ookinete which penetrates the mosquito midgut to establish itself usually just below the basal lamella on the outer surface of the midgut. Over the following 10 days or so the zygote, now referred to as an oocyst, continues its development which culminates with the release of several thousand sporozoites into the hemocoel. The sporozoites migrate to the salivary glands to become the agents of infection to the vertebrate host.

The circumstances under which a malarious individual becomes infectious, or fails to become infectious, to a mosquito are complex. Various problems concerning gametocyte production and infectivity in malaria have been previously discussed in the excellent review by Bishop (1955). In this chapter we have attempted to analyze or develop specific concepts concerning infectiousness in malaria. We have drawn upon literature dealing with malaria in various laboratory animals including birds, rodents, and monkeys, as well as in humans, both under laboratory conditions and in populations exposed to natural malaria transmission.

II. AVIAN MALARIA (*Plasmodium gallinaceum*)

A. Blood Infections of *Plasmodium gallinaceum*

Blood infections of *P. gallinaceum* in chickens are characterized by synchronous growth of the asexual parasites with a cycle length of 36 hours (Giovannola, 1938). Peaks of schizogony take place at midday and midnight on alternate days. In sporozoite-induced disease, the blood infection is preceded by two distinct phases of exoerythrocytic schizogony in the cells of the reticuloendothelial system, the second of which gives rise to the blood infection (Garnham, 1966).

The course of asexual parasitemia in chickens may be dependent upon several variables: the age and probably the strain of bird; the manner of induction, i.e., by inoculation of sporozoites or parasitized blood; and probably also the strain and laboratory history of the parasite. The acute phase of a blood-induced infection (parasitemia > 1%) lasts between 5 and 10 days. At the peak of parasitemia, typically 50% or greater, the infection enters the period of so-called crisis during which morphologically abnormal parasites prevail. During the crisis period of 2–4 days, the parasitemia falls generally quite rapidly to less than 1%. The birds continue to harbor parasites until long after recovery from the acute phase of infection but are refractory to superinfection (Garnham, 1966).

Sporozoite-induced infections are consistently milder than those induced by blood inoculation (Eyles, 1952b; Gwadz, 1976). In such infections, the peak of parasitemia is generally not more than 10% and rarely exceeds 20%.

B. Gametocyte Production by *Plasmodium gallinaceum*

Gametocytes arise not only from merozoites released by blood stage schizonts but also directly from exoerythrocytic schizonts (Adler and Tchernomoretz, 1943). Consequently, gametocytes appear in the bloodstream at the same time as the asexual parasites. The time required for morphological maturation of gametocytes of *P. gallinaceum* was shown by Adler and Tchernomoretz (1943) to be about 40 hours. This is also the time period suggested by the results of Hawking *et al.* (1969) for the functional maturation of microgametocytes of *P. gallinaceum* as indicated by their ability to exflagellate. After reaching maturity, the gametocytes appear to remain functional for less than 24 hours. During the

rising phase of the parasitemia, gametocytes represent a rather constant fraction
of the total parasites of 2–5%.

C. Infectiousness of Normal Chickens Infected with *Plasmodium gallinaceum*

1. Course of Infectiousness

Sporozoite- and blood-induced infections of *P. gallinaceum* are characterized
by distinct patterns of infectiousness to mosquitos. In blood-induced infections,
infectiousness increases with parasitemia until 1–2 days before the peak of the
blood infection (Fig. 1a). At this time and during the 2- to 3-day period of crisis,
infectiousness declines steadily (Cantrell and Jordan, 1946; Huff and Marchbank, 1955; Huff *et al.*, 1958; Carter *et al.*, 1979a). Similar patterns of
infectiousness have been shown for pigeons, turkeys, and canaries infected with
P. fallax and *P. cathemerium* (Huff and Marchbanks, 1955). In the blood-
induced infections of *P. gallinaceum* studied by Cantrell and Jordan (1946), the
peak of parasitemia marked the beginning of a rapid fall in the number of
gametocytes relative to the asexual parasites (Fig. 2a). The infectivity of the
remaining gametocytes also began to decline sharply 1 day before peak
parasitemia but returned to normal by the second and third day after the peak
(Fig. 2a).

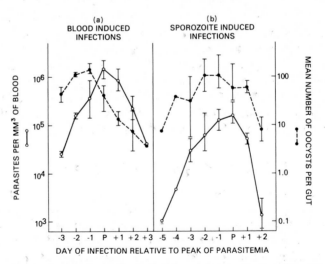

FIG. 1. Parasite densities in the blood of chickens infected with *P. gallinaceum* and oocyst
densities in *A. aegypti* mosquitoes fed on the same birds during infection, expressed daily in relation
to the day of peak parasitemia. (a) Blood-induced infections; data derived from Cantrell and Jordan
(1946). (b) Sporozoite-induced infections; data derived from Eyles (1951). Results from four birds
are represented in each study and are expressed as the range about a geometric mean.

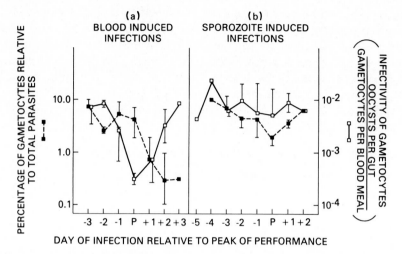

FIG. 2. Percentage of gametocytes relative to total blood parasites in chickens infected with *P. gallinaceum* and infectivity of gametocytes to *A. aegypti* mosquitoes fed on the same birds during infection, expressed daily in relation to the day of peak parasitemia. Data from the same sources and expressed in the same way as in Fig. 1.

In sporozoite-induced infections of *P. gallinaceum*, infectiousness remained proportional to parasitemia throughout the blood infection (Eyles, 1951) (Fig. 1b). Neither the proportion of gametocytes nor their infectivity to mosquitoes changed significantly during or following the peak of parasitemia (Fig. 2b).

Data from blood-induced (Cantrell and Jordan, 1946) and sporozoite-induced

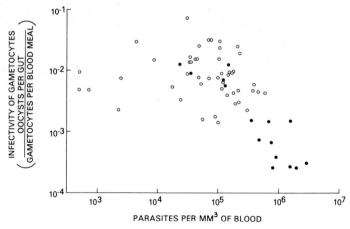

FIG. 3. Infectivity of gametocytes of *P. gallinaceum* to *A. aegypti* mosquitoes in relation to the density of asexual parasites in the blood of infected chickens. ●, Blood-induced infections; data from Cantrell and Jordan (1946). ○, Sporozoite-induced infections; data from Eyles (1951).

(Eyles, 1951) infections of *P. gallinaceum* are combined in Fig. 3 to illustrate the relationship between gametocyte infectivity and parasite densities in the blood. At densities above about 10^5 parasites/mm³ (equivalent to 5–10% parasitemia), infectivity of the gametocytes begins to decrease steadily with increasing parasitemia. At densities above about 10^6 parasites/mm³, the infectivity of the gametocytes is severely impaired. Such densities are characteristic of the peak of blood-induced infections but are rarely encountered in those induced by sporozoite inoculation.

2. Factors Determining the Infectivity of Gametocytes

Loss of infectivity of gametocytes of *P. gallinaceum* could result from a variety of conditions including (1) depletion of nutrients or factors necessary for infectivity of gametocytes, (2) formation of toxic substances, (3) production of antibodies or other immunological agents. Such conditions could affect gameto-cyte infectivity either by direct damage to the gametocytes while still in the circulation or by their effects on the gametocytes after ingestion by a mosquito.

Virtually nothing is known of the requirements of gametocytes during their habitation in the blood. Huff *et al.* (1958) administered various substances including coenzyme A, ferrous sulfate, sodium glutathione, calcium pantothe-nate, and sucrose to chickens infected with *P. gallinaceum*. None of these materials led to any change in infectiousness to mosquitoes. Knowledge of toxic or immunological factors which affect circulating gametocytes is equally lack-ing. Gametocytes appear to suffer morphological damage following peak parasitemia in blood-induced infections (Cantrell and Jordan, 1946; Eyles, 1952b), but the origin of such damage is unknown.

Rather more evidence is available concerning factors affecting gametocyte infectivity after their ingestion by mosquitoes. Washed, gametocyte/infected RBCs fed to mosquitoes in physiological saline retained only 25% of the infectiv-ity of defibrinated whole blood (Eyles, 1952a). Infectivity of the washed cells was almost completely restored by the addition of serum drawn from normal chickens and dialyzed against 1% sodium chloride. Although addition of glucose to the saline had a slight restorative effect, neither albumin nor the serum dialy-sate led to any improvement in gametocyte infectivity. These results suggest that the development of gametocytes in the mosquito is supported by certain non-dialyzable, presumably protein, components but does not depend upon any of the dialyzable components of serum.

Humoral factors associated with the period of peak parasitemia in blood-induced infections were shown by Eyles (1952b) to reduce the infectivity of gametocytes in the mosquito. Gametocyte-carrying RBCs were resuspended in various sera and fed to mosquitoes through a membrane. Compared to serum from normal birds, that taken from chickens 1 day after the peak of a blood-induced infection caused marked suppression of the infectivity of gametocytes to mosquitoes. Serum taken from peak parasitemia in a sporozoite-induced infection had no suppressive effect. Infectiousness of blood taken during the peak of a blood-induced infection was partially restored by resuspending it in normal serum. Such results indicate that humoral factors present during the peak of blood-induced infections are detrimental to the development of gametocytes in the mosquito. It is unclear, however, whether these factors are of immunological or other origin. Our studies (Carter *et al.*, 1979b) have shown that antibodies associated with suppression of infectiousness in immunized birds are not present at the peak of a blood infection in unimmunized birds.

D. Gamete Immunization against *Plasmodium gallinaceum*

1. Reduction in Infectiousness by Artificial Immunization

Except for the removal of gametocytes from the circulation during the period of crisis there is no evidence that immunity to the sexual stages is significantly involved in determining infectiousness to mosquitoes during acute *P. gallinaceum* infection in normal chickens. Passive transfer of serum from birds which had recovered from the acute phase of infection to birds with rising parasitemias of *P. gallinaceum* or inoculation of gametocytes into recovered birds also failed to reduce infectivity of gametocytes to mosquitoes (Huff *et al.*, 1958).

Other experiments described in the same report (Huff *et al.*, 1958) suggested that appropriate active immunization could, on the other hand, result in marked suppression of infectiousness to mosquitoes. The material used for immunization in these studies was Formalin-killed parasitized blood. Turkeys were immunized by five successive intravenous inoculations, each of 4 ml of blood parasitized with *P. fallax* beginning 2 days before and continuing for 2 days after challenge with live parasites. During the subsequent blood infection, infectiousness to mosquitoes was dramatically reduced compared to that of unimmunized birds. Neither the course of the asexual parasitemia nor the gametocytemia differed significantly from that of the controls. Similar results were obtained when chickens were immunized by daily intravenous inocula of 3.5 ml of Formalin-killed *P. gallinaceum*-infected blood for 3 days prior to live challenge. The peak infectiousness of the immunized birds was reduced by 90% compared to that of the controls. Neither the asexual parasitemia nor the gametocytemia differed greatly from that of the controls.

The approach of artificial immunization with parasitized blood formed the basis of the more extensive study by Gwadz (1976). Formalin-killed or x-irradiated chicken blood parasitized with *P. gallinaceum* was inoculated intravenously into chickens at weekly intervals for up to 5 weeks prior to live challenge. Such a procedure led to a dramatic reduction in infectiousness to mosquitoes following subsequent challenge.

Another approach to artificial immunization was introduced by Carter and Chen (1976). Extracellular gametes of *P. gallinaceum* were used for immunization with the expectation that antibodies against these stages might neutralize the gametes after their release in the mosquito midgut and thus sterilize the infection in the mosquito. X-irradiated preparations of partially purified micro- and macrogametes of *P. gallinaceum* were administered to chickens in three weekly intravenous inoculations. The numbers of oocysts developing in mosquitoes fed during subsequently induced blood infections were reduced by 99.99–100% below control levels.

2. Comparative Immunogenicity of Gametocyte- and Gamete-Containing Preparations

Comparative studies of materials used for immunization have demonstrated large differences in their relative effectiveness in reducing infectivity to mosquitoes. Based on a standard schedule of three weekly intravenous inoculations, Carter *et al.* (1979a) have shown that whole *P. gallinaceum* parasitized blood has an effect only when large amounts (approximately 10^{10} cells in total) are administered. However, much smaller amounts of blood were effective in reducing subsequent infectiousness when the extracellular gametes were released prior to inoculation. Preparations containing partially purified gametes of both sexes were the most effective immunogens in eliminating infectiousness during subsequent blood infection. Highly purified preparations of either microgametes or macrogametes (including unexflagellated microgametocytes) were poorly effective compared to the mixed gametes. The possibility exists, therefore, that antigens of gametes of both sexes may be necessary for effective immunization.

Whether or not gametes of both sexes are necessary, the results of these studies demonstrate that antigens represented on the extracellular gametes of the parasite are those most effective in reducing infectiousness to mosquitoes by artificial immunization.

3. Mechanism of Reduction in Infectiousness following Artificial Immunization

As in the studies by Huff *et al.* (1958), neither the asexual parasitemia nor the gametocytemia were greatly affected by immunization in the studies of Gwadz (1976), Carter and Chen (1976), and Carter *et al.* (1979a). Moreover, gametocytes from immunized birds suffered little intrinsic damage as a result of immunization (Gwadz, 1976) and recovered a normal degree of infectivity when resuspended in nonimmune serum and fed to mosquitoes through a membrane. In similar membrane feeding experiments, serum from immunized birds completely suppressed the infectivity of gametocytes from normal birds. The suppressive factors in immune serum could be recovered with the immunoglobulins precipitated with sodium sulfate.

The effect of immunization was thus shown to be mediated by humoral factors, probably antibodies, but nevertheless to leave the gametocytes circulating in normal numbers and intrinsically undamaged so long as they remained in the bloodstream. These effects of artificial immunization differed from those associated with high parasitemia, which leave the gametocytes themselves functionally impaired in the blood stream and also result in changes in the plasma which impair gametocyte development after their ingestion by a mosquito. Indeed, the results of Gwadz (1976) indicate that a reduction in infectiousness to mosquitoes associated with high parasitemia may be superimposed upon that resulting from immunization. Thus, in birds in which immunization was only partially effective, infectiousness was much lower in relation to the total parasites present at high as compared to low parasitemias.

Examination of the behavior of exflagellating gametocytes in the blood of the birds immunized by Gwadz (1976) showed that the extracellular gametes, unlike the intracellular gametocytes, were directly affected by conditions in the plasma. Emergence of the gametocytes from their host cells and the formation of microgametes (exflagellation) took place initially as seen in normal blood. Almost immediately following their extrusion from the microgametocyte, however, and usually before they became detached from the residual body, the microgametes in immune blood became agglutinated and immobilized. The gamete-agglutinating and immobilizing effect of immune serum was, like its effect in suppressing infectivity to mosquitoes, associated with the immunoglobulin-containing material precipitated with sodium sulfate and could be removed by specific precipitation of the immunoglobulins with mouse antibodies directed against chicken immunoglobulins.

The clear implication of these studies was that specific antibodies from immune birds interacted with the gametes of the malaria parasite to prevent fertilization in the mosquito midgut. This was demonstrated more directly by showing that ookinete formation could be prevented by the addition of immune serum to gametocyte-carrying blood *in vitro*. When immune serum was added prior to or up to the time of exflagellation and fertilization (10–20 minutes after initiating gametogenesis), ookinete formation was completely suppressed. Immune serum had no effect on the subsequent development of the ookinetes when added after the completion of fertilization (Carter *et al.*, 1979b).

4. Elaboration of Antigamete Antibodies during Immunization and Infection

The studies of Carter *et al.* (1979b) showed that two distinct antibody-mediated antigamete reactions could be identified in immune serum (1) a microgamete agglutination (AG) reaction and (2) a microgamete surface fixation (SF) reaction. In the SF reaction, microgametes became attached to the surfaces of slides and coverslips when observed in the presence of immune serum. Almost all birds, whether immunized or not, elaborated AG antibodies during their period of infectiousness. The presence of AG antibodies was not, therefore, associated with a reduction in infectiousness to mosquitoes. The SF antibodies, on the other hand, were invariably present throughout, and usually preceding, the period of the blood infection in immunized birds. These antibodies were never found in the serum of ineffectively immunized or normal birds during their period of infectiousness to mosquitoes.

The active blood infection supplied an important stimulus for the production of antigamete antibodies. The AG antibodies, as already mentioned, were elaborated during infection in normal as well as in immunized birds. The presence of SF antibodies never coincided with the period of acute infection in normal birds, but they often appeared at low titers several days or weeks after recovery from acute infection. In immunized birds, low SF titers were invariably boosted to much higher levels during or following active infection (Carter *et al.*, 1979b).

III. RODENT MALARIA (*Plasmodium yoelii*)

A. Blood Infections of *Plasmodium yoelii*

Plasmodium yoelii is a natural parasite of the African thicket rat, *Thamnomys rutilans*, but it is readily grown in the laboratory mouse, *Mus musculus*. Blood infections in both the natural and the laboratory host are asynchronous; the asexual cycle has been shown, nevertheless, to occupy about 18 hours (Carter and Diggs, 1977). Except in certain highly virulent lines of *P. yoelii*, the blood parasites have a strong preference for reticulocytes. Indeed, in most infections, the height of the parasitemia is restricted by the degree of reticulocytemia. In highly virulent parasite lines, asexual parasitemias may rise rapidly to exceed 80–90%, with death of the rodent host supervening 4–5 days after first infection. Most lines, however, run a comparatively mild course, reaching maximum parasitemias of 10–30% and persisting for 2–3 weeks before falling to low-grade chronic parasitemia (Carter and Diggs, 1977).

B. Gametocyte Production in *Plasmodium yoelii*

Gametocytes of *P. yoelii* are present from the onset of blood infection and are indeed also formed directly from the preerythrocytic schizonts in sporozoite-induced infections (Killick-Kendrick and Warren, 1968). The gametocytes reach maturity within 24 hours and probably survive for less than a day thereafter (Hawking *et al.*, 1972; Mendis and Targett, 1979). Sporozoite-induced infections are, in common with the experience with several other species of malaria parasites, less infectious to mosquitoes than subsequent blood-induced infections. Continuous passage by blood inoculation without intervening mosquito transmission may, however, result in loss of infectivity to mosquitoes within 10 such passages.

C. Infectiousness of Normal Mice Infected with *Plasmodium yoelii*

Although present throughout the period of asexual parasitemia at 0.1–1% of the total parasites, gametocytes are infective to mosquitoes mainly during the second to fifth days of parasitemia (e.g., Mendis and Targett, 1979; Wery, 1968). As may be seen from the data of Mendis and Targett (1979), there is a strong indication that the period of high asexual parasitemia is associated with reduced infectivity of the gametocytes to mosquitoes; at parasitemias above about 10%, infectivity is virtually abolished (see Fig. 3, *P. gallinaceum*). It is interesting to note that in a species of rodent malaria parasite such as *P. chabaudi,* in which the parasites show no preference for young RBCs and parasitemias rise rapidly above 10%, the gametocytes are poorly infective to mosquitoes for about the first 10 days of blood infection. Thereafter, as the host begins to control its infection, they become more infective to mosquitoes (e.g., Wery, 1968).

D. Gamete Immunization against *Plasmodium yoelii*

Immunization of laboratory mice with gametes of the *P. yoelii* subspecies, *P. yoelii nigeriensis,* has been reported to be effective in suppressing the infectivity of gametocytes during a subsequently induced blood infection (Mendis and Targett, 1979). The results of this study are of particular interest, as immunity was achieved by intravenous inoculation without the use of an adjuvant and thus contrasts with experience with *P. knowlesi* in the rhesus monkey (see below). Immunization with material which included asexual parasites in addition to the extracellular gametes enabled the mice to control the asexual infection, while all but one of nine control animals died within 6–7 days. In this respect, the results of immunization of mice with *P. yoelii nigeriensis* are more similar to those with *P. knowlesi* in rhesus monkeys than those with *P. gallinaceum* in chickens in which little effect on the asexual parasitemia was noted. In view of the presence of significant numbers of asexual parasites in the immunizing preparations, however, no conclusions can be drawn regarding the effect of immunization with gametes on the immunity to asexual parasites.

IV. SIMIAN MALARIA

Among the many species of monkey malaria parasites, *P. cynomolgi* and *P. knowlesi* have been most studied in the laboratory. Both species have been usually grown in rhesus monkeys (*Macaca mulatta*).

A. Blood Infections of *Plasmodium cynomolgi* and *Plasmodium knowlesi*

The asexual cycle of the blood stages of *P. cynomolgi* in rhesus monkeys is highly synchronous and occupies 48 hours. Mature schizonts present in the early morning give way to young rings on the afternoon of the same day; large pigmented trophozoites appear during the course of the second day, with the early divisions of schizogony beginning at about midnight. Blood infections are mild; parasitemias rarely rise above 5–10% following either blood or sporozoite inoculation.

Blood infections of *P. knowlesi* in rhesus monkeys run a course strikingly different from that of *P. cynomolgi*. The asexual cycle of *P. knowlesi* is also highly synchronous but lasts only 24 hours. Schizogony occurs at midday. Blood-induced infections usually run a lethal course; parasites multiply in the blood at an almost exponential rate throughout the infection, and the animals die of overwhelming parasitemia unless rescued by appropriate chemotherapy. In sporozoite-induced infections, the parasites first invade the blood after a period of exoerythrocytic development of about 6 days (Garnham, 1966); such infections are rather less virulent than when blood-induced but are, nevertheless, usually fatal unless treated.

B. Gametocyte Production by *Plasmodium cynomolgi* and *Plasmodium knowlesi*

Mature gametocytes of *P. cynomolgi* do not appear in the blood until several days after the first appearance of asexual parasites. This delay may be as long as 9 days in sporozoite-induced infections (Garnham, 1966). According to Garnham (1966), the gametocytes of *P. cynomolgi* require 4 days to reach morphological maturity. Hawking et al. (1966) concluded that the gametocytes of *P. cynomolgi* reached functional maturity after 2½ days and remained infectious for less than 24 hours.

In blood-induced infections of *P. knowlesi,* gametocytes appear in the blood almost immediately following the appearance of the asexual parasites. The gametocytes reach maturity after about 36 hours and remain infectious for about 8 hours (Hawking et al., 1968). Repeated passage of *P. knowlesi* by blood inoculation may result in eventual inability of the parasites to produce gametocytes.

C. Infectiousness of Normal Rhesus Monkeys Infected with *Plasmodium cynomolgi* or *Plasmodium knowlesi*

1. Circadian Changes in Infectiousness

Hawking et al. (1966) found that rhesus monkeys infected with *P. cynomolgi* reached maximum infectiousness to mosquitoes at about midnight on alternate days. A similar pattern of infectiousness was observed by Coatney *et al.* (1971) in a chronic infection of *P. cynomolgi* in a rhesus monkey. Such regular cycles of infectiousness on alternate nights represent the maturation of successive waves of gametocytes produced during the synchronous 48-hour cycle of asexual growth.

A regular pattern of infectiousness of *P. cynomolgi* is not a rule, however. Garnham and Powers (1974) recorded peaks of infectiousness on alternate nights in only one of five monkeys studied. Likewise, the results of R. W. Gwadz (unpublished) give no indication of fluctuations in infectiousness in a regular 2-day cycle. *Plasmodium cynomolgi* infections may become rather poorly synchronous and may also contain broods of parasites reaching maturity on different days. Under these circumstances, mature gametocytes appear in the bloodstream in an erratic or almost continuous fashion, leading to correspondingly continuous infectiousness to mosquitoes.

In rhesus monkeys infected with *P. knowlesi,* infectiousness to mosquitoes reaches a peak at about midnight on each day of the blood infection (Hawking *et al.,* 1968; R. W. Gwadz, unpublished results). Unlike those of *P. cynomolgi,* infections of *P. knowlesi* are almost always highly synchronous; moreover, since the asexual cycle lasts 24 hours, the opportunity for broods of parasites to arise out of phase does not arise. These circumstances, together with the short infectious life of the gametocytes, account for the regular rhythmic infectivity of *P. knowlesi* to mosquitoes.

2. Changes in Infectiousness in Relation to Parasitemia

The infectiousness of gametocytes of *P. cynomolgi* and *P. knowlesi* tends to be highly erratic at any density in the blood. Nevertheless, as the density of the gametocytes increases, infectiousness to mosquitoes tends to rise also. Over the range of parasitemias encountered in *P. cynomolgi,* rarely exceeding about 5%, the density of total parasites in the blood appears to have little effect on the infectivity of the gametocytes to mosquitoes. In infections of *P. knowlesi,* on the other hand, parasitemias rapidly rise above 10%. At such parasite densities the infectiousness of the gametocytes may be severely impaired (R. W. Gwadz, unpublished observations). The infectivity of blood at high parasitemia was sometimes partly restored by resuspending it in normal serum and feeding it to mosquitoes through a membrane. Conversely, the infectivity of blood could be greatly reduced when it was resuspended in serum from monkeys dying of overwhelming parasitemias of *P. knowlesi* (R. W. Gwadz, unpublished results).

Thus, in contrast to *P. cynomolgi* in which high parasitemias are rarely encountered, *P. knowlesi* infections regularly reach high parasite densities associated with impaired infectiousness to mosquitoes. The detrimental effects at high parasitemia could be partly attributed to conditions in the plasma affecting the infectivity of the gametocytes after ingestion by a mosquito. (See also Section II,C,2.)

3. The Role of Immunity in Infectiousness

There are so far no data which suggest that immune mechanisms are involved in modulating the infectivity of gametocytes during the normal course of infection of either *P. cynomolgi* or *P. knowlesi* in rhesus monkeys. Sera from monkeys which had recovered from repeated reinfections with *P. knowlesi* and may indeed have acquired significant immunity against homologous challenge had little effect on the infectivity of *P. knowlesi*-infected blood when presented to mosquitoes through a membrane (R. W. Gwadz, unpublished results). Attempts to demonstrate antibodies to the gametes of *P. knowlesi* during or following infection by direct observation of serum reactions with extracellular gametes have been unsuccessful. Low fluorescent antibody titers have been recorded against air-dried gametes of *P. knowlesi* in some sera taken during or following multiple infections. Such antibodies do not, however, necessarily react with the gamete surface and may, therefore, have little significance in preventing gamete fertilization (see Section V,C,3) (R. Carter, R. W. Gwadz, and I. Green, unpublished results).

Hawking *et al.* (1966) claimed to have demonstrated antibody-mediated suppression of infectivity to mosquitoes during a *P. cynomolgi* infection in a rhesus monkey. Coincident with the peak of parasitemia, the monkey ceased to infect mosquitoes; a few days after the peak the animal became briefly infectious once more. Hawking *et al.* (1966) interpreted these observations by postulating that antigamete antibodies were formed at the peak of parasitemia, which suppressed the infectivity of the gametocytes to mosquitoes; subsequent antigenic variation by the gametocytes was then presumed to have permitted them to become infectious once more. However, these interpretations, quoted by I. N. Brown (1969), Garnham and Powers (1974), and K. N. Brown (1977), were not supported by direct evidence.

D. Gamete Immunization against *Plasmodium knowlesi*

As we have just discussed, there is as yet no evidence that antigamete antibodies play a natural role in modulating the infectivity of simian malaria parasites to mosquitoes. Nevertheless, the results of Gwadz and Green (1978) demonstrated that appropriate artificial immunization of rhesus monkeys with preparations containing extracellular gametes of *P. knowlesi* resulted in total elimination of infectiousness to mosquitoes during subsequently induced blood infection. The site (mosquito midgut), target cells (extracellular gametes of the malaria parasite), mechanism (gamete neutralization by antigamete antibody), and immunogen (gametes of the malaria parasite) involved in such an immunization appear to be analogous to those demonstrated for gamete immunization against *P. gallinaceum* in chickens. The findings from the study of immunization of rhesus monkeys with preparations containing gametes of *P. knowlesi* may be summarized as follows; points of difference as well as similarities between the avian and simian systems will be noted.

1. In marked contrast to the results obtained in chickens, multiple intravenous injections of rhesus monkeys with preparations of *P. knowlesi* gametes and trophozoites had no effect on subsequent infectivity to mosquitoes after a challenge infection with *P. knowlesi*.

2. When similar *P. knowlesi* antigen preparations were emulsified in Freund's complete adjuvant and injected intramuscularly, infectivity to mosquitoes was completely suppressed during subsequent infections. Moreover, most monkeys that received one or two intramuscular injections developed only low-grade parasitemias when challenged with homologous and sometimes with heterologous strain(s) of parasite.

3. Monkeys successfully immunized with gametes developed strong antigamete antibody reactions as shown by fluorescent antibody reactions; sera from such animals also mediated immobilization and AG reactions with *P. knowlesi* gametes *in vitro*.

4. Challenge with a heterologous strain of *P. knowlesi* usually produced a fulminant infection, although the immunized monkeys were still completely unable to infect mosquitoes. Transmission-blocking immunity was thus shown to be effective against gametes of antigenically heterologous strains of *P. knowlesi*. However, immunity did not extend to protection against either the sexual or asexual stages of another species, *P. cynomolgi*.

5. The spleen, which plays an important role in protective immunity against malaria in monkeys, is apparently not involved in the maintenance of transmission-blocking immunity. Thus, when gamete-immunized monkeys, previously resistant to challenge, were splenectomized and rechallenged, all developed fulminant infections regardless of the challenge strain involved. Nevertheless, in spite of the large number of gametocytes produced, none of the monkeys was infectious to mosquitoes.

6. Transmission-blocking immunity is persistent. Intact or splenectomized monkeys show complete immunity against the sexual stages of *P. knowlesi* over 2 years after immunization.

7. Monkeys successfully immunized against the asexual parasites with preparations such as merozoites and trophozoites which do not contain gametes do not produce gamete-specific antibodies, and serum from such animals does not reduce the infectivity of *P. knowlesi* gametocytes to mosquitoes.

V. HUMAN MALARIA

Under natural conditions of transmission of human malaria, the parameters which determine the infectiousness of one individual to another may be summarized as follows (1) the probability of the first individual being infected by a malaria parasite, (2) the time of onset, duration, and intensity of the blood infection and its patterns of recrudescence and relapse, (3) the rate of production of gametocytes at each phase of the infection, (4) the time required for maturation and longevity of the gametocytes as agents infective to mosquitoes, (5) the rate of destruction of gametocytes at each point in the infection, (6) the infectivity of the gametocytes to mosquitoes at each point in the infection, (7) the capacity of local anophelines in relation to the infected individual to become infectious and actively infecting with respect to a second individual.

The present discussion will be concerned with the circumstances relating to the infectiousness of the human host to mosquitoes. While the susceptibility of the mosquito to infection must be taken as an inseparable part of the infectiousness of the human host, a detailed consideration of the role of the vector in malaria transmission is not possible in this chapter. As in previous sections, attention will be directed primarily to a single species of malaria parasite, in this case, *P. falciparum.*

A. Blood Infections of *Plasmodium falciparum*

The disease due to *P. falciparum* is a nonrelapsing malaria and is frequently, in nonimmune individuals, of life-threatening severity. The blood parasites have a synchronous cycle of asexual division of 48 hours. In nonimmune subjects, the first acute bout of infection in the blood lasts for 1–2 weeks following a prepatent period of exoerythrocytic development in the liver of about 6 days. Exoerythrocytic stages do not appear to persist beyond this time (Garnham, 1966). Parasitemia and symptoms decline usually quite rapidly at the end of the first acute phase of the infection, but recrudescences at irregular intervals of 2–4 weeks accompanied by a return of symptoms continue for up to 6 months and with declining frequency for as long as 1 year from the time of initial infection (James *et al.,* 1936; Jeffery and Eyles, 1955; Garnham, 1966). How long the parasites may ultimately persist in the body is unknown. In most isolated cases, symptoms cease completely within 1 year, and the subject appears to be free from disease for life unless exposed to reinfection. This is notably different from the situation in malaria due to *P. vivax* or *P. malariae.* In *P. vivax* relapses due to reinvasion of the blood from persistent exoerythrocytic stages may continue for 2–3 years, while infections with *P. malariae* may persist for life with symptomatic episodes recurring more than 30 years after initial infection (Garnham, 1966). In certain Asian strains of *P. vivax,* the first bout of parasitemia may not occur until 1 year after an infective bite (e.g., Coatney *et al.,* 1971).

In regions of hyperendemic falciparum malaria exposed individuals are subject to repeated infective mosquito bites almost throughout the year from birth onward. Such hyperendemic conditions occur in much of tropical Africa. The incidence of infection rises to almost 100% in children above 1 year of age and falls only slowly to about 50% in adult life as immunity is gradually acquired (e.g., Christophers, 1924; Barber and Olinger, 1931; Davidson and Draper, 1953; Muirhead-Thomson, 1954). The mean density of parasites in the blood of patently infected individuals is generally greatest, however, in children between 6 months and 4 years of age and is on the order of 20–100 times greater than the mean parasite density in adults (e.g., Davidson and Draper, 1953).

B. Production, Maturation, and Longevity of Gametocytes of *Plasmodium falciparum*

The circumstances under which gametocytes of *P. falciparum* are produced are not understood. Available evidence indicates that the rate of production of gametocytes of *P. falciparum* from asexual parasites is not constant. Direct evidence for this was obtained by Smalley (1976) who found that the percentage of rings which developed into gametocytes often varied considerably following successive rounds of schizogony by the asexual parasites. Changing rates of production of gametocytes from asexual parasites are probably controlled by conditions in the blood. Although direct evidence for this is not available, Carter and Miller (1979) have shown that gametocyte production in culture is modulated by environmental conditions. The factors influencing such differences in the rate of gametocyte production are unknown.

The pattern of gametocyte production may vary according to the origin of the blood infection. In the blood-induced infections studied by Shute and Maryon (1951) in nonimmune subjects, the first appearance of gametocytes in the peripheral blood was always 1 or 2 weeks earlier relative to the time of the first symptoms than in sporozoite-induced infections. Boyd and Kitchen (1937), on the other hand, found that the gametocytes of *P. falciparum* appeared at the same time relative to the onset of asexual parasitemia in both sporozoite- and blood-induced infections.

Development of the gametocytes of *P. falciparum* from the young ring to the morphologically mature parasite takes about 10 days (Smalley, 1976; Jensen, 1979). While still in the late ring stage, the young gametocytes become seques-tered in the blood spaces of the spleen and bone marrow (e.g., Marchiafava and Bignami, 1892; Garnham, 1931; Thomson and Robertson, 1935) and reappear in the peripheral circulation as morphologically mature froms or "crescents" only after completion of their 10-day period of development. The gametocytes con-tinue to circulate with an exponential half-life of 3–4 days (Smalley and Sinden, 1977); however, a significant proportion may survive for up to 2–3 weeks (see also Jeffery and Eyles, 1955). In contrast, mature gametocytes of *P. vivax* are present in the peripheral blood within 1 or 2 days of the asexual parasites (Boyd and Kitchen, 1937). The gametocytes of this species are almost certainly short-lived, having a life span of not more than 2–3 days after reaching maturity (Jeffery, 1958).

In blood-induced infections of *P. falciparum* in nonimmune subjects, gameto-cytes are first detectable in the peripheral circulation about 10–14 days after the first appearance of the asexual parasites (Boyd and Kitchen, 1937; Jeffery and Eyles, 1955; Garnham, 1966). The time of appearance of the gametocytes after the first attack, and also following subsequent symptomatic attacks, usually coincides with a period of remission. The gametocytes, however, are clearly little affected by the mechanisms responsible for the rapid removal of the asexual parasites. Low numbers of gametocytes continue to circulate for up to 1 year or even longer after the first acute attack (Jeffery and Eyles, 1954, 1955).

In areas where *P. falciparum* malaria is endemic the mean density of the gametocytes in any group is usually closely related to the mean density of the asexual parasites (e.g., Christophers, 1924; Barber and Olinger, 1931; Thomson, 1935). Thus, nonimmune individuals such as children 6 months to 2 years of age and immigrants from nonmalarious regions not only have the highest parasitemias but also carry the highest densities of gametocytes. Nevertheless, even among adults a significant proportion, on the order of 5%, may at any time carry low densities of gametocytes in areas where *P. falciparum* is hyperendemic (e.g., Muirhead-Thomson, 1954).

C. Infectiousness of *Plasmodium falciparum* Infections to Mosquitoes

1. The Human Reservoir of Infection

The two important questions concerning the human reservoir of malarial infec-tion are (1) who are the individuals comprising the reservoir? (2) What are the circumstances which determine their infectiousness to mosquitoes.

Given the presence of mature gametocytes in the peripheral blood, a suitable starting point is to establish the minimum density of gametocytes capable of infecting mosquitoes—the threshold density. A survey of the results of studies carried out by feeding mosquitoes on *P. falciparum* infections in individuals ranging from experimentally infected nonimmunes to individuals of all ages exposed to holoendemic malaria indicate that this threshold is remarkably low (e.g., Darling, 1912; Kliger and Mer, 1937; Robertson, 1945; Jeffery and Eyles, 1955; Young *et al.*, 1948; Muirhead-Thomson and Mercier, 1952; Muirhead-Thomson, 1954). In general, a gametocyte density in the blood of $1–10/\text{mm}^3$ is infectious to mosquitoes in 5–20% of cases. This result has been obtained with a variety of vector species with *P. falciparum* infections in Europe, Asia, Africa, and the Americas. As the density of gametocytes rises, the proportion of cases infectious to mosquitoes rises to a maximum at densities recorded as about 1000 gametocytes/mm³ (Jeffery and Eyles, 1955; Boyd *et al.*, 1935; Rutledge *et al.*, 1969). In most circumstances, the majority of cases are infectious to mosquitoes at densities on the order of 100 gametocytes/mm³. The threshold of infectivity for gametocytes of *P. vivax* has been recorded at less than 10/mm³ (Boyd and Kitchen, 1937).

In spite of the extraordinarily low threshold density of gametocytes required to infect mosquitoes, the density of gametocytes in the blood is a poor indication of the infectiousness of an individual to mosquitoes. Discrepancies between gametocyte density and infectiousness occur in individuals experiencing their first malarial infection (Jeffery and Eyles, 1955) but appear to be more frequent in individuals who may have experienced several infections. Rutledge *et al.* (1969) found that 8 of 32 individuals exposed to natural *P. falciparum* infection in Thailand failed to infect mosquitoes while circulating gametocytes at densities greater than 1000/mm³. Individuals previously infectious to mosquitoes may become noninfectious, even though circulating an apparently adequate density of gametocytes (Muirhead-Thomson and Mercier, 1952). Certain individuals fail to infect mosquitoes at any time regardless of gametocyte density (Muirhead-Thomson and Mercier, 1952; McCarthy *et al.*, 1978).

The basis of such noninfectiousness of gametocyte carriers is entirely unknown. The only agents known to prevent the infectivity of gametocytes of human malaria to mosquitoes are certain antimalarial drugs (see discussion below). Presumably these were not used in the instances of noninfectiousness referred to above. Positive evidence for the role of immunity in this phenomenon has not so far been forthcoming (see discussion below), although this possibility must remain an open question. Circadian changes in the infectivity of gametocytes of *P. falciparum* proposed by Hawking *et al.* (1971) could not be demonstrated by Bray *et al.* (1976). The only natural circumstances for which there is evidence for an association with reduced infectivity of gametocytes of *P. falciparum* are high asexual parasitemias. Thus, Rutledge *et al.* (1969) found that the infectiousness of gametocyte carriers to mosquitoes tended to fall as the density of the asexual parasites rose above about 1000/mm³ (equivalent to about 0.3% parasitemia). Although the reduction in infectiousness would probably be even higher at greater asexual parasite densities, such effects are not likely to account for total noninfectious cases. Eyles *et al.* (1948) found that, at equivalent gametocyte densities in *P. vivax* infections, asymptomatic carriers tended to be more infectious to mosquitoes than symptomatic carriers. Discrepant ratios of sexes of gametocytes, normally on the order of one male gametocyte to three to five females, were not involved in the cases of noninfectiousness studied by Muirhead-Thomson and Mercier (1952).

Given the presence of at least some gametocytes in the blood, the circumstances under which an individual is infectious to mosquitoes are, therefore, highly variable and generally unpredictable. Who, then, are the individuals infectious to mosquitoes and when are they infectious? In nonimmunes experiencing their first attack of *P. falciparum* malaria, the time of first infectiousness to mosquitoes occurs usually 10–15 days after the first appearance of asexual parasites in the blood (Jeffery and Eyles, 1955; Boyd and Kitchen, 1937). Gametocytes, however, are often detectable at apparently infectious densities 1- or 2 days before this. According to Jeffery and Eyles (1955), this slight delay in infectiousness is due to a period required for complete maturation of the gametocytes in the peripheral blood. The continuing presence of a high, although at this stage of infection usually declining, density of asexual parasites could also contribute to early failure of the gametocytes to infect mosquitoes. In any event, shortly after the first appearance of the gametocytes almost 100% of the nonimmunes studied by Jeffery and Eyles were infectious to mosquitoes and remained so for about 1 month. During subsequent recurrent bouts of asexual parasitemia and clinical symptoms the percentage of cases infectious at any time fell to about 50% by the end of the third month. Even 1 year after the beginning of infection up to 20% of cases remained infectious to mosquitoes, although by this time the percentage was rapidly approaching zero as densities of both asexual parasites and gametocytes fell to undetectable levels. Although gametocyte densities were high (usually greater than $200/mm^3$) during the first month of infection, they were much lower and approached the threshold of infectivity to mosquitoes during the greater period of infectiousness.

The infectiousness of individuals living under conditions of endemic *P. falciparum* malaria has been studied by a number of workers including Barber and Olinger (1931), Robertson (1945), Young *et al.* (1948), Muirhead-Thomson and Mercier (1952), Muirhead-Thomson (1954, 1957), and Rutledge *et al.* (1969). The studies of Muirhead-Thomson (1954, 1957) in particular are informative in illustrating the nature of the human reservoir of infection in populations exposed to hyperendemic *P. falciparum*. These studies were conducted in two similar areas of intense transmission of *P. falciparum* in Ghana (1954) and in Liberia (1957).

In the study in Ghana, the incidence of sexual and asexual parasitemia in various age groups was determined using techniques capable of detecting densities as low as one parasite per cubic millimeter. The incidence of asexual parasites, already 86% in infants less than 1 year of age, reached 100% in children between 1 and 5 years of age and fell slowly through later childhood and adolescence to about 50% in individuals above 15 years of age (Table I). Such figures are characteristic of hyperendemic malaria. The corresponding gametocyte rates were about 40% in infants less than 1 year of age, falling to 26% between 1 and 5 years, to 12–15% between 5 and 15 years, and to about 6% in later life.

In a subsequent study in Liberia, Muirhead-Thomson (1957) set out to determine the infectiousness of different age groups to mosquitoes under similar

TABLE I

Parameters Relating to the Infectiousness of Different Age Groups to Mosquitoes in Human Populations Exposed to Hyperendemic *Plasmodium falciparum* in Africa and the Contribution of Each Age Group to the Human Reservoir of Infection

Age (years)	Percentage of human population represented by each age group[a]	Percentage of individuals with asexual parasites in their blood ($>1/mm^3$)[b]	Percentage of individuals with gametocytes in their blood ($>1/mm^3$)[b]	Percentage of individuals infectious to mosquitoes[c]	Percentage of mosquitoes infected after feeding on infectious individuals[c]	Mean no. of oocysts per gut in infected mosquitoes[c]	Contribution of each age group to human reservoir of infection (expressed as % of total human population)[a,c]
0–1	3	87	40	ND	ND	ND	<3
1–5	12	100	26	28	19	2.0	3
5–15	25	80	13	12	24	2.0	3
Above 15	60	48	6	6	19	3.2	3
							$\sum$ = ~10 = total human reservoir of infection

[a] Data derived from Kuczynski (1948).
[b] Data derived from Muirhead-Thomson (1954).
[c] Data derived from Muirhead-Thomson (1957).

conditions of hyperendemic malaria. His survey, extending over a 12-month period, involved feeding *Anopheles gambiae* on randomly selected members of the native population regardless of parasitemia or gametocytemia. While no feedings were made on infants less than 1 year of age, 28% of children between 1 and 5 years, 12% of those between 5 and 15 years, and 6% of adults above 15 years of age were found to be infectious to mosquitoes (Table 1). Thus, the percentage of each age group infectious to mosquitoes corresponded closely to the percentage found to be carrying gametocytes at any detectable density in the previous study (Muirhead-Thomson, 1954).

When account was taken of the percentage of the population represented by each of the age groups considered [based on data from a demographic survey of West Africa (Kuczynski, 1948), the results of Muirhead-Thomson (1957) indicated that the different age groups contributed about equally to the total number of infectious individuals in the population. For each age group, this contribution represented about 3% of the total population (Table I). Altogether, about 10% of the population was infectious to mosquitoes at any time (seasonal variations were not taken into account). Although not included in this survey, infants less than 1 year of age were no doubt highly infectious to mosquitoes. However, at about 3% of the total human population this group could hardly have contributed much more than any of the older age groups to the total reservoir of infection and probably contributed rather less.

Among mosquitoes feeding upon infectious individuals the percentage which became infected and the mean density of oocysts per infected mosquito were almost identical for each age group, being about 20% and two to three per gut, respectively (Table I); the rate of conversion to sporozoites did not decline with age. Thus, infectious individuals in different age groups infected a similar percentage of mosquitoes which fed upon them; moreover, the mosquitoes acquired gut and gland infections of similar densities. Such results imply that the epidemiological significance of an infectious individual does not depend upon his or her age.

It appears, therefore, that *P. falciparum* gametocyte carriers extend through all age groups under conditions of endemic malaria and that such carriers are more-or-less equally infectious to mosquitoes regardless of age or immune status. In hyperendemic *P. falciparum,* gametocyte densities in carriers of any age are generally less than $100/mm^3$ and commonly approach the threshold of infectiousness (e.g., Muirhead-Thomson, 1954; Davidson and Draper, 1953). Thus, the majority of individuals infectious to mosquitoes under conditions of intense transmission are those with low and often near-threshold densities of gametocytes; most such individuals, at least those above a few years of age, are also probably clinically asymptomatic during the greater period of infectiousness. Asymptomatic low-density gametocyte carriers were implicated as the main human reservoir of *P. falciparum* under conditions of moderate endemicity in South Carolina (Young *et al.*, 1948). Likewise, in the studies of Jeffery and Eyles (1955) on nonimmune subjects the greater period of infectiousness occurred at low gametocyte densities in the absence of clinical symptoms.

2. Vector Susceptibility

A complete analysis of infectiousness of the human host in malaria should take into account the susceptibility of the anopheline vectors to becoming infected and their capacity to transmit the disease to other human beings. Such an analysis would involve an extensive discussion of anopheline bionomics and behavior in relation to the extrinsic phase of development of the malaria parasite (see Mac-Donald, 1973) and is beyond the scope of this chapter. It is important to point out, however, that the human reservoir of infection is not only a function of the distribution of gametocyte densities in different sections of the population and of other characteristics of the human host which determine infectiousness. The true human reservoir of infection is also determined by the degree of exposure of the human population to local anophelines and the many biological characteristics of the mosquitoes which determine their vectorial capacity.

For example, even moderate differences in the threshold density of gametocytes to which different anopheline populations were susceptible could significantly affect the size and distribution of the human population comprising the reservoir of infection. A vector population for which the threshold density was rather high would tend to eliminate low-density carriers from the reservoir of infection; a vector susceptible to a low threshold density, on the other hand, would extend the effective size of the human reservoir of infection. A comparison of the results of various studies reported in the literature indicates that such differences in the gametocyte threshold of susceptibility may occur. Thus, in the studies of Barber and Olinger (1931) the threshold density of gametocytes for infecting *A. gambiae* in a region of hyperendemic *P. falciparum* in Africa appears to have been on the order of 100 gametocytes/mm³. This threshold is at least 10 times greater than that implied in many other studies on *A. gambiae* or other anopheline species.

Clearly other aspects of the human–parasite–anopheline relationship influence the nature of the true human reservoir of infection, including behavioral aspects such as anopheline biting preferences for different age groups, human living conditions, and behavior patterns including the use of antimalarial drugs and perhaps, ultimately, of antimalarial vaccines.

3. Immunity

The gametocytes of *P. falciparum* demonstrate a remarkable capacity for evading destruction by the immune system of the human host. Not only are they able to survive in the peripheral circulation for up to 2–3 weeks but frequently do so at a time when the asexual stages are being vigorously destroyed by the host's immune clearance mechanisms. Moreover, their early development over a 10-day period in the spleen and bone marrow proceeds without apparent disruption by the actively developing immune response to the asexual parasites. In accordance with these observations, Cohen *et al.* (1961) demonstrated that γ-globulin collected from hyperimmune individuals exposed to holoendemic malaria failed to remove the gametocytes of *P. falciparum* when inoculated into heavily infected children, although the asexual parasites were rapidly cleared from the circulation. While gametocyte densities decline with the age of the human host in populations exposed to endemic malaria, they do so at a rate similar to that of the asexual parasites (e.g., Christophers, 1924). There is, therefore, no reason to suppose that increasing immunity acquired with age has any effect on either the rate of gametocyte production from the asexual parasites or the longevity of the gametocytes of *P. falciparum*.

As already discussed, the threshold density of gametocytes and the proportion of gametocyte carriers infectious to mosquitoes are generally much the same under almost all circumstances regardless of age or immune status. This statement requires some qualification, however, in view of the erratic infectiousness of many carriers of high gametocyte densities, including a significant minority who are apparently totally noninfectious to mosquitoes. Although such noninfectious cases are observed among young children as well as among adults (Muirhead-Thomson and Mercier, 1952; Rutledge *et al.*, 1969), they appear to occur more frequently among semiimmune individuals (Rutledge *et al.*, 1969; McCarthy *et al.*, 1978) than among nonimmunes in the early stages of their first *P. falciparum* infection (Jeffery and Eyles, 1955). The possible involvement of some form of immune mechanism in the reduction in the infectiousness of such individuals to mosquitoes cannot be excluded.

Several studies have demonstrated that antibodies to the gametocytes of *P. falciparum* may be present in the serum of semiimmune individuals. The first such report was that by Voller and Bray (1962). Using fluorescein-tagged antibody (FA) these workers demonstrated high titers of antigametocyte antibody in the sera of two Liberians. More recently, Smalley and Sinden (1977), using the FA technique, found antigametocyte antibodies in the serum of two out of seven Gambians infected with *P. falciparum*. No relationship was found, however, between the presence of antigametocyte antibody and either the rate of disappearance of the gametocytes from the circulation or their infectivity to mosquitoes.

Our studies using the FA technique demonstrated the presence of antibodies to gametocytes and microgametes of *P. falciparum* in 37 out of 63 serum samples drawn from Gambians ranging in age from neonates to 73 years (Carter, *et al.*, 1980). Titers against air-dried gametocytes and microgametes were identical or almost so for all sera tested and ranged from 1 : 20 to greater than 1 : 5000. The near identity of titers to gametocytes and microgametes suggests that the antigens recognized were largely similar in both these stages of the sexual parasites. In contrast, titers to air-dried asexual parasites were invariably greater than or equal to, but never less than, those of the same serum against the sexual stages. These results suggested that many antisera recognized antigens specific to the asexual parasites in addition to others probably shared by both stages. There was no indication that any sera recognized antigens unique to the sexual parasites.

A small selection of sera with high FA titers against air-dried parasites were tested against living parasites in wet preparations. With such preparations, high-titer sera reacted strongly to extracellular merozoites (but not to RBCs infected with trophozoites). In contrast, sera with high FA titers to air-dried gametocytes and microgametes failed to react with live extracellular microgametes (or intracellular gametocytes) in wet preparations. These results are consistent with the view that the sera which gave positive reactions against air-dried gametes recognized internal antigens of these stages (exposed by the drying process) but had no specificity for surface antigens of the microgametes in living wet preparations.

The sera were further tested for their effects on the behavior of microgametes of *P. falciparum in vitro* and on the infectivity of gametocytes presented to *A. gambiae* mosquitoes through membranes. Compared to normal serum, from nonimmune American donors, none of the Gambian sera had a very pronounced effect on the behavior of microgametes of *P. falciparum*. Of five Gambian sera tested, all led to moderate suppression of oocyst densities in mosquitoes compared to the nonimmune sera. There was, however, no correlation between the level of reduction and the FA antibody titers against the sexual stages. In no instance was the degree of suppression adequate to account for the total noninfectiousness to mosquitoes found in certain gametocyte carriers discussed above.

Thus, while most individuals living in areas of hyperendemic malaria circulate high titers of antimalarial antibodies as measured by the FA test, there is no evidence that these antibodies have stage specificity for the extracellular gametes of the parasite or that they are detrimental to the capacity of the gametes to infect mosquitoes.

Although we found no evidence for the natural occurrence of antibodies to stage-specific antigens of gametes of *P. falciparum,* these stages appeared to be vulnerable, nevertheless, to phagocytosis following their release into the blood of partially immune individuals. Extracellular gametocytes including those undergoing exflagellation appeared to be the only sexual stages ingested by the phagocytes; neither the free-swimming microgametes (Ross, 1923) not the intracellular gametocytes (Sinden and Smalley, 1976) were affected. The proportion of exflagellating gametocytes of *P. falciparum* ingested by phagocytes was much reduced within the mosquito midgut compared to that recorded *in vitro* (Sinden and Smalley, 1976). Activation of the phagocytic cells, which can migrate more than 40 μm to reach the extracellular gametocytes, may be in response to internal antigens of the parasitized cell released during the process of emergence and exflagellation. Indeed, in air-dried preparations of *P. falciparum,* we observed exflagellating gametocytes surrounded by a cloud of material that gave a highly positive FA reaction with sera positive for the gametocytes themselves (Carter *et al.,* 1980). We have interpreted this material to be parasite antigen released during gametogenesis.

The amount of phagocytosis recorded in mosquitoes by Sinden and Smalley (1976) involved less than 20% of all gametocytes. The phenomenon seems unlikely, therefore, to be of major importance in reducing infectivity of gameto-cytes to mosquitoes. Rutledge *et al.* (1969) found no relationship between the amount of phagocytosis of gametocytes within the mosquito and the infectious-ness of the human subject.

4. Chemotherapy

Antimalarial drugs which are effective to one degree or another against the asexual stages of human malaria parasites differ considerably in their effects on the viability and infectivity of the gametocytes.

8-Aminoquinolines, such as pamaquine and primaquine, are a class of antima-larials which exert a parasitocidal effect against all stages of plasmodium in the vertebrate host. Lethal to both dividing and nondividing stages, these drugs probably represent a form of ''cytoplasmic'' poison. Pamaquine and primaquine rapidly eliminate the infectiousness to mosquitoes of *P. falciparum* gametocytes (Barber *et al.,* 1929; Mackerras and Ercole, 1949b; Jeffery *et al.,* 1956; Burgess and Bray, 1961; Rieckmann *et al.,* 1968, 1969), although primaquine was re-ported by Mackerras and Ercole (1949a) to be somewhat less effective against gametocytes of *P. vivax.* In the studies of Jeffery *et al.* (1956) the gametocytes of *P. falciparum* disappeared from the circulation within 2–4 days after primaquine therapy began. Infectiousness to mosquitoes was eliminated even more rapidly, however, usually within 6–12 hours after the first administration of the drug. Rapid suppression of gametocyte infectivity by 8-aminoquinolines was not associated with the inability of the gametocytes to undergo gametogenesis or fertilization (Barber *et al.,* 1929; Mackerras and Ercole, 1949b). Nor did primaquine affect sporogonic development if administered to mosquitoes after feeding on blood carrying gametocytes of *P. vivax* (Terzian *et al.,* 1968). These drugs, therefore, are probably not sporontocidal (i.e., acting after ingestion by the mosquito to prevent sporogonic development) but exert their effects on the infectivity of the gametocytes while they are still in the circulating blood. As a result of such exposure, the gametocytes are unable to establish the sporogonic phase of development in the mosquito.

Quinine and chloroquine are highly effective antimalarials which are, never-theless, apparently toxic only to forms of the parasite dependent upon hemoglo-bin digestion, i.e., asexual blood stage parasites and gametocytes during the early stages of their growth.

For a considerable part of their early development, up to about 5 or 6 days, the gametocytes of *P. falciparum* are susceptible to destruction by chloroquine (Jeffery *et al.*, 1956; Smalley, 1977). Following maturation, however, neither the longevity nor the infectivity of *P. falciparum* gametocytes was effected by chloroquine (Jeffery *et al.*, 1956; Rieckmann *et al.*, 1969; Smalley and Sinden, 1977), quinine (Barber *et al.*, 1929; Mackerras and Ercole, 1949b), or mepacrine (Mackerras and Ercole, 1949b). Quinine and mepacrine were also ineffective against the mature gametocytes of *P. vivax* (Mackerras and Ercole, 1949a). Gametocytes of this species continued to circulate and were infective to mosquitoes in the presence of these drugs for 2–3 days following the disappearance of the asexual parasites. Quinine, chloroquine, and mepacrine failed to prevent sporogonic development when fed to mosquitoes following ingestion of blood carrying gametocytes of *P. vivax* (Terzian *et al.*, 1968).

While effective in destroying gametocytes during their early development, quinine and 4-aminoquinolines are, therefore, without effect on either the longevity or the infectivity of mature gametocytes of human malaria parasites.

Among the most effective antimalarial compounds are specific inhibitors of the plasmodial dihydrofolate reductase such as pyrimethamine and proguanil. By blocking an essential pathway in the parasite leading to the formation of precursors of DNA, these drugs are effective against all stages of the parasite involved in DNA synthesis. Drugs of this group lead to rapid elimination of the asexual blood stages of *P. vivax* and *P. falciparum*.

Proguanil appears to exert no effect on the maturation or longevity of gametocytes of either *P. falciparum* or *P. vivax* after a very early point in their development (Mackerras and Ercole, 1947). Thus, following effective treatment with paludrine (proguanil) of rising parasitemia of *P. falciparum*, the number of mature, healthy gametocytes reached a peak 10–12 days after the beginning of therapy; the gametocytes persisted for about 30 days thereafter. Healthy gametocytes of *P. vivax* also continued to increase in number for 1 day after the beginning of effective therapy against the asexual stages and continued to circulate for 3–4 days thereafter.

Pyrimethamine is ineffective in destroying mature gametocytes of either *P. vivax* or *P. falciparum* but may be somewhat more effective than proguanil against the earliest forms of the gametocytes. Thus, Srivastava *et al.* (1953) found that gametocytes of *P. vivax* persisted in undiminished numbers during the first 2 days of pyrimethamine therapy, during which time the asexual parasites were being rapidly cleared; by the third day, however, the gametocytes were themselves largely eliminated. The same workers found that gametocytes of *P. falciparum* reached their peak within 5–6 days after the initiation of treatment with pyrimethamine (or 10–12 days following proquanil), suggesting that early forms of the gametocytes of this species may have been eliminated by the drug.

In spite of the inability of pyrimethamine and proquanil to eliminate gametocytes of either *P. vivax* or *P. falciparum,* these drugs are, nevertheless, highly effective in suppressing their infectivity to mosquitoes. Both pyrimethamine (Foy and Kondi, 1952; Shute and Maryon, 1954; Jeffery *et al.,* 1956) and proguanil (Fairley, 1946; Mackerras and Ercole, 1947; Ramakrishnan *et al.,* 1952) are effective in suppressing the infectivity of gametocytes of *P. falciparum* and *P. vivax* within 1–2 hours of administration. After a single dose of proguanil, suppression of the infectivity of gametocytes of *P. falciparum* was of short duration, 1–3 days; higher drug doses or prolonged courses of treatment extended the effect for up to 10 days after the termination of treatment (Fairley, 1946; Mackerras and Ercole, 1947). Proguanil had no effect on the ability of gameto- cytes of *P. falciparum* to undergo exflagellation or fertilization (Fairley, 1946). Both pyrimethamine and proguanil, unlike 8-aminoquinolines, suppressed sporogonic development of *P. vivax* when administered to mosquitoes following a blood meal (Terzian *et al.,* 1968).

Dihydrofolate reductase inhibitors therefore, appear to be truly sporontocidal but not gametocytocidal. Gametocytes of *P. falciparum* are neither destroyed nor rendered permanently noninfectious by the presence of these drugs in the bloodstream; their effect is probably exerted within the mosquito itself following the ingestion of gametocytes and drug together. It is interesting to note that strains of *P. falciparum* whose asexual stages are resistant to pyrimethamine are also resistant to its sporontocidal action (Laing, 1956; Burgess and Young, 1959).

Competitive inhibitors of *p*-aminobenzoic acid metabolism such as sulfones and sulfonamides are comparatively weak schizontocidal antimalarials. Where tested, such compounds have been found to exert no effect on either the viability (Findlay *et al.,* 1946; Laing, 1965; Powell *et al.,* 1967) or the infectivity of gametocytes of human malarias to mosquitoes (Laing, 1965; Terzian *et al.,* 1968).

VI. CONCLUSIONS

The primary components of infectiousness of the vertebrate host in malaria are the presence of gametocytes in the peripheral blood, their infectivity to mosquitoes, and the susceptibility of the prevalent vectors to infection.

Patterns of gametocyte production, maturation time, and longevity in the peripheral circulation vary according to the species of parasite and the nature of the infection. In species such as *P. gallinaceum* and *P. yoelii,* gametocytes are known to be formed directly from exoerythrocytic merozoites following sporozoite-induced infection, and gametocyte production continues from the earliest stage of the blood infection. There is some evidence, however, that with certain species of parasite there may be a delay of several days during the early phase of blood infection before gametocytes are formed in appreciable numbers following sporozoite inoculation, e.g., *P. cynomolgi* and *P. falciparum*. In blood-induced infections, gametocyte production is in progress from an early time in the infection in most species, e.g., *P. gallinaceum, P. yoelii, P. knowlesi, P. cynomolgi,* and *P. falciparum.*

Gametocytes of *P. gallinaceum, P. yoelii,* and *P. knowlesi* mature rapidly, within 1–2 days, and remain infectious for less than 12 hours. Gametocytes of *P. cynomolgi* appear to require a little longer to reach maturity, about 4 days, but their infectious life is also short, being less than 1 day. In *P. vivax,* gametocyte maturation and infectious life probably occupy not more than 3 or 4 days. Rapid maturation and short-lived infectivity thus appear to be characteristic of the gametocytes of most malaria parasites. Those of *P. falciparum,* however, are exceptional. Gametocytes of this species require 10 days to reach maturity. Maturation takes place in the blood spaces of the spleen and bone marrow, and only the mature forms are generally found in the peripheral blood. After their appearance in the peripheral blood, mature gametocytes remain infective for many days or weeks. During this time and from an early stage in their development they appear to be unaffected by immune mechanisms capable of rapidly clearing the asexual parasites from the circulation.

Gametocytes of *P. falciparum* and *P. vivax* may be infectious to mosquitoes at densities as low as 1–10/mm^3 of blood; maximum infectiousness is reached between 100 and 1000/mm^3. Nevertheless, even at high densities, the infectiousness of gametocyte carriers to mosquitoes is exceedingly variable for reasons which are generally obscure. High asexual parasitemias tend to be associated with impaired infectivity of gametocytes in several species, e.g., *P. gallinaceum, P. yoelii, P. knowlesi,* and *P. falciparum.* Such impairment becomes detectable as parasitemias rise above 0.1–1%, and gametocyte infectivity may be severely curtailed at parasitemias above 20–30%. The effect seems to be associated with toxic or inhibitory conditions produced in the blood at high parasitemias but does not appear to involve immune mechanisms mediated by antibodies specific to the sexual stages of the parasites. Indeed, available evidence suggests that neither direct antibody-mediated mechanisms nor phagocytosis of sexual stages after their release in the mosquito midgut are significantly involved in reducing the infectivity of gametocytes under natural circumstances. Nevertheless, in *P. falciparum* malaria, the incidence of noninfectious gametocyte carriers appears to be higher among semiimmune individuals than among those experiencing their first infection. A role for immunity in modulating the infectivity of gametocytes under natural conditions of malaria transmission cannot, therefore, be excluded.

In human populations exposed to endemic *P. falciparum* malaria, gametocyte densities decline with age in association with lower asexual parasitemias and increasing immunity to the asexual stages. Even under hyperendemic conditions, however, gametocyte densities in the oldest and most immune sections of the population are often sufficient to be infectious to mosquitoes. Thus, although young children having the lowest levels of immunity and highest parasitemias are unquestionably the most infectious group, the human reservoir of infection extends through all age groups among which the infectious and generally asymptomatic adults are an important part. Under conditions of less intense transmission, the degree of immunity in the adult population is correspondingly lower, and the contribution of this group to the reservoir of infection increases. In stable endemic malaria, the human reservoir of infection consists primarily of asymptomatic carriers with low gametocyte densities regardless of the intensity of transmission. In hyperendemic malaria, the reservoir appears to represent about 10% of the total population at any time.

The infectivity of gametocytes may be suppressed artificially by means of chemotherapy or by appropriate forms of immunization. Certain antimalarial drugs are either directly gametocytocidal (8-aminoquinolines such as primaquine and pamaquine) or sporontocidal, i.e., prevent development of the parasites within the mosquito (e.g., pyrimethamine and proguanil). Quinine, chloroquine, and mepacrine, while destroying gametocytes of *P. falciparum* during their earlier stages of development, have no effect on the longevity or infectivity of mature gametocytes.

Immunization with preparations containing gametes of the malaria parasite leads to highly effective suppression of infectiousness to mosquitoes during subsequent blood infection in three laboratory systems, *P. gallinaceum* in chickens, *P. knowlesi* in the rhesus monkey, and *P. yoelii* in the laboratory mouse. Such immunization results in the elaboration of gamete-specific antibodies. When a mosquito ingests gametocyte-carrying blood containing such antibodies, the gametes are neutralized in the mosquito midgut almost immediately following their release during gametogenesis; fertilization is prevented, and the infection in the mosquito is sterilized. The immunity appears to be specific to the sexual stage. Monkeys immunized with preparations of asexual parasites alone do not produce antigamete antibodies, and their sera do not reduce the infectivity of gametocytes to mosquitoes. Nevertheless, in immunized chickens, blood infection leads to a marked elevation of titers of antigamete antibodies. It is not yet known whether blood infection has a similar effect in immunized monkeys.

The primary established difference between gamete immunization in chickens and mice, on the one hand, and in monkeys on the other, is the requirement for an adjuvant in the latter. Chickens and mice may be effectively immunized without adjuvant by intravenous inoculation of gametes of *P. gallinaceum* and *P. yoelii,* respectively. This stratagem is entirely ineffective in immunizing rhesus monkeys with gametes of *P. knowlesi;* in this system the most effective procedure involves intramuscular inoculation with Freund's complete adjuvant.

REFERENCES

Adler, S., and Tchernomoretz, I. (1943). The extra-erythrocytic origin of gametocytes of *Plasmodium gallinaceum*. Brumpt, 1935. *Ann. Trop. Med. Parasitol.* **37**, 148–151.

Barber, M. A., and Olinger, M. J. (1931). Studies on malaria in southern Nigeria. *Ann. Trop. Med. Parasitol.* **25**, 461–508.

Barber, M. A., Komp, W. H. W., and Newman, B. M. (1929). The effect of small doses of plasmochin on the viability of gametocytes of malaria as measured by mosquito infections. *Public Health Rep.* **44**, 1409–1421.

Bishop, A. (1955). Problems concerned with gametogenesis in Haemosporidiidea, with particular reference to the genus *Plasmodium*. *Parasitology* **45**, 163–185.

Bishop, A., and McConnachie, E. W. (1960). Further observations on the *in vitro* development of the gametocytes of *Plasmodium gallinaceum*. *Parasitology* **50**, 431–448.

Boyd, M. F., and Kitchen, S. F. (1937). On the infectiousness of patients infected with *Plasmodium vivax* and *Plasmodium falciparum*. *Am. J. Trop. Med.* **17**, 253–262.

Boyd, M. F., Stratman-Thomas, W. K., and Kitchen, S. F. (1935). On the relative susceptibility of *Anopheles quadrimaculatus* to *P. vivax* and *P. falciparum*. *Am. J. Trop. Med.* **15**, 485–493.

Bray, R. S., McCrae, A. W. R., and Smalley, M. E. (1976). Lack of a circadian rhythm in the ability of the gametocytes of *Plasmodium falciparum* to infect *Anopheles gambiae*. *Int. J. Parasitol.* **6**, 399–401.

Brown, I. N. (1969). Immunological aspects of malaria infection. *Adv. Immunol.* **11**, 267–349.

Brown, K. N. (1977). Antigenic variation in malaria. *In* "Immunity to Blood Parasites of Animals and Man" (L. H. Miller, J. A. Pino, and J. J. McKelvey, Jr., eds.), Chapter 1, pp. 5–25. Plenum, New York.

Burgess, R. W. and Bray, R. S. (1961). The effect of a single dose of primaquine on the gametocytes, gametogony and sporogony of *Laverania falcipara*. *Bull. W.H.O.* **24**, 451–456.

Burgess, R. W., and Young, M. D. (1959). The development of pyrimethamine resistance by *Plasmodium falciparum*. *Bull. W.H.O.* **20**, 37–46.

Cantrell, W., and Jordan, H. B. (1946). Changes in the infectiousness of gametocytes during the course of *Plasmodium gallinaceum* infections. *J. Infect. Dis.* **78**, 153–159.

Carter, R., and Chen, D. H. (1976). Malaria transmission blocked by immunization with gametes of the malaria parasite. *Nature (London)* **263**, 57–60.

Carter, R., and Diggs, C. (1977). Plasmodia of rodents. *In* "Parasitic Protozoa" (J. P. Kreier, ed.), Vol. 3, Chapter 27, pp. 368, 430–432. Academic Press, New York.

Carter, R., and Miller, L. H. (1979). A method for the study of gametocytogenesis by *Plasmodium falciparum* in culture: Evidence for environmental modulation of gametocytogenesis. *Bull. W.H.O.*, 57, Suppl. 1, 38–67.

Carter, R., Gwadz, R. W. and McAuliffe, F. M. (1979a). *Plasmodium gallinaceum:* Transmission blocking immunity in chickens. I. Comparative immunogenicity of gametocyte and gamete containing preparations. *Exp. Parasitol.* **47**, 185–193.

Carter, R., Gwadz, R. W., and Green, I. (1979b). *Plasmodium gallinaceum:* Transmission blocking immunity in chickens. II. The effect of antigamete antibodies *in vitro* and *in vivo* and their elaboration during infection. *Exp. Parasitol.* **47**, 194–208.

Carter, R., Gwadz, R. W., Green, I., (1980). In preparation.

Christophers, S. R. (1924). The mechanism of immunity against malaria in communities living under hyperendemic conditions. *Indian J. Med. Res.* **12**, 273–294.

Coatney, G. R., Collins, W. E., Warren, M., and Contacos, P. G. (1971). "The Primate Malarias." U. S. Dept. of Health, Education and Welfare, Washington, D.C.

Cohen, S., McGregor, I. A., and Carrington, S. (1961). Gamma-globulin and acquired immunity to human malaria. *Nature (London)* **192**, 733-737.

Darling, S. T. (1912). "Studies in Relation to Malaria," pp. 17-24. Isthmian Canal Commission Press.

Davidson, G., and Draper, C. C. (1953). Field studies of some of the basic factors concerned in the transmission of malaria. *Trans. R. Soc. Trop. Med. Hyg.* **47**, 522-535.

Eyles, D. E. (1951). Studies on *Plasmodium gallinaceum*. I. Characteristics of the infection in the mosquito *Aedes aegypti*. *Am. J. Hyg.* **54**, 101-112.

Eyles, D. E. (1952a). Studies on *Plasmodium gallinaceum*. II. Factors in the blood of the vertebrate host influencing mosquito infection. *Am. J. Hyg.* **55**, 276-290.

Eyles, D. E. (1952b). Studies on *Plasmodium gallinaceum*. III. Factors associated with the malaria infection in the vertebrate host which influence the degree of infection in the mosquito. *Am. J. Hyg.* **55**, 386-391.

Eyles, D. E., Young, M. D., and Burgess, R. W. (1948). Studies on imported malarias. 8. Infectivity to *Anopheles quadrimaculatus* of asymptomatic *Plasmodium vivax* parasitemia. *J. Natl. Malar. Soc.* **7**, 125-133.

Fairley, N. H. (1946). Researches on Paludrine (M 4888) in malaria: An experimental investigation undertaken by the L. H. Q. medical research unit (A. I. F.), Cairns, Australia. *Trans. R. Soc. Trop. Med. Hyg.* **40**, 105-162.

Findlay, G. M., Maegraith, B. G., Markson, J. L., and Holden, J. R. (1946). Investigations in the chemotherapy of malaria in West Africa. V. Sulphonamide compounds. *Ann. Trop. Med. Parasitol.* **40**, 358-367.

Foy, H. and Kondi, A. (1952). Effect of Daraprim on the gametocytes of *Plasmodium falciparum*. *Trans. R. Soc. Trop. Med. Hyg.* **46**, 370.

Garnham, P. C. C. (1931). Observations on *Plasmodium falciparum* with special reference to the production of crescents. *Kenya East Afr. Med. J.* **8**, 2-21.

Garnham, P. C. C. (1966). "Malaria Parasites and other Haemosporidia." Blackwell, Oxford.

Garnham, P. C. C., and Powers, K. G. (1974). Periodicity of infectivity of plasmodial gametocytes: The "Hawking phenomenon." *Int. J. Parasitol.* **4**, 103-106.

Giovannola, A. (1938). Il *Plasmodium gallinaceum* Brumpt, 1935, i cosi ditti corpi *Toxoplasma*-simili el alcune inclusioni di probabile natura parassitaria ni globuli bianchi del *Gallus gallus*. *Riv. Parassitol.* **2**, 129-142.

Gwadz, R. W. (1976). Malaria: Successful immunization against the sexual stages of *Plasmodium gallinaceum*. *Science* **193**, 1150-1151.

Gwadz, R. W., and Green, I. (1978). Malaria immunization in rhesus monkeys: A vaccine effective against both the sexual and asexual stages of *Plasmodium knowlesi*. *J. Exp. Med.* **148**, 1311-1323.

Hawking, F., Worms, M. J., Gammage, K., and Goddard, P. A. (1966). The biological purpose of the blood cycle of the malaria parasite *Plasmodium cynomolgi*. *Lancet* **2**, 422-424.

Hawking, F., Worms, M. J., and Gammage, K. (1968). 24- and 48-hour cycles of malaria parasites in the blood: Their purpose, production and control. *Trans. R. Soc. Trop. Med. Hyg.* **62**, 731-765.

Hawking, F., Worms, M. J., and Gammage, K. (1969). Duration of the mature gametocytes of *P. gallinaceum*. *Trans. R. Soc. Trop. Med. Hyg.* **63**, 421.

Hawking, F., Worms, M. J. and Gammage, K. (1971). Evidence for cyclic development and short lived maturity in gametocytes of *Plasmodium falciparum*. *Trans. R. Soc. Trop. Med. Hyg.* **65**, 549-559.

Hawking, F., Gammage, K., and Worms, M. J. (1972). The asexual and sexual circadian rythms of *Plasmodium vinckei chabaudi*, of *P. berghei* and of *P. gallinaceum*. *Parasitology* **65**, 189-210.

Huff, C. G., and Marchbank, D. F. (1955). Changes in infectiousness of malarial gametocytes. I. Patterns of oocyst production in seven host-parasite combinations. *Exp. Parasitol.* **4,** 256–270.

Huff, C. G., Marchbank, D. F., and Shiroishi, T. (1958). Changes in infectiousness of malarial gametocytes. II. analysis of the possible causative factors. *Exp. Parasitol.* **7,** 399–417.

James, S. P., Nicol, W. D., and Shute, P. G. (1936). Clinical and parasitologic observations on induced malaria. *Proc. R. Soc. Med., Sect. Trop. Dis. Parasitol.* **29,** 879–894.

Jeffery, G. M. (1958). Infectivity to mosquitoes of *Plasmodium vivax* following treatment with chloroquine and other antimalarials. *Am. J. Trop. Med. Hyg.* **7,** 207–211.

Jeffery, G. M., and Eyles, D. E. (1954). The duration in the human host of infections with a Panama strain of *Plasmodium falciparum*. *Am. J. Trop. Med. Hyg.* **3,** 219–224.

Jeffery, G. M., and Eyles, D. E. (1955). Infectivity to mosquitoes of *Plasmodium falciparum* as related to gametocyte density and duration of infection. *Am. J. Trop. Med. Hyg.* **4,** 781–789.

Jeffery, G. M., Young, M. D., and Eyles, D. E. (1956). The treatment of *Plasmodium falciparum* infection with chloroquine, with a note of infectivity to mosquitoes of primaquine- and pyrimethamine-treated cases. *Am. J. Hyg.* **64,** 1–11.

Jensen, J. B. (1979). Observations on gametocytogenesis in *Plasmodium falciparum* from continuous cultures. *J. Protozool.* **26,** 129–132.

Killick-Kendrick, R., and Warren, M. (1968). Primary exoerythrocytic schizonts of a mammalian *Plasmodium* as a source of gametocytes. *Nature (London)* **220,** 191–192.

Kligler, I. J., and Mer, G. (1937). Studies on the effect of various factors on the infection rate of *Anopheles elutus* with different species of *Plasmodium*. *Ann. Trop. Med. Parasitol.* **31,** 71–83.

Kuczynski, R. R. (1948). "Demographic Survey of the British Colonial Empire," Vol. 1. Oxford Univ. Press, London and New York.

Laing, A. B. G. (1956). Proguanil resistance: Extension to the gametocytes of *Plasmodium falciparum*. *Trans. R. Soc. Trop. Med. Hyg.* **50,** 496–504.

Laing, A. B. G. (1965). Sporogony in *Plasmodium falciparum* apparently uneffected by sulphorthomidine (Fanasil). *Trans. R. Soc. Trop. Med. Hyg.* **59,** 357–358.

McCarthy, V. C., Clyde, D. F., and Woodward, W. E. (1978). *Plasmodium falciparum:* Responses of a semi-immune individual to homologous and heterologous challenges and non-infectivity of gametocytes in *Anopheles stephensi*. *Am. J. Trop. Med. Hyg.* **27,** 6–8.

Macdonald, G. (1973). "Dynamics of Tropical Disease" (L. J. Bruce-Chwatt and V. J. Glanville, eds.), Oxford Univ. Press, London and New York.

Mackerras, M. J., and Ercole, O. N. (1947). Observations on the action of Paludrine on malarial parasites. I. The action of Paludrine on *Plasmodium vivax*. II. The action of Paludrine on *Plasmodium falciparum* gametocytes. *Trans. R. Soc. Trop. Med. Hyg.* **41,** 365–376.

Mackerras, M. J., and Ercole, Q. N. (1949a). Some observations on the action of quinine, atebrin and plasmoquine on *Plasmodium vivax*. *Trans. R. Soc. Trop. Med. Hyg.* **42,** 443–454.

Mackerras, M. J., and Ercole, Q. N. (1949b). Observations on the action of quinine, atebrin and plasmoquine on the gametocytes of *Plasmodium falciparum*. *Trans. R. Soc. Trop. Med. Hyg.* **42,** 455–463.

Marchiafava, E., and Bignami, A. (1892). "Sulle febbri malariche estivo-autumnnali." E. Loescher & Co., Rome.

Mendis, K. N., and Targett, G. A. T. (1979). Immunization against gametes and asexual erythrocytic stages of rodent malaria parasite. *Nature (London)* **277,** 389–391.

Micks, D. W., de Caires, P. F., and Franco, L. B. (1948). The relationship of exflagellation in avian plasmodia to pH and immunity in the mosquito. *Am. J. Hyg.* **48,** 182–190.

Muirhead-Thomson, R. C. (1954). Factors determining the true reservoir of infection of *Plasmodium falciparum* and *Wuchereria bancrofti* in a West African village. *Trans. R. Soc. Trop. Med. Hyg.* **48,** 208–225.

Muirhead-Thomson, R. C. (1957). The malarial infectivity of an African village population to mosquitoes (*Anopheles gambiae*): A random xenodiagnostic survey. *Am. J. Trop. Med. Hyg.* **6,** 971–979.

Muirhead-Thomson, R. C., and Mercier, E. C. (1952). factors in malaria transmission by *Anopeles albimanus* in Jamaica. Part I. *Ann. Trop. Med. Parasitol.* **46,** 103–116.

Nijhout, M. M. (1979). *Plasmodium gallinaceum:* Exflagellation stimulated by a mosquito factor. *Exp. Parasitol.* **48,** 75–80.

Nijhout, M. M., and Carter, R. (1978). Gamete development in malaria parasites: Bicarbonate dependent stimulation by pH *in vitro. Parasitology,* **76,** 39–53.

Powell, R. D., DeGowin, R. L., and McNamara, J. V. (1967). Clinical experience with sulphadiazine and pyrimethamine in the treatment of persons infected with chloroquine-resistant *Plasmodium falciparum. Ann. Trop. Med. Parasitol.* **61,** 396–408.

Ramakrishnan, S. P., Young, M. D., Jeffrey, G. M., Burgess, R. W., and McLendon, S. B. (1952). The effect of single and multiple doses of Paludrine upon *Plasmodium falciparum. Am. J. Hyg.* **55,** 239–245.

Rieckmann, K. H., McNamara, J. V., Frischer, H., Stockert, T. A., Carson, P. E., and Powell, R. D. (1968). Gametocytocidal and sporontocidal effects of primaquine and of sulphadiazine with pyrimethamine in a chloroquine-resistant strain of *Plasmodium falciparum. Bull. W. H. O.* **38,** 625–632.

Rieckmann, K. H., McNamara, J. V., Kass, L., and Powell, R. D. (1969). Gametocytocidal and sporontocidal effects of primaquine upon two strains of *Plasmodium falciparum. Mil. Med.* **134,** Spec. Issue, 802–819.

Robertson, J. D. (1945). Notes on the gametocyte threshold for infection of *Anopheles gambiae* Giles, 1902, and *Anopheles melas* Theobald, 1903, in West Africa. *Ann. Trop. Med. Parasitol.* **39,** 8–10.

Ross, R. (1923). "Memoirs." Murray, London.

Rutledge, L. C., Gould, D. J., and Tantichareon, B. (1969). Factors affecting the infection of anophelines with human malaria in Thailand. *Trans. R. Soc. Trop. Med. Hyg.* **63,** 613–619.

Shute, P. G., and Maryon, M. (1951). A study of gametocytes in a West African strain of *Plasmodium falciparum. Trans. R. Soc. Trop. Med. Hyg.* **44,** 421–438.

Shute, P. G., and Maryon, M. (1954). The effect of pyrimethamine (Daraprim) on the gametocytes and oocysts of *Plasmodium falciparum* and *Plasmodium vivax. Trans. R. Soc. Trop. Med. Hyg.* **48,** 50–63.

Sinden, R. E., and Croll, N. A. (1975). Cytology and kinetics of microgametogenesis and fertilization in *Plasmodium yoelii nigeriensis. Parasitology* **70,** 53–65.

Sinden, R. E., and Smalley, M. E. (1976). Gametocytes of *Plasmodium falciparum:* Phagocytosis by leucocytes *in vivo* and *in vitro. Trans. R. Soc. Trop. Med. Hyg.* **70,** 344–345.

Smalley, M. E. (1976). *Plasmodium falciparum* gametocytogenesis *in vitro. Nature (London)* **264,** 271–272.

Smalley, M. E. (1977). *Plasmodium falciparum* gametocytes: The effect of chloroquine on their development. *Trans. R. Soc. Trop. Med. Hyg.* **71,** 526–529.

Smalley, M. E., and Sinden, R. E. (1977). *Plasmodium falciparum* gametocytes: Their longevity and infectivity. *Parasitology* **74,** 1–8.

Srivastava, R. S., Chakrabarti, A. K., and Mukherjee, S. K. (1953). Therapeutic trial of pyrimethamine (Daraprim) in human malaria. *Indian J. Malar.* **7,** 5–12.

Terzian, L. A., Stahler, N., and Dawkins, A. T., Jr. (1968). The sporogonous cycle of *Plasmodium vivax* in *Anopheles* mosquitoes as a system for evaluating the prophylactic and curative capabilities of potential antimalarial compounds. *Exp. Parasitol.* **23,** 56–66.

Thomson, J. G. (1935). Malaria in Nyasaland. *Proc. R. Soc. Med.* **28,** 391–404.

Thomson, J. G., and Robertson, A. (1935). The structure and development of *Plasmodium fal-ciparum* gametocytes in the internal organs and the peripheral circulation. *Trans. R. Soc. Trop. Med. Hyg.* **29,** 31–40.

Voller, A., and Bray, R. S. (1962). Fluorescent antibody staining as a measure of malarial antibody. *Proc. Soc. Exp. Biol. Med.* **110,** 907–910.

Wery, M. (1968). Studies on the sporogony of rodent malaria parasites. *Ann. Soc. Belge Med. Trop.* **48,** 1–137.

Young, M. D., Hardman, N. F., Burgess, R. W., Frohne, W. C., and Sabrosky, C. W. (1948). The infectivity of native malarias in South Carolina to *Anopheles quadrimaculatus. Am. J. Trop. Med.* **28,** 303–311.

Appendix 1

Prospects for Development of Vaccines against *Plasmodium falciparum* Infection

Carter L. Diggs

I. INTRODUCTION

The possibility of developing vaccines which prevent malaria, especially disease due to *Plasmodium falciparum,* has recently received increasing attention (Cohen, 1978; NMRI/USAID/WHO Workshop on the Immunology of Malaria, 1979). This increase in interest is due in part to the promising results of immunization experiments (Sadun *et al.,* 1969; Mitchell *et al.,* 1977; Siddiqui, 1977; Siddiqui *et al.,* 1978; Reese *et al.,* 1978; Wellde *et al.,* 1979) but has gained major impetus from the successful continuous cultivation of *P. falciparum in vitro* (Trager and Jensen, 1976; Haynes *et al.,* 1976), thus making the possibility

Malaria, Vol. 3.

of production of a suitable immunogen much more credible. In spite of these developments, major problems exist in the conceptualization, design, and implementation of a practical vaccination scheme. Opinions regarding the gravity and complexity of these difficulties very widely; at the extremes, there are those who feel that practical vaccines are only a few years or perhaps even months away and there are skeptics who believe that vaccination may never be practical. The purpose of this chapter is to summarize our progress in this area and to attempt the formulation of a realistic assessment of our current position.

The notion of artificial immunization against malaria was entertained during the first half of this century by a number of prominent scientists. Jules Freund, using the complete adjuvant which he developed, successfully immunized ducks against *P. lophurae* (Freund *et al.*, 1945a; Thomson *et al.*, 1947) and monkeys against *P. knowlesi* (Freund *et al.* 1945b, 1948). Another group, which included Michael Heidelberger, Manfred Mayer, and A. S. Alving (Heidelberger *et al.*, 1946a,b), attempted to immunize humans against *P. vivax* using Formalin-treated vaccine; this resulted in essentially no modification of disease on challenge.

The advent of apparently very adequate methods of malaria control inhibited work leading toward artificial immunization for a number of years. However, with the development of chloroquine-resistant *P. falciparum* (Powell *et al.*, 1963; Box *et al.*, 1963; Young *et al.*, 1963), interest was again sparked. Encouragement was engendered by such findings as the dramatic antiparasitic effect of IgG from immune Gambian adults when administered to children with *P. falciparum* infections (Cohen *et al.*, 1961). The efforts since this renaissance of interest have been well documented in a series of monographs which resulted from workshops on malaria, the first four sponsored by the United States Army (Sadun, 1964, 1966, 1969, 1972) and the two most recent by several agencies (USAID/WHO Workshops on the Biology and *in Vitro* Cultivation of Malaria Parasites, 1977; NMRI/USAID/WHO Workshop on the Immunology of Malaria, 1979). In the section to follow, a brief review of the experience to date with immunization against *P. falciparum* will be presented. Although much information of value has been acquired using nonhuman parasite models, these are considered to be less directly relevant for present purposes than the human pathogens themselves.

II. EXPERIMENTAL IMMUNIZATION AGAINST *Plasmodium falciparum* BLOOD STAGES

Immunization against *P. falciparum* blood forms was studied more than a decade ago, shortly after *Aotus trivirgatus,* the owl monkey, was demonstrated to be a useful experimental host for *P. falciparum* (Geiman and Meagher, 1967).

Following up previous work using rodent models, Sadun and his co-workers (1969) used irradiated parasitized erythrocytes as the immunogen in these studies. Owl monkeys which had been allowed to develop high parasitemia were used as donors. Parasitized erythrocytes from these animals were washed, irradiated (20 krads) using a ^{60}Co source, and administered intravenously into uninfected recipients. In these experiments it was necessary to give four injections at weekly intervals in order to induce significant immunity. These early experiments were hampered by intercurrent infection in a number of animals, but the demonstration of induced immunity was clear. Two of seven immunized animals developed no parasitemia at all, but the other five developed low-grade parasitemia and four of these eventually died. Thus three of the seven immunized animals survived at least 150 days even though low-grade parasitemia was observed in one. Thirteen control animals, four of which received irradiated normal erythrocytes, all died with high parasitemia, although one animal exhibited a delay in the development of parasitemia. It should be noted that no adjuvant was used in this study.

More recently, additional information has been obtained on artificial immunization of the owl monkey against *P. falciparum*. Mitchell *et al.* (1977) reported on the immunization of three monkeys with a merozoite preparation derived from short-term culture of *P. falciparum;* complete Freund's adjuvant was used in this study. All three animals exhibited parasitemia but survived challenge.

Using a schizont antigen, Siddiqui (1977) successfully immunized three owl monkeys, again using complete Freund's adjuvant, with the result that one of the three animals exhibited no parasitemia and all three survived.

Wellde *et al.* (1979) presented additional information on the efficacy of irradiated parasitized erythrocytes. In this study, three owl monkeys were immunized. One showed no parasitemia at all, a second exhibited low-grade parasitemia but survived, whereas the third exhibited only low-grade parasitemia but died after surviving for more than a month.

Reese *et al.* (1978) collected a merozoite-rich fraction from continuous cultures of *P. falciparum* and used it to immunize three monkeys using muramyl dipeptide as adjuvant. All three animals exhibited modified parasitemia as compared to the controls, with one monkey clearing all detectable parasites by 30 days after challenge. In another experiment, three animals given a similar preparation in complete Freund's adjuvant showed some evidence of immunity as compared to the controls.

Siddiqui also reported experiments in which muramyl dipeptide, in conjunction with liposomes, was used with *P. falciparum* antigens to immunize owl monkeys. All three immunized animals survived (Siddiqui *et al.*, 1978).

The experience with artificial immunization of owl monkeys against *P. falciparum* is summarized in Table I. This table does not include regimens which were tried but which demonstrated no evidence of a difference in response from

TABLE I

Immunization of Owl Monkeys against *Plasmodium falciparum*[a]

Data	Sadun et al. (1969)	Wellde et al. (1978)	Mitchell et al. (1977)	Siddiqui (1977)	Reese et al. (1978)	Siddiqui et al. (1978)		Total
Adjuvant	None	None	Freund's complete	Freund's complete	Freund's complete	MDP	MDP-liposomes	
No. of monkeys immunized	7(13)	3(3)	3(1)	3(2)	3(3)	3(3)	4(3)	26(28)
No. in which detectable parasitemia was prevented	2(0)	1(0)	0(0)	1(0)	0(0)	0(0)	0(0)	4(0)
No. with parasitemia <10%	7(0)	3(0)	3(0)	3(0)	0(0)	1(0)	2(0)	12(0)
No. of survivors	3(0)	2(0)	3(1)	3(0)	0(0)	1(0)	4(1)	16(2)

[a] Numbers in parentheses refer to the number of control, nonimmunized monkeys in each category. MDP, Muramyl dipeptide.

the concurrently studied controls; all the animals included showed at least some delay in the development of parasitemia. It is of interest that only 4 of the 26 animals developed no parasitemia at all, the obvious optimal result. On the other hand, 16 of the 26 did survive after challenge. In contrast to these results, survival in control groups was the exception, with only two animals of the 28 studied surviving.

Comparisons among the various reports can only result in the crudest of generalizations, since many variables including, most importantly, the quality and quantity of antigen administered, differ among the various experiments considered. However, it is interesting that, in two of the three experiments in which all the immunized animals survived, one control animal also survived. The possibility that relatively low host susceptibility and/or virulence of the challenge organisms influenced survival of the immunized animals must be considered. It is also of interest that both the best and the worst result from the point of view of survival were both obtained with complete Fruend's adjuvant. Although there is little doubt that the likelihood of successful immunization will be enhanced by the use of this agent, additional data will be required for its documentation, particularly since in no instance has a parallel study with separate groups of animals, with and without adjuvant, been reported.

III. IMMUNIZATION OF HUMANS AGAINST SPOROZOITE-INDUCED MALARIA

Whereas blood form immunogens have been evaluated only in monkeys, *P. falciparum* sporozoites have been shown to be capable of immunizing man against subsequent challenge. This has been demonstrated in two separate laboratories (Clyde *et al.*, 1973, 1975; Rieckmann *et al.*, 1974, 1979a). Since parenteral administration of sporozoite suspensions to man is not currently feasible because of bacterial contaminants present in such preparations, irradiated sporozoites were given via mosquito bite. Infected mosquitoes were irradiated to inactivate the sporozoites and then fed on volunteers. After exposure of the volunteers to large numbers of bites from irradiated mosquitoes, repeated challenges of the volunteers were made, sometimes demonstrating failure of the immunization procedure but sometimes demonstrating efficacy. In each case, immunity was assessed by the absence of parasitemia after challenge with viable sporozoites. A total of six humans have been immunized against *P. falciparum* and one against *P. vivax* by this method. Results in a single human volunteer (Clyde *et al.*, 1975) illustrate the salient features of these experiments (Fig. 1). This individual was immunized against both *P. falciparum* and *P. vivax* during the course of the more than 500 days of observation. Circumsporozoite precipitin (CSP) tests were performed on his serum initially, at which time they were

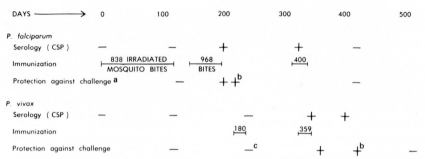

FIG. 1. Immunization of a human volunteer against sporozoite-induced malaria (Clyde *et al.*, 1975). a. + = Immunity on challenge (no infection), − = no evidence of immunity (patent infection on challenge). b. Heterologous strain. c. Patent infection due to failure of irradiation to inactive sporozoites.

negative, and then serially throughout the study. The bites from 838 irradiated *P. falciparum*-infected mosquitoes were sustained by the volunteer, after which time the CSP test remained negative. At this time he was challenged by the bites of mosquitoes infected with *P. vivax,* a heterologous species of parasite, and as a result developed parasitemia. This was arrested by chemotherapy, and he was then bitten by *P. falciparum*-infected mosquitoes and also developed parasitemia as a result of this challenge; this episode of parasitemia was also cured by chemotherapy. After this first attempt at immunization, the volunteer sustained 968 bites of irradiated mosquitoes over the next approximately 50 days. At this point the CSP test was positive, and on challenge with *P. falciparum* no parasitemia resulted. After chemotherapy, the volunteer was challenged with a heterologous strain of *P. falciparum,* also without development of parasitemia, thus demonstrating cross-strain immunity to the parasite. Shortly thereafter, a series of immunizations with irradiated *P. vivax*-infected mosquitoes was instituted. Malaria developed as a result of one of these bites, presumably because of the failure of irradiation to inactivate the organisms. During this time, the *P. vivax* CSP test remained negative. Later, an additional 359 *P. vivax*-infected mosquito bites were sustained, resulting both in a positive CSP test and in resistance to challenge with infectious organisms. In the meantime, the CSP test to *P. falciparum* had become negative, and challenge with *P. falciparum* resulted in a patent infection. This was cured, and the volunteer was challenged with a heterologous strain of *P. vivax,* to which he was immune. Approximately 100 days later, however, a final challenge resulted in a patent infection with the original homologous strain of *P. vivax,* demonstrating that the immunity to this parasite had also waned. Confirmation of the infectivity of the challenge dose was documented in each case by a parallel challenge of nonimmunized controls.

This detailed consideration of a single volunteer illustrates the fact that immunity is species-specific but strain nonspecific in this system. It also demonstrates the transient nature of the immunity induced against both *P. falciparum* and *P. vivax*. The lack of a practical delivery system for the immunogen is clear from this case. The large number of mosquito bites needed for immunization suggests that the amount of antigen required is relatively large, although no real quantitative information is available.

Although only blood stage and sporozoite immunogens have been used to immunize experimental animals or man against *P. falciparum* or other human malaria parasites, a new approach to immunization against malaria deserves mention. Immunization against the gametes of *P. gallinaceum* and *P. knowlesi* is a procedure which markedly inhibits subsequent infectivity of mosquitoes fed on the immunized animals (Gwadz *et al.*, 1979a). This interesting approach would not protect the individual immunized any more (or any less) than his or her nonimmunized peers who share the same attacking anopheline population; antibody inactivates the gametes after their development within the mosquito gut. Future developments in this field will be of great interest.

IV. PREREQUISITES FOR VACCINES FOR HUMAN USE

Until recently, there had been little serious discussion of the problems to be encountered in the development of practical malaria vaccines. The most recent WHO workshop began deliberations on this subject in earnest (McGregor, 1979; Powell, 1979). In consideration of the qualities required for an experimental vaccine for human use, the following five points stand out:

1. The availability of immunogen which can be prepared in large amounts in a reproducible fashion.
2. An immunogen free of microbial contaminants, pyrogens, toxins, and potentially dangerous antigens.
3. A stable immunogen, a single batch of which can be used over a period of time without serious deterioration.
4. An assay or assays capable of measuring the potency of the immunogen either in terms of some correlate of efficacy and/or in chemical terms.
5. An immunogen which has been demonstrated to be efficacious in an animal model.

It will be instructive to consider progress toward each of these prerequisites with respect to both blood stage and sporozoite immunogens of *P. falciparum* in view of the experience summarized above and in view of insights gained from model systems. Again, this is best done by separate consideration of blood stages and sporozoites.

A. Currently Available Blood Stage Immunogens

As regards blood stage immunogens, whole cells have been used in all the work with *P. falciparum* (cited above), although cell extracts have been used in model systems, notably *P. knowlesi* in the rhesus monkey (Schenkel *et al.* 1973). Merozoites are considered by most authorities to be a major target of the immune response. This opinion is based on evidence from a variety of sources. The classic studies of Cohen *et al.* (1961), implicating a role for immune serum in immunity against *P. falciparum* in humans, demonstrated that no abrupt diminution in the number of parasitized erythrocytes in the circulation occurred immediately after the administration of immune serum, but rather that, in the next generation, the number of parasites was much lower than that observed in controls. Similarly, in the *P. knowlesi* system, the inhibition of incorporation of radioactive amino acids by immune serum is not operative against the intracellular parasites but, again, is observable after extracellular exposure of the merozoites to immune serum (Cohen *et al.*, 1969). Furthermore, direct observations of the interaction of merozoites with serum from monkeys immune to *P. knowlesi* indicate that they are agglutinated and thus prevented from entering erythrocytes (Miller *et al.*, 1975). Evidence of an indirect nature using hyperimmune serum against *P. berghei* also favors the merozoite as the target cell (Chow and Kreier, 1972; Diggs and Osler, 1975). In all these cases, the immune serum is derived from humans or experimental animals either immunized by natural infection and recovery or by artificial procedures which mimic the immunity seen in the convalescent situation. Conceivably immunogens which result in an immune status in which entirely different targets are attacked may be forthcoming, but little evidence that this will be the case is currently available. Worthy of mention, and certainly further investigation, is the observation that the knobs on the exterior surface of erythrocytes infected with *P. falciparum* (and certain other malaria parasites) bind antibody from animals immune to challenge (Kilejian *et al.*, 1977). It should also be mentioned that the schizonts of *P. knowlesi* are agglutinated by immune serum, but this is not generally believed to be of functional significance under *in vivo* conditions (Brown and Hills, 1973).

Since merozoites are likely targets of the immune response, by inference, these stages might be expected to be a prime source of the appropriate immunogens for protective immunization. A rather large literature attempting to evaluate the relative efficacy of merozoites, schizonts, trophozoites, and extracts of parasites has developed, but only one study has made an attempt to compare directly various immunogens in controlled parallel experiments (Rieckmann *et al.*, 1979b). In this study, no evidence that merozoites were in fact superior to schizonts was obtained. Merozoites therefore remain a very likely source of the appropriate immunogens, but for theoretical reasons rather than through compelling evidence. In fact, immunity against *P. knowlesi* has been observed in animals immunized with trophozoites only (R. W. Gwadz, personal communication, 1979). It may be that the pertinent antigens are surface constituents of merozoites, but they may also be present in other stages of the parasite life cycle.

The use of whole merozoites derived from *P. falciparum* culture for the preparation of a candidate human vaccine holds promise, but implementation will be difficult. The technology of recovery of *P. falciparum* merozoites from culture is just now being developed. A variety of factors contribute to the problem, among them the lack of synchrony of *P. falciparum* cultures and the relatively low total parasitemias (percentage of erythrocytes parasitized) generally sustainable in *P. falciparum* cultures as opposed to the acutely *P. knowlesi*-infected rhesus monkey, the usual source of parasites for the preparation of merozoites of this organism (Mitchell *et al.*, 1977). Evaluation of the quality of merozoites of *P. falciparum* after collection is difficult, since few markers are available. Merozoites of *P. falciparum* obtained from asynchronous cultures seem to be of poor quality based on morphological criteria (J. D. Haynes, personal communication, 1979).

B. Blood Stage Antigen Safety

The safety of merozoite vaccines for human use must be considered from several points of view. The probable contamination with erythrocyte stromata must be monitored, probably by immunochemical means and, if a significant degree of contamination exists after moderate measures of purification (differential centrifugation, etc.), a serious obstacle to human use may be encountered. Widespread immunization against blood group substances is clearly not acceptable when possible consequences such as transfusion reactions, hemolytic disease of the newborn, and autoimmune hemolytic anemia are considered.

A safety hazard of equal or greater importance is that due to the incorporation of adventitous human pathogens in vaccines prepared from pools of human erythrocytes and serum. Although difficult, solutions to the serum problem can be envisioned in a number of ways including the use of sera of other than human origin and the development of serum-free culture media. The necessity for using human erythrocytes, however, is perhaps a more serious problem. It appears that a treatment which results in the inactivation of hepatitis and other agents will be required. Whether or not this will result in the inactivation of pertinent immunogens is an important consideration.

C. Stability of Blood Stage Antigens

If merozoites of suitable quality in sufficient quantity could be obtained, the method of storage for optimal stability would need to be worked out. It is encouraging that *P. falciparum* merozoites can be stored in the frozen state and subsequently serve as immunogens for the induction of functional protective immunity (Mitchell *et al.*, 1977).

D. Blood Stage Antigen Potency Assays

Although information on the efficacy of the crude preparations now in use has been obtained from the 26 animals described above, it is unlikely that preparations which are true candidates for human use will bear a sufficiently close resemblance to these crude preparations to allow predictions of their efficacy. It is therefore crucial that assays be developed for evaluating the likelihood that candidate antigens will be efficacious. At the moment, several laboratories are developing growth inhibition assays for assessing the potency of immune serum (Campbell *et al.*, 1979; J. D. Chulay, personal communication, 1979). Such assays will be valuable in candidate antigen evaluation and development. However, this assumes that the most relevant effector mechanism of immunity against malaria is humoral, an assumption which may not be warranted. Continued investigations of immune mechanisms, especially with new antigens, are clearly required.

In addition to bioassays of potency, chemical characterization and the use of chemical analysis in controlling the quality of candidate vaccines will be of great importance. In fact, it may be necessary to use highly purified antigens in vaccine formulations in order to circumvent problems of degradation due to endogenous hydrolases (J. D. Haynes, personal communication, 1979) as well as of toxic contaminants. Much work is obviously necessary before a useful purified preparation derived from *P. falciparum* will be available. An example of such a material has been described in the *P. lophurae* system. A histidine-rich protein has been obtained in highly purified form and has been shown to be an effective immunizing agent (Kilejian, 1978).

E. Efficacy of Blood Stage Immunogens in Humans

Although less than completely effective, antigens derived from *P. falciparum* blood stages are clearly capable of inducing striking protection of owl monkeys against challenge as documented above. It is not known whether similar results will be obtained in humans. Artificial immunization of humans with nonreplicating *P. falciparum* blood stage immunogens has not been attempted. However, immunity acquired during active infections has been carefully documented (Powell *et al.*, 1972). Immunity induced in owl monkeys by active infection which is allowed to proceed to only a limited extent before termination by chemotherapy resembles in extent immunity in humans similarly immunized (K.

H. Rieckmann, personal communication, 1979). These considerations suggest that humans will also respond well to nonreplicating *P. falciparum* immunogens.

Another factor which must be dealt with is the possible heterogeneity of antigenic types of *P. falciparum*. Although there is good evidence of immunity to heterologous challenge after monkeys have first experienced immunization and challenge with the homologous parasites (Mitchell *et al.,* 1977), no systematic study of strain differences has thus far been feasible. Such an analysis is most readily envisioned in terms of *in vitro* correlates of immunity rather than extensive experimentation using primates.

In nonhuman systems, notably *P. knowlesi* in the rhesus monkey, there is good evidence for variation in the antigens of parasites during the immune response (Brown, 1971). A similar phenomenon is a plausible explanation for the prolonged, low-grade, chronic infections often observed in animals immunized against *P. falciparum* after challenge, or in those undergoing naturally occurring chronic infection. Whether or not this is the case needs to be determined. If antigenic variation does exist, it will be important to assess the degree of heterologous immunity induced by immunization with organisms of a single antigenic type. It has been suggested that priming with malaria parasites of a given antigenic type will enhance the subsequent immune response to a heterologous type (Brown, 1971), but no information is available regarding *P. falciparum*.

F. Sporozoite Immunogen Availability and Safety

At present, immunization against sporozoite challenge has been accomplished only with intact cells, both in the human experiments cited above and in extensive study of rodent models (Nussenzweig *et al.,* 1969, 1972b). To date the only source of sporozoites is mosquitoes and, although much progress has been made in the purification of sporozoites (Wood *et al.,* 1979), significant numbers of bacteria and yeasts still contaminate even the best preparations. It appears that a definite safety hazard exists which may limit or even preclude the use of mosquito-derived sporozoites in vaccines. Disinfection of the preparations is probably achievable, but the impact on retention of immunogenicity of the various procedures required is thus far not known. The use of chemically defined, highly purified antigens appears to be as desirable a goal here as in the case of blood stage immunogens.

The feasibility of production of sufficiently large numbers of sporozoites from mosquitoes to be useful in practical immunization schemes has been addressed, and it has been concluded that feasibility would be for limited numbers of recipients, such as for example marine troops during short-term operations in endemic areas; other approaches would be necessary for more extensive applications. *In vitro* production of sporozoites appears to be a goal which will be achieved only at some undetermined time in the future. Gametocytes can be produced *in vitro* from erythrocyte cultures of *P. falciparum* (Carter and Miller, 1979), but there is unexplained strain variation, and differentiation of cultures toward gametocyte production thus far cannot be controlled or predicted. Even if it were possible to develop gametes *in vitro* with regularity, subsequent development of the parasite into zygotes and then into oocytes and sporozoites would involve formidable difficulties, although some notable promising results have been obtained (review by Vanderberg *et al.*, 1977).

G. Stability of Sporozoites

Sporozoites can be successfully cryopreserved for extended periods of time as determined by infectivity to recipients after retrieval (Jeffery and Rendtorff, 1955). Thus it is theoretically feasible to store irradiated sporozoite immunogens under these conditions. The quantitative aspects of recovery, as well as the precise cryopreservation and holding conditions, are being exhaustively investigated (Leef *et al.*, 1979).

H. Potency Assays for Sporozoite Immunogens

The adequacy of potency assays for sporozoite vaccines has not been established. The production of antibodies appears to correlate with immunity in the human experiments (Clyde *et al.*, 1975), but in rodent models this correlation does not always hold using sporozoite-neutralizing activity (SNA) and CSP testing as the indicators (Spitalny and Nussenzweig, 1973). Whereas both SNA and CSP reactions probably involve the surface coat of the organism, and therefore are reasonable indicators of the immune response of this potentially important immunogen, the meaning of fluorescent antibody methods in general is less clear. Where antibodies to internal components are detected, the relevance to protection is tenuous indeed. Recently an immunofluorescence technique has been described which allows the detection of antibodies directed against the surface of the organism with minimal interference from internal antigens (Nardin and Nussenzweig, 1979). This appears to be a very useful test for antibodies reactive with the putatively important surface antigens.

Since the effector mechanisms involved in immunity against sporozoites are not clear, the relevance of antibody to protection is a topic of some uncertainty. Where T cell-deficient mice cannot be successfully immunized with the sporozoites of *P. berghei,* mice treated with anti-μ to abolish the B-cell response can sustain an otherwise lethal innoculum after sporozoite immunization (Chen *et al.*, 1977). It is thus clear that antibody-independent mechanisms of immunity are operative. However, since sporozoites can be neutralized by antibody (Nussenzweig *et al.*, 1969), and passive transfer of immune serum results in prolongation of the prepatent period after sporozoite challenge (Nussenzweig *et al.*, 1972a), it seems likely that antibody-mediated inactivation of sporozoites is also involved in the resistance of actively immunized animals. Further insight into these phenomena will be needed to clarify the requirements for potency assays.

I. Efficacy of Sporozoite Immunization

As discussed above, immunization of humans against sporozoite-induced *P. falciparum* infection has been documented. The immunity is transient. It is possible that longer-term immunity can be induced by variations in antigen dose, adjuvant, etc. If not, the usefulness of sporozoite vaccination will be limited. This is particularly so since, based on the study of model systems after immunity has waned, resulting infections are just as severe as in unimmunized individuals (Nussenzweig *et al.*, 1972b). This result is predictable, since there is no cross-immunity between sporozoites and blood stages. Once erythrocytic infection is initiated, unmodified disease ensues.

V. CONCLUSIONS

It is apparent from the considerations just discussed that serious problems exist in the development of vaccines against malaria using either blood stage or sporozoite immunogens. If adequate amounts of antigens, either particulate or soluble, can be collected through methods now in use, if there is an adequate method for the evaluation of their potency, if they are stable for at least a year, and if they are efficacious in preventing malaria on challenge in owl monkeys or other susceptible subhuman primates, the question of safety for human use will still be a major consideration. Careful quality control, to include immunochemical estimates of the concentrations of erythrocyte antigen contaminants (in the case of blood stage preparations), and an evaluation of the persistence of living microorganisms will be minimal requirements. Even with such surveillance, small amounts of such contaminants will be difficult to rule out, and this may limit the utility of these preparations. Theoretically, alternatives exist which, although extending the estimates of time to achievement markedly, nevertheless engender optimism with respect to eventual achievement of the goal. I refer to recombinant DNA technology, with its potential for allowing the large-scale production of proteins and presumably eventually glycoproteins of any desired structure through use of the appropriate genetic information cloned in a suitable host microorganism. Problems of contamination of the immunogen with unacceptable adventitious material and limitations on the quantity of material which can be practically obtained can be overcome, in theory, by this approach (Itakura *et al.*, 1977). Prerequisite to these far-reaching achievements is a determination of the structure of the relevant antigens, a task which is just now beginning. Good progress has been made with the *P. knowlesi* system with respect to the blood stages (Deans and Cohen, 1979) and, as mentioned above, in the case of *P. lophurae,* a discrete protein has been identified which can be used as an immunogen in inducing protection (Kilejian, 1978). Encouraging progress is being made in studies on the immunochemistry of sporozoite surface antigens (Nardin and Nussenzweig, 1980). These developments, it appears, exemplify the problems which should occupy our major attention until they are adequately solved.

A major advance has recently been made in the chemical characterization of functionally important sporozoite antigens. A monoclonal antibody has been prepared against a *P. berghei* surface antigen of apparent molecular weight 44,000; this antibody neutralizes sporozoite infectivity (Yoshida *et al.*, 1980).

ACKNOWLEDGMENTS

I am grateful to Phil Russell and David Haynes who made suggestions, and to Mrs. Mary Watson who typed the manuscript.

REFERENCES

Box, E. D., Box, Q. T., and Young, M. D. (1963). Chloroquine resistant *Plasmodium falciparum* from Porto Velho, Brazil. *Am. J. Trop. Med. Hyg.* **12,** 300–304.

Brown, K. N. (1971). Protective immunity to malaria parasites, a model for the survival of cells in an immunologically hostile environment. *Nature (London)* **230,** 163–167.

Brown, K. N., and Hills, L. A. (1973). Antigenic variation and immunity to *Plasmodium knowlesi:* Antibodies which induce antigenic variation and antibodies which destroy parasites. *Trans. R. Soc. Trop. Med. Hyg.* **68,** 139–142.

Campbell, G. H., Mrema, J. E., O'Leary, T. R., Jost, R. C., and Rieckmann, K. H. (1979). *In vitro* inhibition of growth of *Plasmodium falciparum* by aotus serum. *Bull. W.H.O.* **57,** Suppl. 1, 219–225.

Carter, R., and Miller, L. H. (1979). Evidence for environmental modulation of gametocytogenesis in *Plasmodium falciparum* in continuous culture. *Bull. W.H.O.* **57,** Suppl. 1, 37–52.

Chen, D. H., Tigelaar, R. E., and Weinbaum, F. I. (1977). Immunity to sporozoite-induced malaria infection in mice. I. The effect of immunization of T and B cell-deficient mice. *J. Immunol.* **118,** 1322–1327.

Chow, J., and Kreier, J. P. (1972). *Plasmodium berghei:* Adherence and phagocytosis by rat macrophages *in vitro. Exp. Parasitol.* **31,** 13–18.

Clyde, D. F., Most, H., McCarthy, V. C., and Vanderberg, J. P. (1973). Immunization of man against sporozoite-induced falciparum malaria. *Am. J. Med. Sci.* **266,** 169–177.

Clyde, D. F., McCarthy, V. C., Miller, R. M., and Woodward, W. E. (1975). Immunization of man against falciparum and vivax malaria by use of attenuated sporozoites. *Am. J. Trop. Med. Hyg.* **24,** 397–401.

Cohen, S. (1978). Development of a malaria vaccine. *J. R. Soc. Med.* **71**, 476–478.

Cohen, S., McGregor, I. A., and Carrington, S. P. (1961). Gamma globulin and acquired immunity to human malaria. *Nature (London)* **192**, 733–737.

Cohen, S., Butcher, G. A., and Crandall, R. B. (1969). Action of malarial antibody *in vitro*. *Nature (London)* **223**, 368–371.

Deans, J. A., and Cohen, S. (1979). Localization and chemical characterization of *Plasmodium knowlesi* schizont antigens. *Bull. W.H.O.* **57**, Suppl. 1, 93–100.

Diggs, C. L., and Osler, A. G. (1975). Humoral immunity in rodent malaria. III. Studies on the site of antibody action. *J. Immunol.* **114**, 1243–1247.

Freund, J., Sommer, H. E., and Walter, A. W. (1945a). Immunization against malaria: Vaccination of ducks with killed parasites incorporated with adjuvants. *Science* **102**, 200–202.

Freund, J., Thomson, K. J., Sommer, H. E., Walter, A. W., and Schenkein, E. L. (1945b). Immunization of rhesus monkeys against malarial infection (*P. knowlesi*) with killed parasites and adjuvants. *Science* **102**, 202–204.

Freund, J., Thomson, K. J., Sommer, H. E., Walter, A. W., and Pisani, T. M. (1948). Immunization of monkeys against malaria by means of killed parasites with adjuvants. *Am. J. Trop. Med.* **28**, 1–22.

Geiman, Q. M., and Meagher, M. J. (1967). Susceptibility of a New World monkey to *Plasmodium falciparum* from man. *Nature (London)* **215**, 437–439.

Gwadz, R. W., Carter, R., and Green, I. (1979a). Gamete vaccines and transmission-blocking immunity in malaria. *Bull. W.H.O.* **57**, Suppl. 1, 175–180.

Gwadz, R. W., Cochrane, A. H., Nussenzweig, V., and Nussenzweig, R. S. (1979b). Preliminary studies on vaccination of rhesus monkeys with irradiated sporozoites of *Plasmodium knowlesi* and characterization of surface antigens of these parasites. *Bull. W.H.O.* **57**, Suppl. 1, 165–173.

Haynes, J. D., Diggs, C. L., Hines, F. A., and Desjardins, R. E. (1976). Culture of human malaria parasites *Plasmodium falciparum*. *Nature (London)* **263**, 767–769.

Heidelberger, M., Prout, C., Hindle, J. A., and Rose, A. S. (1946a). Studies in human malaria. III. An attempt at vaccination of paretics against blood-borne infection with *Pl. vivax*. *J. Immunol.* **53**, 109.

Heidelberger, M., Mayer, M. M., Alving, A. S., Craige, B., Jr., Jones, R., Jr., Pullman, T. M., and Whorton, M. (1946b). Studies in human malaria. IV. An attempt at vaccination of volunteers against mosquito borne infection with *Pl. vivax*. *J. Immunol.* **53**, 113.

Itakura, K., Hirose, T., Crea, R., Riggs, A. D., Heyneker, H. L., Bolivan, F., and Boyer, H. W. (1977). Expression in *Escherichia coli* of a chemically synthesized gene for the hormone somatostatin. *Science* **198**, 1056–1063.

Jeffery, G. M., and Rendtorff, R. C. (1955). Preservation of viable human malaria sporozoites by low temperature freezing. *Exp. Parasitol.* **4**, 445–454.

Kilejian, A. (1978). Histidine-rich protein as a model malaria vaccine. *Science* **201**, 922–924.

Kilejian, A., Abati, A., and Trager, W. (1977). *Plasmodium falciparum* and *Plasmodium coatneyi*: Immunogenicity of "knob-like protrusions" on infected erythrocyte membranes. *Exp. Parasitol.* **42**, 157–164.

Leef, J. L., Strome, C. P. A., and Beaudoin, R. L. (1979). The low temperature preservation of sporozoites of *Plasmodium berghei*. *Bull. W.H.O.* **57**, Suppl. 1, 87–91.

McGregor, I. A. (1979). Basic considerations concerning field trials of malaria vaccines in human populations. *Bull. W.H.O.* **57**, Suppl. 1, 267–271.

Miller, L. H., Aikawa, M., and Dvorak, J. A. (1975). Malaria (*Plasmodium knowlesi*) merozoites: Immunity and the surface coat. *J. Immunol.* **114**, 1237–1242.

Mitchell, G. H., Richards, W. H. G., Butcher, G. A., and Cohen, S. (1977). Merozoite vaccination of douroucouli monkeys against *falciparum malaria*. *Lancet* **1**, 1335–1338.

Nardin, W., Gwadz, R. W., and Nussenzweig, R. S. (1979). Characterization of sporozoite surface antigens by indirect immunofluorescence. *Bull. W.H.O.* **57**, Suppl. 1, 211-217.

NMRI/USAID/WHO Workshop on the Immunology of Malaria (1979). *Bull. W.H.O.* **57**, Suppl. 1.

Nussenzweig, R. S., Vanderberg, J., and Most, H. (1969). Protective immunity produced by the infection of X-irradiated sporozoites of *Plasmodium berghei*. IV. Dose response, specificity, and humoral immunity. *Mil. Med.* **134**, 1176-1182.

Nussenzweig, R. S., Vanderberg, J. P., Sanabria, Y., and Most, H. (1972a). *Plasmodium berghei:* Accelerated clearance of sporozoites from blood as part of immune mechanism in mice. *Exp. Parasitol.* **31**, 88-97.

Nussenzweig, R. S., Vanderberg, J., Spitalny, G. L., Rivera, C. I. O., Orton, C., and Most, H. (1972b). Sporozoite-induced immunity in mammalian malaria: A review. *Am. J. Trop. Med. Hyg.* **21**, 722-728.

Powell, R. D. (1979). Malaria vaccine development. *Bull. W.H.O.* **57**, Suppl. 1, 273-275.

Powell, R. D., Brewer, G. J., and Alving, A. S. (1963). Studies on a strain of chloroquine-resistant *Plasmodium falciparum* from Columbia, South America. *Am. J. Trop. Med. Hyg.* **12**, 509-512.

Powell, R. D., McNamara, J. V., and Rieckmann, K. H. (1972). Clinical aspects of acquisition of immunity to falciparum malaria. *Proc. Helminthol. Soc. Wash.* **39**, 51-66.

Reese, R. T., Trager, W., Jensen, J. B., Miller, D. A., and Tantravahi, R. (1978). Immunization against malaria with antigen from *Plasmodium falciparum* cultivated *in vitro*. *Pro. Natl. Acad. Sci, U.S.A.* **75**, 3665-3668.

Rieckmann, K. H., Carson, P. E., Beaudoin, R. L., Cassells, J. S., and Sell, K. W. (1974). Sporozoite induced immunity in man against an Ethiopian strain of *Plasmodium falciparum*. *Trans. R. Soc. Trop. Med. Hyg.* **68**, 258-259.

Rieckmann, K. H., Beaudoin, R. L., Cassells, J. S., and Sell, K. W. (1979a). Use of attenuated sporozoites in the immunization of human volunteers against falciparum malaria. *Bull. W.H.O.* **57**, Suppl. 1, 261-265.

Rieckmann, K. H., Cabrera, E. J., Campbell, G. H., Jost, R. C., Miranda, R., and O'Leary, T. R. (1979b). Immunization of monkeys with blood stage antigens of *Plasmodium knowlesi*. *Bull. W.H.O.* **57**, Suppl. 1, 139-151.

Sadun, E. H., ed. (1964). Cultivation of plasmodia and immunology of malaria. *Am. J. Trop. Med. Hyg.* **13**, Suppl., 145-241.

Sadun, E. H., ed. (1966). Research in malaria, *Mil. Med.* **131**, Suppl., 847-1272.

Sadun, E. H., ed. (1969). Experimental malaria. *Mil. Med.* **134**, Suppl., 729-1306.

Sadun, E. H., ed. (1972). Basic research in malaria. *Proc. Helminthol. Soc. Wash.* **39**, Spec. Issue, 3-582.

Sadun, E. H., Wellde, B. T., and Hickman, R. L. (1969). Resistance produced in owl monkeys (*Aotus trivirgatus*) by inoculation with irradiated *Plasmodium falciparum*. *Mil. Med.* **134**, Suppl, 1165-1175.

Schenkel, R. H., Simpson, G. L., and Silverman, P. H. (1973). Vaccination of rhesus monkeys (*Macaca mulatta*) against *Plasmodium knowlesi* by the use of non-viable antigen. *Bull. W.H.O.* **48**, 597-604.

Siddiqui, W. A. (1977). An effective immunization of experimental monkeys against a human malaria parasite. *Plasmodium falciparum*. *Science* **197**, 388-389.

Siddiqui, W. A., Taylor, D. W., Kan, S., Kramer, K., and Richmond-Crum, S. M. (1978). Vaccination of experimental monkeys against *Plasmodium falciparum:* A possible safe adjuvant. *Science* **201**, 1237-2139.

Spitalny, G. L., and Nussenzweig, R. S., (1973). *Plasmodium berghei:* Relationship between protective immunity and antisporozoite antibody in mice. *Exp. Parasitol.* **33**, 168-178.

Thomson, K. J., Freund, J., Sommer, H. E., and Walter, A. W. (1947). Immunization of ducks against malaria by means of killed parasites with or without adjuvants. *Am. J. Trop. Med.* **27,** 79–105.

Trager, W., and Jensen, J. B. (1976). Human malaria parasites in continuous culture. *Science* 193, 673–675.

USAID/WHO Workshops on the Biology and *in vitro* Cultivation of Malaria Parasites (1977). *Bull. W.H.O.* **55,** 121–430.

Vanderberg, J. P., Weiss, M. M., and Mock, S. R. (1977). *In vitro* cultivation of the sporogonic stages of *Plasmodium:* A review. *Bull. W.H.O.* **33,** 377–392.

Wellde, B. T., Diggs, C. L., and Anderson, S. (1979). Immunization of *Aotus trivirgatus* against *Plasmodium falciparum* with irradiated blood forms. *Bull. W.H.O.* **57,** Suppl. 1, 153–157.

Wood, D. E., Smrkovski, L. L., McConnell, E., Pacheco, N. D., and Bawden, M. P. (1979). The use of membrane screen filters in the isolation of *Plasmodium berghei* sporozoites from mosquitoes. *Bull. W.H.O.* **57,** Suppl. 1, 69–74.

Young, M. D., Contacos, P. B., Stitcher, J. E., and Millar, J. W. (1963). Drug resistance in *Plasmodium falciparum* from Thailand. *Am. J. Trop. Med. Hyg.* **12,** 305–314.

Yoshida, N., Nussenzweig, R. S., Potocnjak, P., Nussenzweig, V., and Aikawa, M. (1980). Hybridoma produces protective antibodies directed against the sporazoite stage of malaria parasite. *Science* **207,** 71–73.

Appendix 2

The Roles of Vaccination in the Strategy of Malaria Control

R. L. Beaudoin, J. C. Armstrong, and E. McConnell

The three major approaches to vaccination against human malaria employ as immunogens the asexual blood stages, the sporozoites, or the gametes of malaria parasites. Diggs (this volume, Appendix 1) has discussed the major developmental problems associated with each of these approaches. Here we offer a viewpoint on the role of malaria vaccination in general, from the perspective of the whole malaria management problem, and suggest some specific, rather limited roles for the three types of vaccine under consideration.

The first malaria vaccine experiments were reported nearly 70 years ago (Sergent and Sergent, 1910), even before the etiology of malaria as an infectious disease was universally accepted. Despite the partial successes shown by these and subsequent experiments in animals, vaccination of humans against malaria was not seriously considered until quite recently, and some of the earlier reservations still persist today. First, immunity to malaria has been observed to develop slowly and incompletely in man, even in hyperendemic areas, and the assumption has followed that artificial vaccination would not substantially improve on the immunity induced by repeated, severe, natural infections. Second, vaccination of any sort in the areas affected by malaria would involve immense logistic problems and demand sustained high levels of acceptability within the target populations. Third, the costly development of a vaccine to serve as an adjunct or alternative to the inexpensive and effective insecticides and drugs which have been used so successfully to eradicate malaria from large areas of the world has seemed patently unnecessary. These three points exemplify, respectively, the scientific, administrative, and economic objections raised against heavy investment in malaria vaccine development programs.

During the past decade, however, a series of unfortunate circumstances has permitted the resurgence of malaria on a scale that has ended all expectations of

Malaria, Vol. 3

global eradication within the foreseeable future. In parts of the world where the prospects of eradication once seemed brightest, economic constraints have forced the premature relaxation of malaria surveillance, and the disease has again become highly endemic. Elsewhere, the progress of malaria eradication has been interrupted by political turmoil. At the same time, confidence in the feasibility of eradication has been eroded by increasingly widespread reports of mosquito resistance to insecticides and parasite resistance to antimalarial drugs.

Malaria vaccination has suddenly gained serious worldwide attention because of the breakdown of eradication programs. The concept of malaria vaccination fills a void left by the loss of hope for success by these programs through traditional methods alone.

The funding of malaria vaccine research will create more than just the hope for a modern, sophisticated weapon against the disease. It will also attract a wide range of new talent and imagination to the contest against malaria. The effects of this infusion of fresh hope and new skills will be wasted, however, if the vaccination concept is allowed to preempt traditional methods of malaria eradication and control. Malaria vaccines must be viewed as reinforcements rather than replacements for vector control and chemotherapy. Where, then, are these reinforcements needed?

All the presently projected malaria vaccines consist of *Plasmodium falciparum* immunogens and would probably be of no use in areas where only vivax malaria occurs, as in parts of Mexico and Peru. In the Amazon basin and in tropical Africa, where falciparum malaria is predominant, it is debatable whether mass vaccination or, for that matter, any other activity should be undertaken that would seriously disrupt the conditions of stable malaria until such time as the prospects for malaria eradication in these areas are greatly improved. Malaria vaccines may have their greatest potential value where the conditions of stable malaria have already been disrupted or never existed and where drug-resistant parasites coexist with insecticide-resistant vectors. Vaccines would also be useful where the short-term economic burden of an all-out effort toward malaria eradication could be justified by a reasonable expectation of success.

As already pointed out by Diggs (1979), many technical problems remain to be solved before any of the malaria vaccines under development can be assigned realistic roles in either control or eradication programs. We may hope that, by the time vaccines are generally available, some countries will have achieved eradication by traditional methods. For the near future, though, it appears that priority should be given to the development of anti-falciparum vaccines to be used for the control of malaria in carefully selected populations. Specifically, then, how may the three vaccine types be matched with appropriate target populations for the control of falciparum malaria?

Blood stage-, sporozoite-, and gamete-based vaccines are *not* mutually competitive approaches to malaria control any more than vaccination per se is competitive with the use of insecticides and chemotherapeutic agents. Blood stage vaccines are expected to eliminate mortality and reduce morbidity by inducing a degree of immunity comparable to the premunition observed among survivors in highly endemic areas. Sporozoite vaccines, on the other hand, are expected to induce complete but relatively short-term protection from patent falciparum malaria. Finally, gamete vaccines are being designed to interrupt the falciparum life cycle by blocking transmission from infected humans to vector mosquitoes.

Target populations for a blood stage vaccine might include families participating in agricultural development and resettlement programs. Many of these programs, in effect throughout the malarious world, move participants from overcrowded, nonendemic areas to areas where they encounter malaria for the first time in their lives. Transients such as tourists, bus and truck drivers, and others on brief visits to malarious areas would be better protected, perhaps, by sporozoite vaccines; and revaccination at intervals might be advisable for temporary residents such as teachers and health workers. Of course, neither the permanent nor the temporary newcomers to an endemic area would require vaccination unless local strains of *P. falciparum* were resistant to the available antimalarial drugs.

Administration of blood stage vaccines to the indigenous populations of endemic areas may involve hazards, or at least raise questions. For example, will the vaccination of infants produce suppression of parasitemias or induce immunological tolerance? And will the vaccination of older children and adults in hyperendemic areas enhance antiparasite immunity or provoke autoimmune disease? Perhaps these and similar questions are just as relevant to vaccination with sporozoite- and gamete-based preparations.

From a malariologist's point of view, the idea of protecting definitive hosts (mosquitoes) from infection by intermediate hosts (man) is both attractive and epidemiologically sound. Successful vaccination of humans against falciparum gametes would abort transmission regardless of the female anopheline's indoor or outdoor feeding and resting behavior or her response to insecticides. In special circumstances, the gamete vaccine could be employed to hinder reintroduction of falciparum malaria. Large numbers of seasonal laborers moving from malarious to malaria-freed areas might be given a gamete vaccine to prevent infection of mosquitoes at the destination. This tactic would have value even in the absence of chloroquine resistance, because falciparum gametocytes remain infective for some time after the carrier is cured with chloroquine. It remains to be seen how this novel approach will be received by medical research human use committees, since volunteer subjects would derive no direct benefit from a gamete vaccine.

Many additional uses for each of the three types of vaccines may be imagined. The examples of target populations given above are intended to illustrate the distinctive and valuable, yet, in our opinion, somewhat limited roles these vaccines might play in the total strategy of malaria control.

The hard lessons offered by the collapse of the global malaria eradication campaign deserve careful study if we are to avoid repetition of past errors. One of the mistakes of that campaign was the failure to recognize that the missionary zeal motivating the administrators of malaria eradication services did not always carry out to the field. In many places, neither the purveyors nor the recipients of antimalaria services were adequately educated for the campaign and, despite dramatic successes, the drudgery of domicile spraying was met with increasing hostility and recalcitrance. Simply stated, the service was often imposed on people, and the imposition was often resented. A similar fate for malaria vaccination programs can be avoided by making available safe and effective vaccines for informed and willing recipients through the agencies and personnel of integrated health care delivery systems. The creation and maintenance of these systems should precede control or eradication programs in parts of the world where malaria is firmly entrenched.

Premature and exaggerated claims for malaria vaccines are a disservice. It will take time to develop the vaccines, time to evaluate their safety and efficacy, and more time to determine their proper roles in the strategy of malaria eradication and control. An Ethiopian adage states: A long walk around the ravine is better than two leaps across.

ACKNOWLEDGEMENT

This work was supported by the Naval Medical Research and Development Command, Work Unit No. ZF58.524.009.0072. The opinions or assertions contained herein are the private ones of the authors and are not to be construed as official or reflecting the views of the U.S. Navy or the naval service at large.

REFERENCE

Sergent, E., and Sergent, E. (1910). Sur l'immunité dans le paludisme des oiseaux. Conservation *in vitro* des sporozoites de *Plasmodium relictum*. Immunité relative obtenue par inoculation de ces sporozoites. *C. R. Acad. Sci.* **151**, 407–409.

Appendix 3

Prospects for Malaria Blood Stage Vaccine

Karl H. Rieckmann

The results of recent studies with blood stage antigens of *Plasmodium falciparum* indicate that such antigens can induce varying degrees of partial immunity in *Aotus trivirgatus* monkeys (see Table I by Diggs, this volume, Appendix 1). This is an encouraging finding because the development of clinical immunity following drug suppression of falciparum infections in *Aotus* monkeys appears to be similar to that observed in the human host. With the continuous cultivation of *P. falciparum* in human erythrocytes (Trager and Jensen, 1976), it is now possible to use blood stages of this species as a source of antigen for immunization studies and to conserve this scarce experimental simian host for the assessment of various antigens and immunization schedules.

The antigenic stability of parasites maintained in continuous culture may, of course, be different from that of parasites obtained directly from *in vivo* sources. Findings from our laboratory indicate that *viable* parasites, obtained from a continuous culture of 3 months' duration, can induce an immunity in *Aotus* monkeys comparable to that observed with parasites obtained from another monkey (Rieckmann *et al.*, 1978). The immunity induced by *nonviable* cultured parasites (Reese *et al.*, 1978) may possibly be less than that induced by parasites obtained directly from a simian host (Mitchell *et al.*, 1977; Siddiqui, 1977; Siddiqui *et al.*, 1979; Wellde *et al.*, 1979). Changes on the surface of infected erythrocytes (loss of "knobs") have now been observed in three strains maintained in continuous culture for over a year (Langreth *et al.*, 1979) and, although the implications of this change with regard to the antigenicity of parasites have not yet been determined, the possibility that prolonged continuous culture of parasites may alter the immunogenicity of malaria antigens should be kept in mind.

The antigen preparations used in these studies contained host erythrocyte

Malaria, Vol. 3

material and, in most instances, antigens were derived from parasite suspensions in which schizonts predominated over other developmental stages. Erythrocyte contaminants will have to be excluded from antigenic preparations used eventually for human vaccination. As intracellular parasites do not appear to be more immunogenic than extracellular parasites, it might be preferable to pursue further immunization studies with merozoites released spontaneously from erythrocytes rather than to attempt the freeing and separation of intracellular parasites from their host cells. The harvesting of cultured merozoites, adequate in quantity and quality and free of erythrocyte debris, still remains to be achieved. When this is accomplished, studies with *Aotus* monkeys should be carried out to identify with certainty that merozoites, and not contaminating parasitized erythrocyte material, are responsible for the limited protection observed after immunization with various antigenic preparations.

The recent evaluation of adjuvants, used in conjunction with parasite antigens, indicates that alternative, less toxic adjuvants will probably replace Freund's complete adjuvant in assessing the efficacy of various antigenic preparations. Although such investigations have been useful, it is conceivable that the purified antigens or antigen fractions used eventually in human studies may not require the concomitant administration of adjuvants. If adjuvants, however, are still needed to induce protection against malaria, it is likely that a greater selection of even more improved adjuvants will be available and, at that time, the most suitable one can be chosen.

The inavailability of animal models as supplements to the *Aotus–P. falciparum* system is delaying the prospect of obtaining a blood stage vaccine. The search for readily available, inexpensive animal models for evaluating the efficacy of human malaria antigens should receive high priority (Jiang, 1978). In addition, investigations must be pursued to improve the breeding in captivity of simian models, such as the *Aotus* monkey. Until recently, the successful breeding of these monkeys was considered a difficult proposition. However, in the small *Aotus* colony maintained at our facility, there has been an average of one live birth (with 95% survival) per parent pair per year for the past two years. Despite such encouraging findings, *Aotus* monkeys will be relatively scarce during the next few years, and they will have to be used very judiciously in the assessment of candidate vaccines. The development of potentially useful antigens will, therefore, depend heavily on the availability of *in vitro* methods for evaluating chemically defined antigens or antigen fractions and to narrow down the candidate antigens that will eventually be tested in the simian model. Evaluation, characterization, and purification of antigens can be accomplished by developing a number of different procedures, such as growth inhibition assays (Campbell *et al.*, 1979; Reese and Motyl, 1979), cell hybridization procedures (Melchers *et al.*, 1978), immunoelectrophoretic analysis (Deans and Cohen, 1979), and reticulocyte cell-free systems (Eggitt *et al.*, 1979). It is probably true that without intensified efforts to utilize alternate approaches to *in vivo* evaluation of antigenic preparations, the prospects for developing a vaccine suitable for human use are quite remote.

The problems which still have to be surmounted before candidate vaccines can be tested in human volunteers have been outlined by Diggs, this volume, Appendix 1, and general conditions pertaining to the eventual conduct of such studies have been reviewed recently by Cohen and Mitchell (1978), McGregor (1979), and Powell (1979). Human studies for determining the safety and immunoprophylactic value of a potential vaccine can, of course, only be started after extensive preclinical evaluation of the toxicity and efficacy of a well-standardized antigenic preparation. Clinical studies would have to be carried out, in the first instance, with nonimmune volunteers at clinical malaria research centers where exposure to infection can be well controlled and documented. By defining the duration of protection after single or multiple exposure to homologous or heterologous strains of *P. falciparum,* important information will become available which will be critical in the planning and design of further preclinical studies and of field trials. The drastic decline in the number of clinical malaria centers during recent years will adversely affect our prospects for obtaining a malaria vaccine, and efforts should be made to reverse this trend.

Evaluation of an antigenic preparation under epidemiologically well-defined field conditions would be the next logical step in the development of a prospective antimalarial vaccine. Field trials should involve both nonimmune individuals moving into endemic areas and long-term residents of such areas who have probably acquired varying degrees of partial immunity to the disease. The response of adults and children to vaccination may be anticipated to a certain extent from preclinical studies with animals of various ages, obtained from an *Aotus* breeding colony, that have either been exposed or not exposed to malaria and from clinical studies with nonimmune and partially immune volunteers. The antimalarial activity of a vaccine to be used in a field trial should, preferably, be sufficiently pronounced to prevent the onset of clinical disease after exposure to infection. The level of parasitemia usually observed after challenge of *Aotus* monkeys immunized with crude antigenic preparations would be too high to prevent the development of acute symptoms of malaria in nonimmune or even partially immune persons. Without a significant reduction in the malaria morbidity rate, many communities would not be receptive to the administration of a vaccine against falciparum malaria. Similarly, potentially useful antigen preparations of *P. vivax* or *P. malariae* would have to suppress parasites to a level below the relatively low-grade parasitemia usually observed during the course of a vivax or quartan infection.

A safe and effective malaria vaccine, if and when it becomes available, would undoubtedly be a powerful tool for improving the control of malaria infections. It is highly unlikely, however, that such a vaccine will replace traditional antimalarial measures or that it will be the final answer to the many problems facing us in the control and eradication of this disease. Enthusiasm for the potential value of a malaria vaccine must always be tempered by a realistic appraisal of what can be practically achieved in many of the malarious areas of the world.

REFERENCES

Campbell, G. H., Mrema, J. E., O'Leary, T. R., Jost, R. C., and Rieckmann, K. H. (1979). *In vitro* inhibition of growth of *Plasmodium falciparum* by *Aotus* serum. *Bull. W.H.O.* **57** (Suppl. 1), 219–225.

Cohen, S., and Mitchell, G. H. (1978). Prospects for immunization against malaria. *Curr. Top. Microbiol. Immunol.* **80,** 97–137.

Deans, J. A., and Cohen, S. (1979). Localization and chemical characterization of *Plasmodium knowlesi* schizont antigens. *Bull. W.H.O.* **57** (Suppl. 1), 93–100.

Eggitt, M. J., Tappenden, L., and Brown, K. N. (1979). Synthesis of *Plasmodium knowlesi* polypeptides in a cell free system. *Bull. W.H.O.* **57** (Suppl. 1), 109–113.

Jiang, J. (1978). *Plasmodium:* Experimental animals for human malaria and research needs. *Exp. Parasitol.* **46,** 339–352.

Langreth, S. G., Reese, R. T., Motyl, M. R., and Trager, W. (1979). *Plasmodium falciparum:* Loss of knobs on the infected erythrocyte surface after long-term cultivation. *Exp. Parasitol.* **48,** 213–219.

McGregor, I. A. (1979). Basic considerations concerning field trials of malaria vaccines in human populations. *Bull. W.H.O.* **57** (Suppl. 1), 267–271.

Melchers, F., Potter, M., and Warner, N. L. (1978). Lymphocyte hybridomas. *Curr. Top. Microbiol. Immunol.* **81,** 1–246.

Mitchell, G. H., Richards, W. H. G., Butcher, G. A., and Cohen, S. (1977). Merozoite vaccination of douroucouli monkeys against falciparum malaria. *Lancet* **1,** 1335–1338.

Powell, R. D. (1979). Malaria vaccine development. *Bull. W.H.O.* **57** (Suppl. 1), 273–275.

Reese, R. T., and Motyl, M. R. (1979). *In vitro* inhibition of *Plasmodium falciparum* growth with immune sera from monkeys and man. *63rd Annu. Meet. Fed. Am. Soc. Exp. Biol.* Abstract No. 5540, p. 1275.

Reese, R. T., Trager, W., Jensen, J. B., Miller, D. A., and Tantrayahi, R. (1978). Immunization against malaria with antigen from *Plasmodium falciparum* cultivated *in vitro. Proc. Nat. Acad. Sci. U.S.A.* **75,** 5665–5668.

Rieckmann, R. H., Mrema, J. E., and Campbell, G. H. (1978). Malaria immunity induced by infection with cultured parasites of *Plasmodium falciparum. J. Parasitol.* **64,** 750–752.

Siddiqui, W. A. (1977). An effective immunization of experimental monkeys against a human malaria parasite, *Plasmodium falciparum. Science* **197,** 388–389.

Siddiqui, W. A., Taylor, D. W., Kan, S. C., Dramer, K., Richmond-Crum, S. R., Kotani, S., Shiba, T., and Kusumoto, S. (1979). Immunization of experimental monkeys against *Plasmodium falciparum;* use of synthetic adjuvants. *Bull. W.H.O.* **57** (Suppl. 1), 199–203.

Trager, W., and Jensen, J. B. (1976). Human malaria parasites in continuous culture. *Science* **193,** 673–675.

Wellde, B. T., Diggs, C. L., and Anderson, S. (1979). Immunization of *Aotus trivirgatus* against *Plasmodium falciparum* with irradiated blood forms. *Bull. W.H.O.* **57** (Suppl. 1), 153–157.

Appendix 4

Manufacturing Aspects of Antiplasmodial Vaccine Production

Robert G. Brackett

Approaches to antiplasmodial vaccination have been categorized by the forms within the life cycle for which they are targeted, i.e., sporozoites, gametocytes, and merozoites. My emphasis will be on the latter, a merozoite vaccine, however, the concepts I will put forth bear on all vaccines regardless of their form.

At the joint World Health Organization–Agency for International Development Workshop held in Bethesda, Maryland, in October 1978, a group met with the intention of setting forth plans and strategies for clinical field studies for assessing malaria vaccines. It was the recommendation of this group that vaccines considered for use in man should be prepared in a facility dedicated to the manufacture of human biologicals rather than in a research laboratory.

This position was taken because of the recognition that the success or failure of the first and all subsequent field evaluations will be very important to the ultimate success or failure of the vaccine approach to the control of malaria. Thus production and control testing should be carried out only by highly qualified vaccine producers (commercial or governmental) and at facilities approved by the appropriate regulatory authorities.

The research scientist's interest, goals, and objectives are diverse. He or she may be interested in obtaining basic knowledge which will contribute to the understanding of malaria as a disease or in obtaining knowledge in such an area as pathology, immunology, biochemistry, or biology of the parasite. The development scientist may take basic knowledge and, by applying known procedures and methods, convert it to a practical, useful product. The manufacturer's task is to make the product in a consistent and reliable manner and to test it to ensure that it meets designated specifications. This is the case whether the product is an experimental one or a product which is "tried and true."

Whether the product is a drug or a biological, the primary consideration of the

Malaria, Vol. 3
Copyright © 1980 by Academic Press, Inc.
All rights of reproduction in any form reserved.
ISBN 0-12-426103-5

manufacturer is its safety and efficacy. These concerns are also shared by the regulatory health authorities and must be kept in mind by research and development scientists as they conduct their phase of the work toward a new vaccine.

Strain selection is a crucial element in the manufacture of any safe and effective vaccine. The first consideration is to devise a suitable system of nomenclature for identifying various strains. To this end Jensen and Trager (1978) in a recent paper have suggested a uniform system of designation. This system can be adapted or modified, or alternates chosen, but we need a system for strain identification.

The history of the strain should be carefully kept in each laboratory when there is a serious possibility that the strain might become a candidate for vaccine production. This history should include details of the origin of the isolate and the type and quality of substances, substrates, and etc., to which the strain is exposed. For example, records should be kept of the donors of erythrocytes and serum used for the *in vitro* propagation of the parasite. The number of passages, conditions of growth, and other manipulations to which the parasite was subjected must also be recorded. The characteristics of the strain must be well established. This is usually done only when a strain has been clearly identified as a vaccine candidate. Such characterization provides a method for checking the identity and validity of the strain and avoids mix-ups which could have a serious impact on our main concerns—safety and efficacy.

One method which has been used extensively in the manufacture of vaccines is the seed lot concept. However, its application should not only be implemented when manufacture of a vaccine is imminent. Rather seed lots should be preserved on first isolation and at frequent times during vaccine development. I have cautioned on this point before, but I think it is worthy of restatement. Each laboratory should preserve and store stocks of parasites at passage levels as close to the initial isolation as possible. Research should be conducted on parasites carried in continuous culture only for a limited number of passages, and then the continuous culture should be abandoned, with a return to the original master stock. This will ensure consistency of the culture and avoid unrecognized modifications. Langreth has presented data (Langreth and Reese, 1979) proving that alterations occur in P. falciparum in continuous cultures. In my laboratory we have observed that treatment of *in vitro* cultured *P. falciparum* with sorbitol to induce partial synchrony can exert a selective pressure on the parasites in culture. What effect modifications such as these might have on the antigenic characteristics of the parasite and the immunological competence of the vaccine remains to be seen. Unless one's objective is intentionally to alter the parasite, for instance, to develop attenuated strains, continuous passage should be avoided, as it may introduce unrecognized and misleading modifications of the parasite, which are costly to the researcher and totally unacceptable to the vaccine manufacturer and the ultimate recipient.

Once a candidate vaccine strain is selected, it is desirable to find characteristics for which one can easily test. These are termed markers. Numerous examples of useful genetic markers are described in the literature on attenuated live virus vaccine research. For example, the *in vitro* "t_{50}" marker for thermal sensitivity and the *in vivo* monkey neurovirulence marker of poliovirus vaccines (Kantoch, 1978) are genetic markers used by vaccine manufacturers.

Selection of a cell substrate acceptable for production of human vaccine is a major concern. The ideal situation is to have a master lot of cells which have been well characterized and shown to be free of adventitious agents. This is not possible when erythrocytes are the cell substrate. The next best thing is to have a "stable" of suitable donors from which to obtain red blood cells. The Bureau of Biologics of the Food and Drug Administration in the United States has established guidelines for red blood cell donors whose cells are to be used to immunize plasma donors in order to make anti-Rho (D) globulin (Federal Register, 1978). The requirements are demanding. They emphasize laboratory testing of donors cells and sera and a proved record of transfusions free of hepatitis.

It is difficult to see how carefully selected erythrocyte donors can provide enough cells to meet the extensive worldwide needs for malaria vaccines. I, therefore, feel it is important to continue the search for other cell substrates, such as tissue cultures in which plasmodia can be propagated.

The vaccine manufacturer must ensure that the product is free from adventitious agents and extraneous antigens. This requirement is closely tied to the previous one, the need for a clean cell substrate, but it extends beyond to all components of the growth medium, stabilizer, etc.

We have an excellent illustration of the types of problems which may arise during vaccine preparation from the experience with the live attenuated yellow fever vaccine (17-D) developed by Theiler in 1937. This vaccine made a very remarkable contribution to mankind because it lacked the neurotoxicity of the French Dakar strain used earlier. However, several problems were experienced when it was used in Brazil and by the United States military in the early years of World War II. Three types of problems occurred with some batches of this vaccine: (1) failure to immunize, (2) postvaccinal encephalitis, and (3) illness and death from infectious hepatitis. The first two problems were attributed to modifications which had occurred in the virus. These were solved by switching to a seed lot system. The source of infectious hepatitis was traced to the use of heat-inactivated human serum as a vaccine stabilizer. When human serum was omitted from the vaccine, the hepatitis problem was solved. More than 100 million doses have been administered since without hepatitis occurring (Saenz, 1971). Allergenic side reactions which may cause postvaccinal encephalitis still occur because of the chicken antigens in the vaccine. Live virus yellow fever vaccine (17 D) is also notorious because of its contamination with avian leukosis virus. This adventitious agent was present in the vaccine for the first 30 years of its manufacture. Fortunately, so far no adverse effects from this viral contaminant have been recognized.

If one is lulled by the fact that I have reached back in history for this example, recall the more recent discovery of live SV40 in polio- and adenovirus vaccines or look at a paper published this year in Cancer Immunology and Immunotherapy describing chemoimmunotherapy of stage III breast carcinoma with Bacillus Calmette-Guérin and a live allogeneic tumor cell vaccine (Pardridge *et al.*, 1979). In this study, from the University of California at Los Angeles, 4 of 10 patients given this therapy developed hepatitis B virus infection, which was traced to an infected human serum used to grow the tumor cells for the vaccine.

Substitutes for human serum for cultivation of *falciparum* parasites are possible. In my laboratory we have had good results using rabbit serum for the *in vitro* growth of *P. falciparum*. However, this solution to the hepatitis problem associated with human serum only adds another source of extraneous protein antigen, which we want to avoid. Further, the idea of providing the required amounts of rabbit serum for a worldwide vaccine program is somewhat overwhelming. Clearly other solutions must be sought. Methods must be devised for harvesting merozoites free of erythrocyte antigens, or a method must be devised for the separation of antigens from contaminating erythrocyte antigens.

Potency tests must be developed which will reflect the immunogenicity of the vaccine. This is no easy task with any vaccine. For example, influenza vaccines have been available for about 30 years, and we are still changing potency tests. Last year many countries switched from the chick cell agglutination test to single radial diffusion and immunoelectrophoresis (Laurell) techniques for measuring hemagglutinin. With malaria the problem of developing a meaningful potency test is complex, because thus far antibody to the parasite, as measured by a number of serological techniques, has failed to show a positive correlation with protection (Miller *et al.*, 1977).

Reference standards will have to be developed. The importance of developing such standards at an early stage in the development of all biologicals was acknowledged in the recommendations from the 1976 International Conference on the Role of the Individual and the Community in the Research, Development, and Use of Biologicals (Cockburn, 1978).

The lack of toxicity of the vaccine must be established by appropriate *in vivo* tests in at least two species. Not only the vaccine but the adjuvant's freedom from toxicity must be established. We are all aware of the problems with Freund's complete adjuvant, but the safety of new adjuvants must be extensively tested before evaluation in man. For example, the promising new adjuvant muramyl dipeptide (MDP) has been reported in a personal communication from Edgar Ribi, National Institutes of Health, to have significantly enhanced the endotoxic shock and lethality of gram-negative endotoxins in guinea pigs when given intravenously. A recent study of commercial vaccines by Geier *et al.* (1978)

showed that 16 of 20 samples contained >0.1 ng of endotoxin, thus we should proceed cautiously in evaluating this new and promising adjuvant.

Researchers must consider the cost of vaccines, for if raw materials, production, and purification costs are too high, the vaccine will not be used in developing countries.

In conclusion, let me say that we are making excellent progress, but we have many problems to overcome before we will have a vaccine ready for clinical trials in man. Recognition of the concerns I have expressed as a manufacturer and early efforts to solve these problems will shorten the time until we have a safe and effective vaccine for malaria.

REFERENCES

Cockburn, W. C. (1978). The role of the individual and community in the research, development, and use of biologicals. *WHO Chron.* **32**, 283–285.

Federal Register (1978). Guidelines for immunization of source plasma (human) donors. *Fed. Regist.* **43**, No. 88, 19461.

Geier, M. R., Stanbro, H., and Merril, C. R. (1978). *Appl. Environ. Microbiol.* **36**, 445–449. Endotoxins in commercial vaccines.

Jensen, J. B., and Trager, W. (1978). *Plasmodium falciparum* in culture: Establishment of additional strains. *Am. J. Trop. Med. Hyg.* **27**, 743–746.

Kantoch, M. (1978). Markers and vaccines. *Adv. Virus Res.* **22**, 259–311.

Langreth, S. G., and Reese, R. T. (1979). Loss of antigenicity of *Plasmodium falciparum*-infected erythrocyte surface after long-term culture of the parasite. *Proc. Int. Conf. Malar. Babesiosis, 1979.*

Miller, L. H., Powers, K. G., and Shinoishi, T. (1977). *Plasmodium knowlesi:* Functional immunity and anti-merozoite antibodies in rhesus monkeys after repeated infection. *Exp. Parasitol.* **41**, 105–111.

Pardridge, D. H., Sparks, F. C., Goodnight, J. E., Spears, I. K., and Morton, D. L. (1979). Chemoimmunotherapy of stage III breast carcinoma with BCG and a live allogeneic tumor cell vaccine. *Cancer Immunol. Immunother.* **5**, 217–220.

Saenz, A. C. (1971). Yellow fever vaccines: Achievements, problems, needs. *Proc. Int. Conf. Appl. Vaccines Against Viral, Rickettsial, Bacter. Dis. Man, Pan Am. Health Org.* No. 226, 31–34.

Theiler, M., Smith, H. H. (1937). Use of yellow fever virus modified by *in vitro* cultivation for human immunization *J. Exper. Med.* **65**, pp. 787–800.

Appendix 5

The Agency of International Development Program for Malaria Vaccine Research and Development

Edgar A. Smith and James M. Erickson

The Agency for International Development (AID) was pleased to be one of the sponsors of the International Conference on Malaria and Babesiosis. The records are replete with evidence of hunger and human suffering that occur as a result of these diseases. The research efforts and expenditures that have been put forth are extensive, yet we still do not have viable solutions in hand.

AID has supported research on malaria immunity and vaccination since 1966, beginning with a single contract with the University of Illinois. This project was designed to determine the feasibility of developing a vaccine against human malaria and involved the testing of sporozoite and erythrocytic antigens and the *in vitro* cultivation of these parasite stages. After several years of investigation, the biological feasibility of vaccination against malaria was convincingly demonstrated. In 1972, the project was moved to the University of New Mexico, and a subcontract was established with Rush Memorial Institute to develop a monkey–human malaria model system.

The agency sponsored a malaria vaccine workshop through the National Academy of Sciences in 1974 to examine the state of the art of malaria immunology and vaccine research. The workshop was highly successful in (1) reviewing the current status of research on malaria immunity and vaccination and identifying research needs, (2) providing AID with a basis for a more specific focus on research approaches and priorities, and (3) stimulating increased interest and cooperation among scientists working in this area.

Following this workshop, AID brought together a group of consultants to assist in developing a strategy for malaria vaccine research by advising the agency regarding the elements of malaria vaccine research in terms of priority

Malaria, Vol. 3
Copyright © 1980 by Academic Press, Inc.
All rights of reproduction in any form reserved.
ISBN 0-12-426103-5

research needs, institutional facilities, expertise, and interest. This proposed strategy was approved by the agency's research advisory committee in November 1975. The strategy proposed several priorities:

1. *In vitro* production of erythrocytic antigens which involved (a) the continuation of the work in progress and (b) the development as rapidly as possible of additional projects utilizing the available facilities and experience of tissue culture experts not already involved in malaria research.

2. Increased concentration on erythrocytic antigen research, shifting appropriately in emphasis to merozoite antigen. This included (a) testing in monkeys and continuing investigations of the characteristics, administration, effects, toxicity, and other features of the antigenic materials and their application, and (b) the study of adjuvants, which was considered an important element in the research on erythrocytic antigens.

3. Continuation of work on sporozoite antigens but deemphasized in comparison with work on erythrocytic forms. This included (a) research on *in vitro* production, and (b) basic studies on sporozoite immunization.

4. In addition to the above, but with lower priority, consideration was given to possible developments in attenuated strains, the use of organisms other than malaria, and similar alternative methodology which might become worthy of support.

With these priorities established, the agency placed an advertisement in *Commerce Business Daily* which resulted in the selection and funding of four additional research projects on *in vitro* cultivation of malaria parasites at (1) Rockefeller University, (2) the University of Hawaii, (3) Parke-Davis, Co., and (4) New York University.

In terms of *in vitro* culture of parasites, the Rockefeller University project headed by William Trager achieved within the first year a significant breakthrough. The University of Hawaii project has focused on the production of parasites *in vitro* at high parasitemia; the Parke-Davis, Co. project has taken a different approach by utilizing various cell lines for the cultivation *in vitro* of malaria parasites.

The breakthrough by William Trager in the continuous culture of parasites *in vitro* prompted the agency to advertise a second time for contractors to work on special areas of study of *in vitro* cultivation of the erythrocytic stages of malaria parasites as follows:

1. Testing the immunogenicity of parasites produced *in vitro*.
2. Purification of the antigen produced (with special attention given to removal of host red cell membranes).
3. Increasing the yield of parasites in relation to red cells.
4. Culturing different strains and/or species of malaria parasites.

5. Improving the synchrony of the asexual erythrocytic cycle during culture.

6. Developing reproducible methods for *in vitro* cultivation of gametocytes and subsequent infection of mosquitoes.

7. Developing methods for harvesting erythrocytic parasite antigens.

About 25 responses to this Request for Proposal were received and, after intensive review, two projects were selected, one at New York University and one at Parke-Davis, Co. At the present time, the collaborating network on malaria immunity and vaccination includes the 10 following projects. (a) *In vitro* cultivation of malaria parasites—six projects including Rockefeller University, University of Hawaii, Parke-Davis and Company (two projects), Walter Reed Army Institute of Research, and the Gorgas Institute in Panama. (b) Testing of erythrocytic stage antigens—two projects, one at the University of New Mexico and one at the National Institute of Health in Bogota, Colombia, funded through Pan-American Health Organization. (c) Sporozoite immunity research—two projects, both at New York University.

In June 1978, an AID workshop was held at the University of New Mexico to update the 1975 strategy and review the forward progress of the collaborative network. Problems and priorities identified in the previous strategy statement of 3 years ago were still considered valid but, because of the breakthrough at Rockefeller University in developing a continuous-culture system and because of the degree of progress on several associated problems, a reordering of priorities and a more careful delineation of the problems were necessary. The expert consultant team considered the highest priorities for future activities to be as follows:

1. Continuation of improvement of the continuous-culture system with particular reference to eliminating components not suitable for producing an antigen to be used in man. This would include replacement of components in short supply such as *Aotus* serum and red cell supporting components.

2. Characterization and purification of antigenic material.

3. Other secondary objectives as follows:

a. Development of *in vitro* correlates based on cellular or humoral responses which would provide a test for immunity.

b. Development of better synchrony in continuous cultures.

c. Development of an alternative model system to permit use of the large numbers of animals needed for greater statistical validity in certain studies.

d. Study of geographically distinct strains of malaria with respect to their biological and biochemical characteristics both *in vivo* and *in vitro*.

e. Encouragement of the elimination of unnecessary duplication but support of planned replication of significant findings.

f. Insistence on the publication of confirmatory studies whether results are positive or negative.

g. Promotion of a program of exchange through observation visits and/or work visits between project personnel of appropriate laboratories, including some outside the AID network.

h. Continuation of the present level of support of sporozoite immunity research.

i. Deferral of any expansion of effort in the development of a suitable adjuvant for the present.

j. Improvement of the supply of monkeys, including the development of breeding facilities.

Appendix 6

The Great Neglected Diseases of Mankind

Kenneth S. Warren

Parasitology is a biological discipline concerned largely with two quite separate groups of organisms—single-celled protozoa and the multicellular metazoa of which the helminths form the most important group. As a specialist in tropical medicine my major research interest has been schistosomiasis, which certainly is the most important of the helminth infections. Malaria is unquestionably the most important of the protozoan infections—"important" is simply defined here as having a relatively high prevalence of infection and disease as measured by mortality and morbidity. When the title of this chapter was mentioned to Dr. Julius Kreier, he concurred with the idea, but then stated that "the neglected diseases most certainly do not include malaria." This is certainly true when malaria is compared to its fellow parasitic infections (for instance, malaria receives $4 million per annum from the World Health Organization Tropical Diseases Research Program, while schistosomiasis and the others are allotted from one-half to one-eighth as much). When malaria is compared with the major diseases of the developed world, however, we see a different picture: while research on this protozoan infection of approximately 300 million people receives at most $20 million from all sources, cancer, an affliction of 10 million people, is provided with more than $800 million by the United States government alone.

The Great Neglected Diseases of Mankind is a new program at the Rockefeller Foundation, having received the approval of the board of trustees in December 1977. In the recent past, however, the foundation's Division of Health Sciences was engaged principally in a program dealing with the massive growth in world population. The imminent retirement of four members of the health sciences team left the president, John H. Knowles, with the problem of deciding the future direction of this division of The Rockefeller Foundation. Considering the history of the foundation and the relative lack of constraints upon voluntary organizations, this could have been in many different directions including health care

ISBN 0-12-426103-5

delivery, medical education, or biomedical research, and could have been directed to either the national or the global scene. John Knowles (1976, 1977) finally decided on a primary focus on the major diseases of the forgotten three-quarters of the world's people in the developing countries and afforded me the great privilege of directing that effort. In a piece of fancy footwork Knowles was able to have his cake and eat it too by bringing into the foundation in May of 1978 an eminent figure in the field of reproductive biology, Sheldon J. Segal, to head a separate Population Division.

The appointment of a tropical medicine specialist was in line with the traditional interests of the Rockefeller Foundation. The foundation began with a major global hookworm control campaign. Over the years it has played a significant role in the control of malaria and yellow fever for which a foundation officer, Max Theiler, received a Nobel prize. In the last 40 years, however, the foundation has developed major programs in other areas. For example, The Conquest of Hunger Program of the Agricultural Sciences Division fostered the "green revolution" for which one of its officers, Norman Borlaug, received a Nobel prize. As the foundation's interest developed in agricultural sciences, population, and other areas, so its involvement in programs in health sciences waned. By the time John H. Knowles, of Massachusetts General Hospital, was appointed president in the early 1970s, Health was no longer a specific program, and was included in an area called Allied Interests. One of Knowles' first acts was to add the name of Health to the Population Program which was then called Population and Health. At the time of my arrival at the foundation in July 1977, annual expenditures in the area of health other than those related directly to the Population Program were less than 2% of the entire disbursements of the foundation and were devoted largely to an excellent field research program on schistosomiasis on the island of St. Lucia. It is worthy of note, however, that a major grant during that period permitted the founding of a Division of Geographic Medicine at Case Western Reserve University in 1974. In the Spring of 1976, Knowles was lured to Cleveland as the first annual lecturer in Geographic Medicine.

The Division of Geographic Medicine was organized as an integral part of the Department of Medicine, having the same status as the Divisions of Cardiology, Hematology, Gastroenterology, etc. (Warren, 1976). Each of the individuals in the division was expected to develop a collaborative clinical or epidemiological program with an institution in the tropics and to work there for 2–4 months annually. In the remainder of the time in the United States no more than 2 months was spent on general and specialty ward rounds, the rest of the year being devoted largely to laboratory research. Interestingly enough this difficult challenge was well met by a cadre of bright young individuals from Egypt, Australia, and of course, Cleveland. Furthermore, they were all articulate and, when they presented their work to Knowles, he was agreeably surprised by the quality of their investigations. Just before Knowles left Cleveland he asked the director of the division whether he might be interested in joining the Rockefeller Foundation. Several months later the director received a phone call from the president asking him to pay a visit to New York. The ensuing discussion resulted in a rough outline of the program which was subsequently called The Great Neglected Diseases of Mankind.

It is unquestionable that both financial neglect and lack of interest by the scientific establishment of the developed world in the last 40 years have resulted in a lower quantity and quality of work on the major diseases of the less developed countries. During this period, however, there has been a burgeoning of molecular biology, immunology, and biochemistry leading to vaccines and chemotherapeutic agents for control of the infectious diseases prevalent in the industrial world. In addition, vast sums of money and enormous efforts have been expended on those presently intractable problems, atherosclerosis and cancer. Recently, however, outstanding scientists have been attracted by the opportunities for rapid advances in knowledge afforded by the great neglected diseases, and by a new spirit of humanitarianism. Capitalizing on this situation the foundation, by moving rapidly and providing long-term support, has been able to build a critical mass of research units in departments of medicine and research institutes throughout the world. These include divisions of geographic or tropical medicine at Case Western Reserve University, Tufts University, the University of Virginia, the University of Washington, Oxford University, and the Biomedical Research Center for Infectious Diseases in Cairo, Egypt. Immunology units have been formed at Harvard University, the Walter and Eliza Hall Institute, the Universities of Stockholm and Uppsala and the Weizmann Institute, and pharmacology units are in action at the Rockefeller University, Case Western Reserve University, the Centro de Investigation y de Estudios Azanzados in Mexico City and Mahidol University in Bangkok. All these groups spend approximately 30% of their time in collaborative research in the developing world with countries such as Kenya, Egypt, Sudan, India, Guatemala, Brazil, Malaysia, Gambia, Indonesia, and Papua, New Guinea. The investigators work largely on bacterial diarrheas and helminth and protozoan infections; with respect to the latter, three of the units are currently working on different aspects of malaria.

The Walter and Eliza Hall Institute has been using a cell sorter for isolating parasitized cells in their attempts to purify malarial antigens, Oxford University is studying the mechanism of protection of sickle cell anemia against malaria, the Swedish Universities are studying immunoregulation in murine malaria, and Rockefeller University is planning experiments on unique ways of producing repository drugs for the prophylaxis of malaria. Furthermore, we have recently inaugurated a new research career development award for young investigators, and a recipient of one of these awards, Anil Jayawardena, is working on the mechanisms of immunity against malaria at Yale University and Rupert Schmidt-Ulrich at Tufts University is studying malaria membranes. At this point it is important to observe that one of the major purposes of the program is to attract the brightest young investigators to this field by providing the critical mass needed for a viable career track.

Now that the great neglected diseases program is well on its way, I am happy to say that our network has essentially been accepted by the World Health Organization as a donation in kind and that the Rockefeller Foundation has been accorded the honor of being elected to the Joint Coordinating Board of the Tropical Diseases Research Programme. We are also particularly pleased that Adetokunbo Lucas, director of the WHO program, has agreed to be a member of the advisory board to the Rockefeller Foundation network.

In the midst of all of these clinical, immunological, and pharmacological developments we have become concerned with the future of fundamental biological investigation on parasitism. A study of the situation is being planned, and there is a possibility of significant support for education and research in this area. At this point I should mention the great spirit of collaboration which has developed among the officer-biologists of the Divisions of Health Sciences, Agricultural Sciences, and Population of the foundation. Parasitism is a major global problem for human medicine, veterinary medicine, and agriculture. Solution of some of the problems of parasitism will effect industrial and agricultural development and population growth. Thus, the work of these three divisions of the foundation are inextricably bound to "the well-being of mankind throughout the world."

Finally, I would like to point out that, in spite of the vast difficulties lying ahead, malariologists are better off than schistosomologists. With respect to vector control, insecticides, particularly in the palmy days when DDT was fully effective and available, are far better than molluscicides. For the most part chemotherapeutic agents used in this area are rapidly effective and nontoxic in contrast to antischistosomal drugs, and excellent means of prophylaxis now exist in most parts of the world in contrast to nonexistent programs for prophylaxis for schistosomes. In the area of experimental vaccines, three are currently available, antigametocyte, antimerozoite, and antisporozoite, while only one (irradiated cercaria), which is merely partially effective, is available for schistosomologists. Nevertheless, I know that great problems still exist, with vectors resistant to insecticides and parasites becoming refractory to antimalarial drugs. I believe that malaria is still the most important disease in the world and that financially it is still one of the great neglected diseases of mankind.

REFERENCES

Knowles, J. H. (1976). American medicine and world health 1976. *Ann. Intern. Med.* **84,** 483–485.
Knowles, J. H. (1977). Rationale for increased United States interest in international health. *Trans. Am. Climat. (Clin.) Assoc.* **89,** 67–76.
Warren, K. S. (1976). The division of geographic medicine. *J. Trop. Med. Hyg.* **79,** 189–190.

Index

A

Adenylate kinase, 39
Adjuvant, 167–168, 234, 236, 237, 239, 243, 250–251, 254, 256, 292, 322
  Freund's complete, 121, 141–142, 208, 217, 233, 238, 251–252, 301, 302, 303, 328
Agar diffusion, of antibody precipitation, 80–83
Age-specificity, of malaria, 282–284
Agency for International Development, malaria vaccine research and development program, 331–334
Agglutination, of erythrocyte, 20, 21, 42
Agglutination test, 76–78, 122
L-Alanyl-D-isoglutamine, 250–251
Amino acid, 41
p-Aminobenzoic acid, 290
4-Aminoquinoline, 232, 289
8-Aminoquinoline, 288
Ammonium chloride, 25, 31
Ammonium sulfate, 12
Anaplasmosis, 33
Anemia, hemolytic, 75, 138, 139–140
Anopheles balabacensis, 241, 244
Anopheles gambiae, 285, 287
Anopheles stephensis, 187
Anopheline, 232, 285
Antibody, action mechanisms, 127–131
  action site, 128
  antiblood stage response, 74–101
  antiexoerythrocyte response, 73–74
  antigamete response, 271–272, 276–277, 286–288
  antisporozoite response, 67–73, 171–177, 184–187, 191–194
  binding, 128
  cytophilic, 115, 120, 136–137, 139
  inhibition of erythrocyte penetration, 129–131
  opsonic, 136–137, 139

  production, 93–95, 113, 122–123, 125
  profile, 96
  protective, 72–73, 75, 123, 125–127, 129
  species specificity, 176–177, 185–186, 191–192, 193
  stage specificity, 175–176, 192, 193
Antigen, blood stage, 231–257, 307–309, 321–324
  characterization, 169–171, 182–184, 190–191
  competition, 117
  complement fixing, 13, 15, 17, 34–35
  identification, 35–37, 171, 183–184
  isolation, 34–41
  labile, 10, 11, 45, 46, 81
  localization, 169–171, 183
  plasma content, 43–46
  preparation, 8–13, 165–168
  presentation, 114, 115, 118, 120, 148
  recognition, 114
  resistant, 10, 11, 45, 46, 81
  soluble, 124, 144
  species specificity, 36, 37, 72, 143–144, 192
  stable, 10, 45, 46, 81
  storage, 83, 307–308
  variant, 42
Antigen antibody reaction, 36, 45–46
  effect of complement, 131
  immunoassay, 67–101, 123–125
  lymphocyte regulation, 118–122
  macrophage regulation, 114–118
  protective, 125–127
Antigenic analysis, of *Plasmodium* extract, 35–37
Antigenic maturation, of sporozoite, 182, 183, 190
Antiglobulin, 76
Antisera, use in erythrocyte lysis, 25–27